Advances in Stem Cells

Advances in Stem Cells

Edited by Ashton Silk

hayle
medical

New York

Hayle Medical,
750 Third Avenue, 9ᵗʰ Floor,
New York, NY 10017, USA

Visit us on the World Wide Web at:
www.haylemedical.com

ISBN: 978-1-63241-867-8

Cataloging-in-Publication Data

Advances in stem cells / edited by Ashton Silk.
    p. cm.
Includes bibliographical references and index.
ISBN 978-1-63241-867-8
1. Stem cells. 2. Stem cells--Research. 3. Cells. I. Silk, Ashton.
QH588.S83 A28 2020
616.027 74-dc23

Table of Contents

Preface.. VII

Chapter 1   **Effect of Compression Loading on Human Nucleus Pulposus-Derived Mesenchymal Stem Cells**.. 1
Hang Liang, Sheng Chen, Donghua Huang, Xiangyu Deng, Kaige Ma and Zengwu Shao

Chapter 2   **The Differential Effects of Leukocyte-Containing and Pure Platelet-Rich Plasma on Nucleus Pulposus-Derived Mesenchymal Stem Cells: Implications for the Clinical Treatment of Intervertebral Disc Degeneration**.................... 11
Jun Jia, Shan-zheng Wang, Liang-yu Ma, Jia-bin Yu, Yu-dong Guo and Chen Wang

Chapter 3   **Differentiation of Human Embryonic Stem Cells to Sympathetic Neurons: A Potential Model for Understanding Neuroblastoma Pathogenesis**.................................... 23
Jane Carr-Wilkinson, Nilendran Prathalingam, Deepali Pal, Mohammad Moad, Natalie Lee, Aishwarya Sundaresh, Helen Forgham, Peter James, Mary Herbert, Majlinda Lako and Deborah A. Tweddle

Chapter 4   **Characterization of Human Mesenchymal Stem Cells Isolated from the Testis**.................... 35
Letizia De Chiara, Elvira Smeralda Famulari, Sharmila Fagoonee, Saskia K. M. van Daalen, Stefano Buttiglieri, Alberto Revelli, Emanuela Tolosano, Lorenzo Silengo, Ans M. M. van Pelt and Fiorella Altruda

Chapter 5   **Molecular Mechanisms of Transdifferentiation of Adipose-Derived Stem Cells into Neural Cells**.. 43
Liang Luo, Da-Hai Hu, James Q. Yin and Ru-Xiang Xu

Chapter 6   **Icariin Promotes the Migration of BMSCs In Vitro and In Vivo via the MAPK Signaling Pathway** 57
Feng Jiao, Wang Tang, He Huang, Zhaofei Zhang, Donghua Liu, Hongyi Zhang and Hui Ren

Chapter 7   **D-Mannose Enhanced Immunomodulation of Periodontal Ligament Stem Cells via Inhibiting IL-6 Secretion** 66
Lijia Guo, Yanan Hou, Liang Song, Siying Zhu, Feiran Lin and Yuxing Bai

Chapter 8   **Synaptic Plasticity of Human Umbilical Cord Mesenchymal Stem Cell Differentiating into Neuron-like Cells In Vitro Induced by Edaravone** 77
Yunpeng Shi, Chengrui Nan, Zhongjie Yan, Liqiang Liu, Jingjing Zhou, Zongmao Zhao and Depei Li

Chapter 9   **Bioprocessing of Mesenchymal Stem Cells and their Derivatives: Toward Cell-Free Therapeutics**.. 87
Jolene Phelps, Amir Sanati-Nezhad, Mark Ungrin, Neil A. Duncan and Arindom Sen

Chapter 10   **GM1 Ganglioside Promotes Osteogenic Differentiation of Human Tendon Stem Cells** 110
Sonia Bergante, Pasquale Creo, Marco Piccoli, Andrea Ghiroldi, Alessandra Menon,
Federica Cirillo, Paola Rota, Michelle M. Monasky, Giuseppe Ciconte,
Carlo Pappone, Pietro Randelli and Luigi Anastasia

Chapter 11   **Focal Adhesion Kinase and ROCK Signaling are Switch-Like Regulators of Human Adipose Stem Cell Differentiation towards Osteogenic and Adipogenic Lineages** 118
Laura Hyväri, Miina Ojansivu, Miia Juntunen, Kimmo Kartasalo,
Susanna Miettinen and Sari Vanhatupa

Chapter 12   **Zebularine Promotes Hepatic Differentiation of Rabbit Bone Marrow Mesenchymal Stem Cells by Interfering with p38 MAPK Signaling** 131
Yong-Heng Luo, Juan Chen, En-Hua Xiao, Qiu-Yun Li and Yong-Mei Luo

Chapter 13   **Intraparenchymal Neural Stem/Progenitor Cell Transplantation for Ischemic Stroke Animals** 140
Hailong Huang, Kun Qian, Xiaohua Han, Xin Li, Yifeng Zheng, Zhishui Chen,
Xiaolin Huang and Hong Chen

Chapter 14   **The Effects of Platelet-Derived Growth Factor-BB on Bone Marrow Stromal Cell-Mediated Vascularized Bone Regeneration** 150
Maolin Zhang, Wenwen Yu, Kunimichi Niibe, Wenjie Zhang, Hiroshi Egusa,
Tingting Tang and Xinquan Jiang

Chapter 15   **Radiation Induces Apoptosis and Osteogenic Impairment through miR-22-Mediated Intracellular Oxidative Stress in Bone Marrow Mesenchymal Stem Cells** 165
Zhonglong Liu, Tao Li, Si'nan Deng, Shuiting Fu, Xiaojun Zhou and Yue He

Chapter 16   **MicroRNA-132, Delivered by Mesenchymal Stem Cell-Derived Exosomes, Promote Angiogenesis in Myocardial Infarction** 181
Teng Ma, Yueqiu Chen, Yihuan Chen, Qingyou Meng, Jiacheng Sun, Lianbo Shao,
Yunsheng Yu, Haoyue Huang, Yanqiu Hu, Ziying Yang, Junjie Yang and
Zhenya Shen

Permissions

List of Contributors

Index

Preface

This book has been a concerted effort by a group of academicians, researchers and scientists, who have contributed their research works for the realization of the book. This book has materialized in the wake of emerging advancements and innovations in this field. Therefore, the need of the hour was to compile all the required researches and disseminate the knowledge to a broad spectrum of people comprising of students, researchers and specialists of the field.

Stem cells are the cells that differentiate into other cells and divide upon self-renewal to produce more stem cells. There are two types of stem cells, embryonic stem cells and adult stem cells. Progenitor cells and stem cells serve as a repair system by replenishing adult tissues. In the developing embryo, stem cells differentiate into specialized cells- endoderm, ectoderm and mesoderm, and also maintain the normal turnover of regenerative organs like skin, blood and intestinal tissues. Embryonic stem cells are a theoretically potential source for the development of regenerative medicine and tissue replacement. Adult stem cells can be acquired from adipose tissue, blood and bone marrow, as well as from the blood of the umbilical cord after birth. They are used in medical therapies such as in bone marrow transplantation. They can also be artificially grown and differentiated into specialized cells. Stem cell therapy helps to treat and prevent diseases or conditions. Some of the diseases where stem cell treatment holds potential include Parkinson's disease, diabetes, osteoarthritis, spinal cord injury repair, rheumatoid arthritis, cancer, amyotrophic lateral sclerosis, etc. This book is a valuable compilation of topics, ranging from the basic to the most complex advances in stem cells. It explores all the important aspects of stem cell therapy in the present day scenario. Scientists and students actively engaged in this field will find this book full of crucial and unexplored concepts.

At the end of the preface, I would like to thank the authors for their brilliant chapters and the publisher for guiding us all-through the making of the book till its final stage. Also, I would like to thank my family for providing the support and encouragement throughout my academic career and research projects.

Editor

Effect of Compression Loading on Human Nucleus Pulposus-Derived Mesenchymal Stem Cells

Hang Liang, Sheng Chen(iD), Donghua Huang, Xiangyu Deng(iD), Kaige Ma(iD), and Zengwu Shao(iD)

Department of Orthopaedics, Union Hospital, Tongji Medical College, Huazhong University of Science and Technology, 1277 Jiefang Avenue, Wuhan 430022, China

Correspondence should be addressed to Kaige Ma; makaige225@hust.edu.cn and Zengwu Shao; szwpro@163.com

Academic Editor: Andrea Ballini

Purpose. Mechanical loading plays a vital role in the progression of intervertebral disc (IVD) degeneration, but little is known about the effect of compression loading on human nucleus pulposus-derived mesenchymal stem cells (NP-MSCs). Thus, this study is aimed at investigating the effect of compression on the biological behavior of NP-MSCs in vitro. *Methods.* Human NP-MSCs were isolated from patients undergoing lumbar discectomy for IVD degeneration and were identified by immunophenotypes and multilineage differentiation. Then, cells were cultured in the compression apparatus at 1.0 MPa for different times (0 h, 24 h, 36 h, and 48 h). The viability-, differentiation-, and differentiation-related genes (Runx2, APP, and Col2) and colony formation-, migration-, and stem cell-related proteins (Sox2 and Oct4) were evaluated. *Results.* The results showed that the isolated cells fulfilled the criteria of MSC stated by the International Society for Cellular Therapy (ISCT). And our results also indicated that compression loading significantly inhibited cell viability, differentiation, colony formation, and migration. Furthermore, gene expression suggested that compression loading could downregulate the expression of stem cell-related proteins and lead to NP-MSC stemness losses. *Conclusions.* Our results suggested that the biological behavior of NP-MSCs could be inhibited by compression loading and therefore enhanced our understanding on the compression-induced endogenous repair failure of NP-MSCs during IVDD.

1. Introduction

Intervertebral disc (IVD) degeneration is among the most important contributors to low back pain, leading to patient disability and heavy financial burdens globally [1, 2]. Currently, conservative and surgical operations are the main treatments for IVD degeneration. However, these treatments are not long-lasting and effective for the limitation that they cannot reverse the structural and mechanical function of IVD tissues [3]. Stem cell-based therapies have shown an exciting perspective for IVD repair recently [4]. In different animal models of disc degeneration, which are established by annular puncture or nucleus aspiration, transplantation of exogenous mesenchymal stem cells (MSCs) has improved the evaluation scores of radiographs, magnetic resonance images (MRI), and histological analysis [5–7]. In a pilot study

[8], ten patients suffering from chronic back pain and positively diagnosed with lumbar disc degeneration were treated by injecting autologous expanded bone marrow MSCs into the nucleus pulposus (NP) area. The results indicated the feasibility, safety, and clinical efficacy of the treatment.

Apart from exogenous stem cell transplantation, endogenous stem cell stimulation and recruitment are also essential ways to repair IVD degeneration and play a key role in endogenous repair [9]. Evidence has been found in latest researches that nucleus pulposus mesenchymal stem cells (NP-MSCs) exist naturally in the IVD [10, 11] and participate in IVD regeneration [9]. The aim of NP-MSC therapy is to make NP-MSCs differentiate into nucleus pulposus-like cells and stimulate disc cells maintaining IVD homeostasis. Although activating the endogenous NP-MSCs could be an attractive strategy for endogenous repair, it is hard to maintain the number of viable and functional NP-MSCs under an adverse microenvironment in IVD [12]. It was reported that the viability and proliferation rate of NP-MSCs were significantly inhibited under hypoxia [13], and acidic conditions could decrease the extracellular matrix (ECM) synthesis and stem cell-related gene expression of NP-MSCs [14]. Mechanical loadings [15], including compression, shear, torsion, and flexion, are another essential factors that influence the fate of NP-MSCs.

The IVD functions as a shock absorber, and external forces on the spine lead to intense stresses that act on the IVD. From a mechanical point of view, disc cells and progenitor cells embedded in the different areas are exposed to wide ranges of mechanical loadings [16]. Inappropriate or excessive compressive force stimulus applied to intervertebral discs (IVDs) is an important contributing factor in the progress of disc degeneration. We have reported that apoptosis and necroptosis could be induced by compression at a magnitude of 1 MPa in rat NP cells previously [17, 18]. However, to our best knowledge, there have been no studies focusing on the effect of compression loading on human NP-MSCs so far. Therefore, the present study is aimed at exploring the effect of compression on the biological behavior of NP-MSCs in vitro.

2. Methods

2.1. Isolation and Culture of NP-MSCs.
NP tissues were donated by five patients undergoing lumbar discectomy for lumbar disc hernia, and the ages of those five patients are 42, 49, 45, 41, and 40, respectively. According to Pfirrmann's MRI (T2WI) Grading Criteria for Disc Degeneration, all the patients were in grade III. All procedures in the present study were approved by the ethics committee of Tongji Medical College of Huazhong University of Science and Technology. NP-MSCs were isolated and cultured as previously described [14]. Briefly, NP tissues were first carefully separated by a dissecting microscope and washed by PBS solution. Secondly, the NP samples were dissected and digested in 0.2% type II collagenase for 12 h at 37°C with 5% CO_2. And then the obtained cells and partially digested tissues were cultured in MSC complete medium (Cyagen, USA) at 37°C in a humidified atmosphere containing 5% CO_2. The media were changed twice a week, and the primary culture was 1 : 3 subcultured when cells reached 80%–90% confluence. NP-MSCs in passage 2 were used in this study.

2.2. Surface Marker Identification of NP-MSCs.
The collected cells were washed and resuspended in PBS and incubated with the following monoclonal antibodies according to the recommendations of ISCT [19]: CD105, CD73, CD90, CD34, CD14, CD19, and HLA-DR. After being incubated for 30 min at 37°C, the cells were washed with PBS and then resuspended in 500 μL PBS to adjust the cell concentration at about 10^6/mL. The labeled cells were examined via flow cytometry (BD LSR II, Becton Dickinson) following standard procedures.

2.3. Multilineage Differentiation.
To assess the multilineage differentiation potential of NP-MSCs, the osteogenic, adipogenic, and chondrogenic differentiation was induced.

For osteogenic differentiation, NP-MSCs were seeded in six-well plates at 2×10^4 cells/cm^2 in normal medium and incubated in osteogenic differentiation medium (Cyagen, USA) at 60%–70% confluence. The inducing conditional medium was changed twice a week. After differentiating for 14 days, the NP-MSCs were used to extract RNA and stained with the Alizarin Red solution, respectively.

For adipogenic differentiation, NP-MSCs were seeded in six-well plates at 2×10^4 cells/cm^2. When the cells grew up to 100% confluence, the medium was changed to adipogenic differentiation medium A (Cyagen, USA). Three days later, the medium was changed to adipogenic differentiation medium B (Cyagen, USA). After 24 h, the medium was replaced back with medium A. The cycle was repeated for 4 times, and the cells were cultured in medium B for additional 7 days. After differentiating, the NP-MSCs were used to extract RNA and stained with Oil Red O.

For chondrogenic differentiation, NP-MSCs were seeded in six-well plates at 2×10^4 cells/cm^2 in normal medium and incubated in chondrogenic differentiation medium (Cyagen, USA) at 60%–70% confluence. The media were changed every 2 to 3 days. After differentiating for three weeks, the NP-MSCs were used to extract RNA and stained with the Alcian blue.

In addition, to evaluate the effect of compression loading on the multilineage differentiation of NP-MSCs, the cells were cultured in a custom-made compression apparatus for different times (0 h, 24 h, 36 h, and 48 h) at a magnitude of 1 MPa as described previously [17, 20]. And the cells were then digested with 0.25% trypsin and seeded in six-well plates for the induced differentiation above.

2.4. Cell Viability Assay (CCK-8).
NP-MSCs were seeded in 96-well plates and cultured in the compression apparatus for different times (0 h, 24 h, 36 h, and 48 h). Cell viability was measured by CCK-8 (Dojindo, Japan) following the manufacturer's protocol. At the appropriate time points, 10 μL CCK-8 solution was added to each well. The plates were then incubated at 37°C with 5% CO_2 for 2 h. The surviving cell counts were determined by absorbance detection at 450 nm with a spectrophotometer (BioTek, USA).

2.5. Colony Formation Assay.
To demonstrate the effect of compression loading on the capacity of colony formation, the NP-MSCs were treated with compression for different times (0 h, 24 h, 36 h, and 48 h). Then, the cells were collected and seeded in six-well plates at the density of 200 cells/well. The medium was changed twice a week. After two weeks, the cells were fixed with 4% paraformaldehyde. Fifteen minutes later, the cells were washed with PBS and stained with 0.1% crystal violet for 15 min. The colonies containing more than 100 cells were counted.

2.6. Wound Healing Assay.
For the wound healing assay, NP-MSCs were seeded in six-well plates with MSC complete medium. When the cells grew to 100% confluence, the

(a)

(b)

(c)

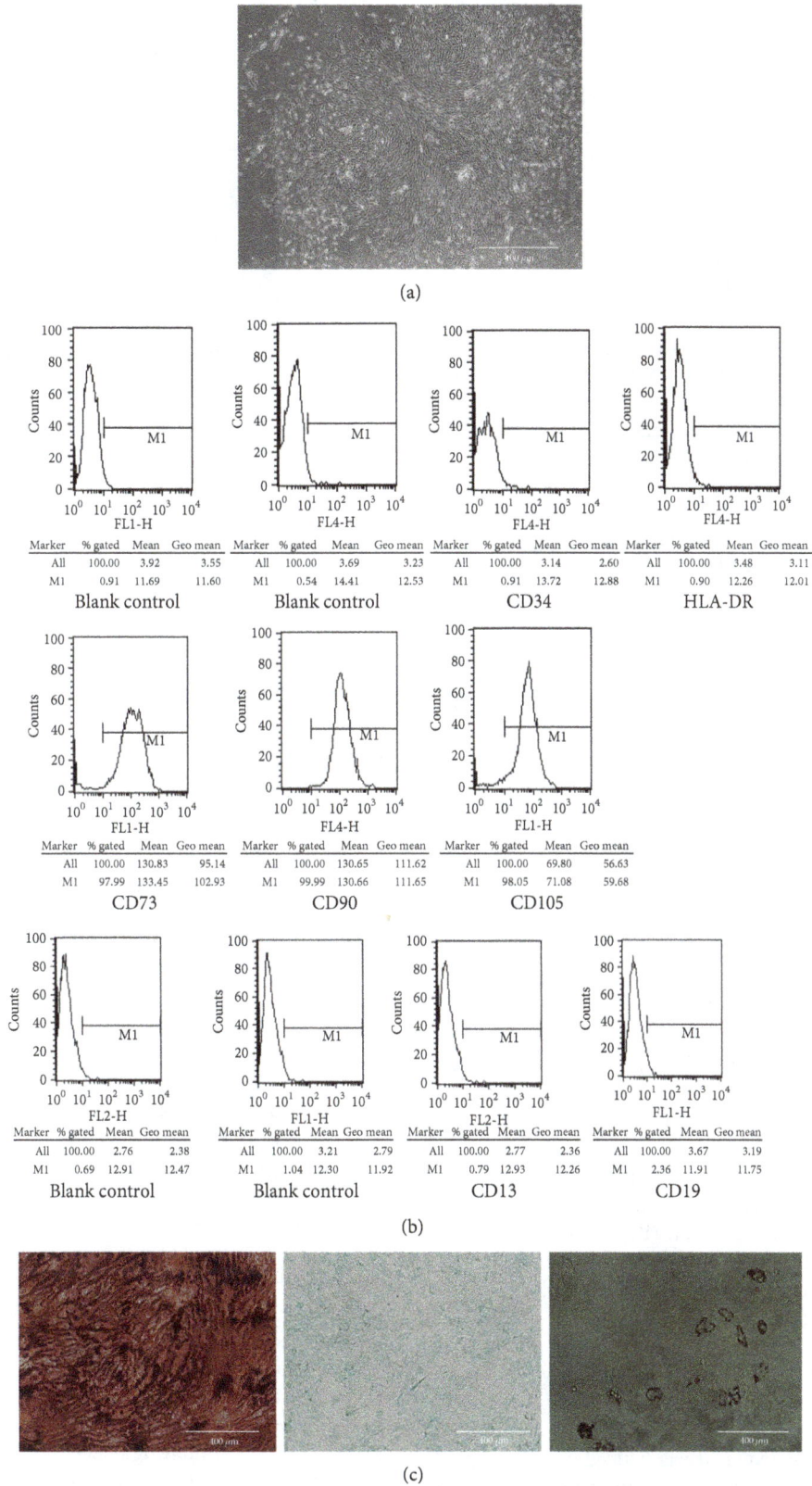

FIGURE 1: The isolated cells fulfilled the criteria of MSC stated by ISCT. (a) The shape of cells isolated from the degenerated IVDs. (b) The MSC-associated surface markers (CD34, CD14, CD19, HLA-DR, CD73, CD90, and CD105) were analyzed by flow cytometry. (c) The induction of osteogenic, chondrogenic, and adipogenic differentiation of the isolated cells.

wound was created by scraping the monolayer cell with a pipette tip, and the medium was replaced with serum-free DMEM-L. Then, the plates were randomly assigned to the compression group or the control group. The photomicrographs were acquired at different time points (0 h, 24 h, 36 h, and 48 h). The migration areas of wound healing were quantified using ImageJ software.

2.7. Transwell Migration Assay. The 24-well plates with 8 μm pore-size transwell inserts were used to assess the migration abilities of NP-MSCs. The cells were adjusted to a density of 10^5 cells/mL with serum-free DMEM-L, and then 200 μL cell suspension was added into the upper chamber and 600 μL DMEM-L with 10% FBS was added into the lower chamber. Subsequently, the cells were treated with compression for different times (24 h, 36 h, and 48 h), and the cells without compression treatment were used as the control. At the appropriate time points, the nonmigrated NP-MSCs were removed and the migrated cells were fixed and stained with crystal violet. The migrated NP-MSCs were counted in five randomly selected optical fields.

2.8. Quantitative Real-Time Polymerase Chain Reaction (QRT-PCR). Total RNA was extracted from NP-MSCs by TRIzol reagent (Invitrogen, USA); then, the RNA was transcribed into cDNA by a reverse transcription kit (Takara,) following the manufacturer's protocol. After reverse transcription, QRT-PCR was performed with the SYBR Premix Ex Taq II according to the manufacturer's instructions (Takara). The $2^{-\triangle\triangle CT}$ method was used to analyze the data, and the housekeeping gene GAPDH was used to normalize the level of mRNA. Primer sequences were as follows: 5′-GTGGACGAGGCAAGAGTTTCA-3′ (forward) and 5′-GGTGCAGAGTTCAGGGAGGG-3′ (reverse) for RUNX2, 5′-CCCATCCCCACTTTGTGATT-3′ (forward) and 5′-ATTCCGCAGGGCAGCAAC-3′ (reverse) for APP, 5′-AGCATTGCCTATCTGGACGAA-3′ (forward) and 5′-GTACGTGAACCTGCTATTGCC-3′ (reverse) for COL2A1, and 5′-AATCCCATCACCATCTTCCAG-3′ (forward) and 5′-GAGCCCCAGCCTTCTCCAT-3′ (reverse) for GAPDH.

2.9. Western Blot Analysis. NP-MSCs were lysed on ice using standard buffer (Beyotime, China), and total protein was extracted by a protein extraction kit (Beyotime, China). The cell lysate was centrifuged at 12,000 ×g for 10 min at 4°C. After protein transfer, the membranes were blocked by nonfat milk and then incubated overnight at 4°C with a rat polyclonal antibody against cleaved Sox2, Oct4, and GADPH (Abcam, 1 : 3000). After washing several times, the membrane was incubated with secondary antibodies for 1 h at room temperature. Finally, the immunoreactive membranes were visualized via the enhanced chemiluminescence (ECL) method following the manufacturer's instructions (Amersham Biosciences, USA).

2.10. Statistical Analysis. All measurements were performed at least three times. The data were presented as mean ± standard deviation (SD). Student's *t*-tests were used in the analysis of two-group parameters. One-way analysis of variance

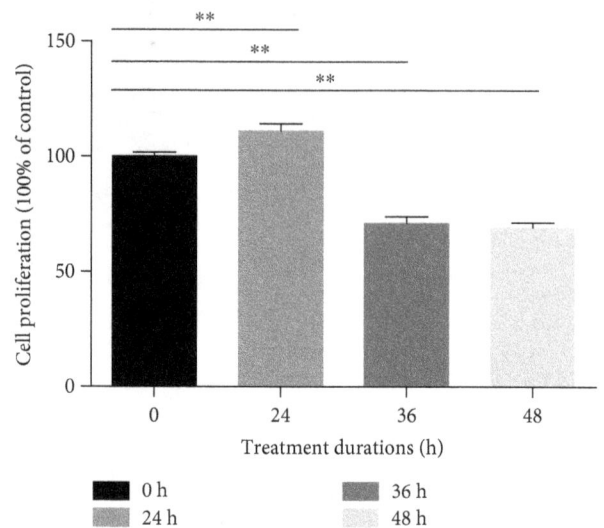

FIGURE 2: CCK-8 assay showed compression loading inhibiting the viability of NP-MSCs (values are presented as means ± SD, $^{**}p < 0.01$ versus control).

(ANOVA) test was used in comparisons of multiple sets of data. $p < 0.05$ were considered statistically significant.

3. Results

3.1. Identification of NP-MSCs. The cells isolated from the degenerated IVDs presented with long spindle-shaped adherent growth and grew in a spiral formation (Figure 1(a)). The MSC-associated surface markers were analyzed by flow cytometry. As shown in Figure 1(b), the isolated cells had high expression levels of markers (CD105, CD73, and CD90) that are normally positive in MSCs and had low expression of markers (CD34, CD14, CD19, and HLA-DR) that are usually negative in MSCs. For osteogenic differentiation, the cells formed highly visible calcium deposits after being induced in osteogenic media for two weeks. In addition, oil droplets were accumulated in the cells and stained with Oil Red O during the adipogenic differentiation. After being induced in chondrogenic media, the cells exhibited strong production of sulfated proteoglycans (Figure 1(c)). The results above showed that the isolated cells fulfilled the criteria of MSC stated by ISCT. Thus, we isolated NP-MSCs, and the cells in passage 2 were used in this study.

3.2. Compression Loading Inhibited the Viability. To evaluate the effect of the compression loading on the viability of NP-MSCs, a CCK-8 assay was performed. As observed in Figure 2, the viability of the NP-MSCs was inhibited by compression and the inhibiting effect was significantly increased as compression time was prolonged except for the time of 24 h, which has shown an increased cell viability. A possible explanation of this phenomenon is that moderate compression may increase the cell viability, but this improvement cannot contribute to the stemness ability of intervertebral disc stem cells (Figure 2, values are presented as means ± SD, $^{*}p < 0.05$ and $^{**}p < 0.01$ versus control).

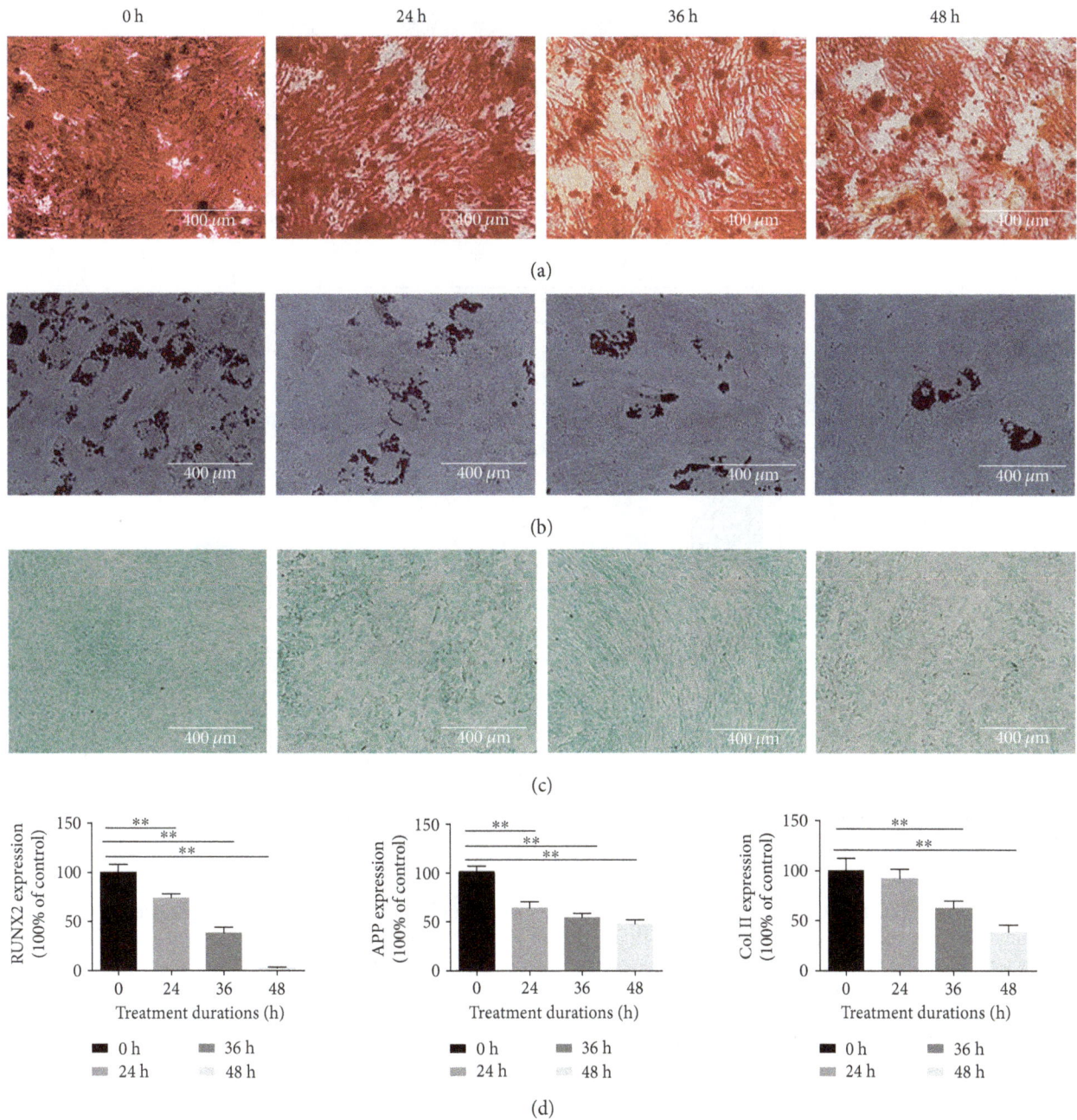

(a)

(b)

(c)

(d)

FIGURE 3: Compression inhibited the multilineage differentiation potential of NP-MSCs. (a) The induction of osteogenic differentiation under the increased compression time from 0 h to 48 h. (b) The induction of adipogenic differentiation under the increased compression time from 0 h to 48 h. (c) The induction of chondrogenic differentiation under the increased compression time from 0 h to 48 h. (d) The expressions of osteogenesis genes (Runx2), adipocyte-specific genes (APP), and chondrocyte-specific genes (Col2) under the increased compression time from 0 h to 48 h (values are presented as means ± SD, $^{**}p < 0.01$ versus control).

3.3. Compression Inhibited the Multilineage Differentiation Potential of NP-MSCs. To determine the effect of the compression loading on the multilineage differentiation potential of NP-MSCs, the osteogenic, adipogenic, and chondrogenic differentiation was induced and the mRNA expressions of Runx2, APP, and Col2 for the osteogenic, adipogenic, and chondrogenic differentiation, respectively, were analyzed. The results showed that the multilineage differentiation was suppressed in accordance with the increased compression time from 0 h to 48 h. For osteogenic differentiation, the mineralized nodules and the expressions of osteogenesis genes (Runx2) significantly decreased in the NP-MSCs with compression treatment (Figures 3(a) and 3(d)). For adipogenic differentiation, the accumulated lipid vacuoles decreased and the expression of adipocyte-specific genes (APP) significantly downregulated (Figures 3(b) and 3(d)). For chondrogenic differentiation, the proteoglycans and the expressions of chondrocyte-specific genes (Col2) obviously decreased (Figures 3(c) and 3(d)). (Figure 3, values are presented as means ± SD, $^{*}p < 0.05$ and $^{**}p < 0.01$ versus control).

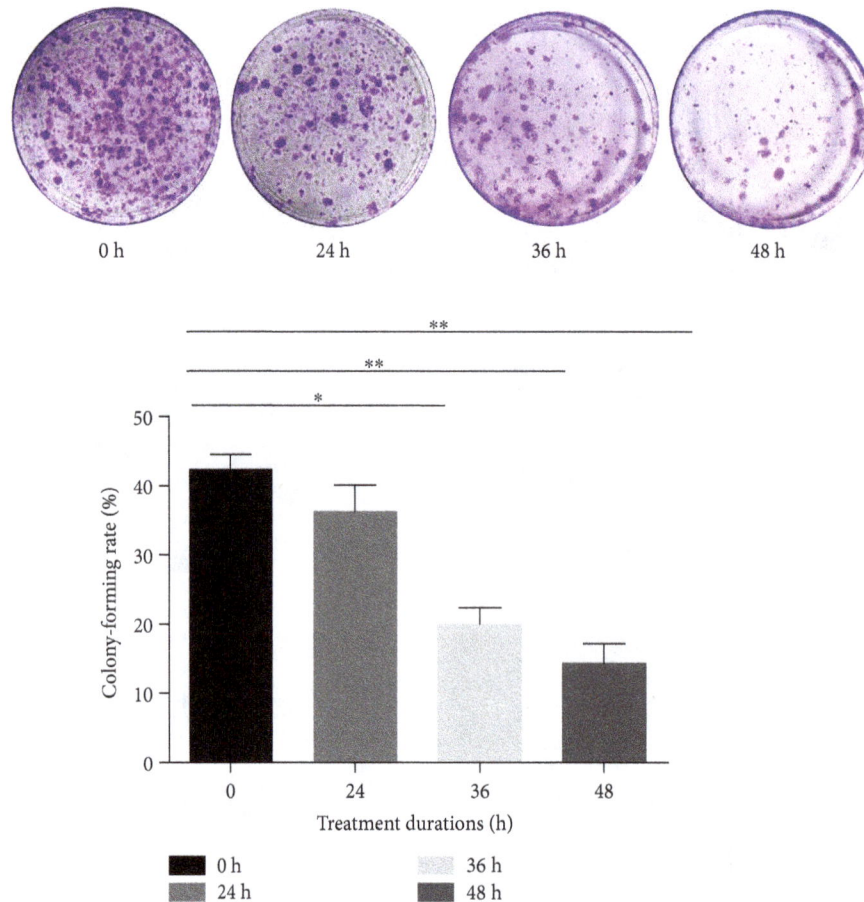

0 h   24 h   36 h   48 h

FIGURE 4: Compression inhibited the capacity of colony formation (values are presented as means ± SD, $^*p < 0.05$ and $^{**}p < 0.01$ versus control).

3.4. Compression Inhibited the Capacity of Colony Formation. The colony-forming ability is a vital factor to evaluate the stemness of NP-MSCs. In the control group, the colony-forming rate was 46%. But in the compression group, the results demonstrated that the colony-forming rate was inhibited by 43.33%, 38.27%, 19.4%, and 14.33% compared to the control at different time points from 24 h to 48 h (Figure 4, values are presented as means ± SD, $^*p < 0.05$ and $^{**}p < 0.01$ versus control).

3.5. Compression Inhibited the Migration Ability. Nondirectional migration ability and directional migration ability were assessed by wound healing assay and transwell migration assay, respectively. As shown in Figure 5, the migration areas and the migrated NP-MSCs were increased over time. However, the migration areas and the migrated NP-MSCs significantly decreased compared to those at different time points from 24 h to 48 h (Figure 5, values are presented as means ± SD, $^*p < 0.05$ and $^{**}p < 0.01$ versus control).

3.6. Compression Decreased the Expression of Stem Cell-Related Genes (Sox2 and Oct4). The genes, including Sox2 and Oct4, were considered the specific genes that maintained the stemness of MSCs. The expression of proteins

(Sox2 and Oct4) was significantly decreased. Protein levels of Sox2 and Oct4 from treated cell lysates were analyzed by Western blotting and normalized against GAPDH levels (Figure 6, values are presented as means ± SD, $^*p < 0.05$ and $^{**}p < 0.01$ versus control).

4. Discussion

Endogenous stem cell repair for IVD degeneration provides a novel strategy to reverse the structure and mechanical function of IVD tissues, and it has excited a great interest to scientists in the past decade. In 2007, Risbud et al. [21] isolated and identified the skeletal progenitor cells from degenerate human disc in vitro, which could express a series of specific surface markers of MSCs and commit to multilineage differentiation. In 2009, Henriksson et al. [22] applied the labeling technique in vivo and demonstrated the existence of slow-cycling cells and stem cell niche in the IVD region. After that, many groups isolated and identified MSCs from the nucleus pulposus, annulus fibrosus, and cartilage endplate [10, 11, 23–30]. In the present study, the cells isolated from NP had the following characteristics: (1) the cells presented with long spindle-shaped adherent growth and grew in a spiral formation; (2) the cells were positive for CD105, CD73, and CD90 and negative for CD34, CD14, CD19, and HLA-

No compression

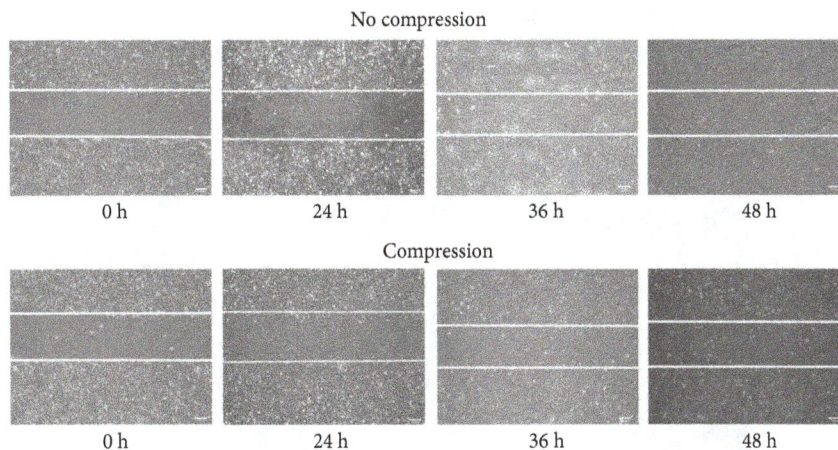

(a)

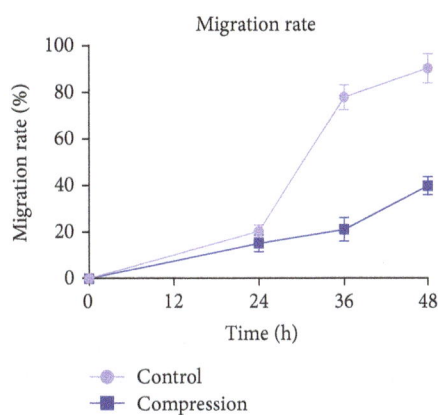

(b)

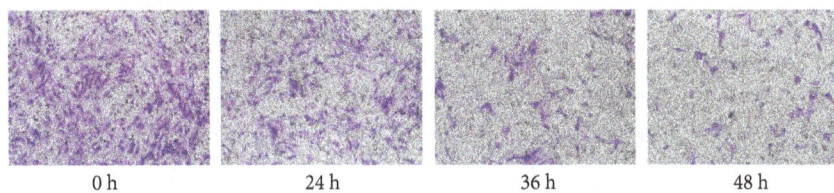

(c)

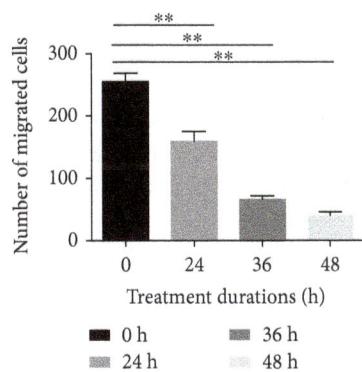

(d)

FIGURE 5: Compression inhibited the migration ability. (a, c) The assessment of nondirectional migration ability by wound healing assay with or without compression from 0 h to 48 h. (b, d) The assessment of directional migration ability by transwell migration assay under compression from 0 h to 48 h (values are presented as mean ± SD, $^{**}p < 0.01$ versus control).

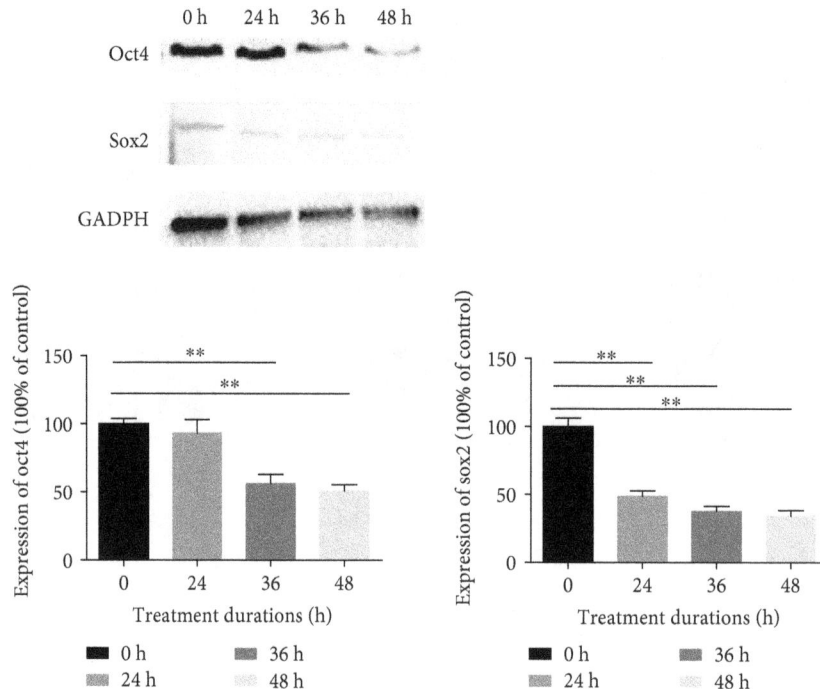

FIGURE 6: Compression decreased the expression of stem cell-related genes (Sox2 and Oct4). The expression of Sox2 and Oct4 was analyzed by Western blotting and normalized against GAPDH levels (values are presented as mean ± SD, $^{**}p < 0.01$ versus control).

DR; and (3) the cells had the multilineage differentiation potential. These characteristics met the criteria stated by the ISCT for MSC.

In the progress of endogenous tissue regeneration, a single stem cell produces two daughter cells: one maintains the stemness to renew itself while the other differentiates to a specific cell to conduct endogenous repair [31]. In terms of endogenous NP-MSC repair for IVD degeneration, one part of NP-MSCs retains the stem cell identity, and another part of NP-MSCs differentiates into nucleus pulposus-like cells and stimulus disc cells to repair the degenerative disc. Therefore, sustaining the number of viable and functional NP-MSCs is vital for maintaining the IVD homeostasis [9]. However, the IVD is avascular and NP-MSCs in the discs have to bear various stresses, including acidity, hypoxia, nutrient deficiency, and hypertonicity and mechanical loads [12]. Although mechanical stress plays an essential role in the progression of IVD degeneration, there have been no studies reporting the effect of compression loading on human NP-MSCs so far. Thus, the current study applied a custom-made compression apparatus for the first time to study the effect of compression loading on the biological behavior of NP-MSCs in vitro.

The results showed that the viability of the NP-MSCs was inhibited by compression except for the time of 24 h, which has shown an increased cell viability. A possible explanation of this phenomenon is that moderate compression may increase the cell viability, but this improvement cannot contribute to the stemness ability of intervertebral disc stem cells. Stem cells may be a special type of intervertebral disc cells which can react to a short time of compression; however, the differentiation ability, migration ability, and

the expression of stem protein have shown a damage when the cells were exposed to the compression of 24 h. We have to say it is interesting and a little strange, but we all know that cell viability cannot be the representative sign of other abilities so this phenomenon needs further research. What is more, the multilineage differentiation potential was also inhibited by compression. But Dai et al. and Kim et al. reported that dynamic compression promoted the proliferation and differentiation of exogenous mesenchymal stem cells [32, 33]. We considered that the conflicting results mainly came from the different modes of compression exerted on cells and the distinct cell types used in the study. In the present study, 1.0 MPa and continuous compression was applied, and NP-MSCs isolated from degenerative NP tissue were used. However, in the study of Dai et al. and Kim et al., lower (17 kPa, 0.2 MPa) and intermittent compression was applied, and viable exogenous MSCs isolated from adipose tissue or bone marrow were used. It was reported that the intradiscal pressure value in a healthy human is around 0.1 MPa in a prone position, 0.5 MPa in a standing position, 1.1 MPa in a flexed position, and even 2.3 MPa in a standing position carrying a weight [15, 34]. Moreover, multiple stress peaks appear under aging and degeneration environment in the IVD [15]. Therefore, our study simulated the effect of excessive compression in degenerative discs on NP-MSCs and emphasized the research of the endogenous repair failure during IVDD.

MSCs can generate colonies when plated at low densities and can also migrate to sites of injury. It has been shown that the colony-forming ability and migration ability are the important biological characteristics of MSCs [35, 36]. The results revealed that compression loading inhibited the colony-forming ability and migration ability. Stem cell-related genes and proteins (Sox2 and Oct4) also play a vital role in maintaining MSC properties [37, 38]. In keeping with our results above, compression loading suppressed the expression of Sox2 and Oct4. All results in this study suggested that inappropriate or excessive compression loading inhibited the biological behavior of NP-MSCs and might be one of the mechanisms of endogenous repair failure for IVD degeneration. Before the IVD tissue-derived MSCs were isolated, many attentions were concentrated on the fate of disc cells and the repair mainly centered around how to supply the disc cells with exogenous cells, growth factors, or biomaterial [16, 39, 40]. Little is known about endogenous stem cells and endogenous repair. The present study investigated the effect of compression on the biological behavior of NP-MSCs in vitro and tried to enhance our understanding on the endogenous repair failure for IVD degeneration. Moreover, it provided a novel method to repair IVD degeneration by activating the endogenous NP-MSCs.

In conclusion, findings from our study demonstrated that the biological behavior of NP-MSCs could be inhibited by compression loading, and it might be one of the mechanisms of endogenous repair failure for IVD degeneration. Further studies discussing the effect of compression on NP-MSCs in vivo and the underlying specific mechanism may be helpful to understand the endogenous repair failure of NP-MSCs during IVD degeneration.

Abbreviations

NP-MSCs:	Nucleus pulposus-derived mesenchymal stem cells
ISCT:	International Society for Cellular Therapy
IVD:	Intervertebral disc
MSCs:	Mesenchymal stem cells
MRI:	Magnetic resonance images
NP:	Nucleus pulposus
ECM:	Extracellular matrix
CCK-8:	Cell viability assay
QRT-PCR:	Quantitative real-time polymerase chain reaction
SD:	Standard deviation
ANOVA:	One-way analysis of variance.

Authors' Contributions

All the authors contribute equally to this paper.

Acknowledgments

The authors want to say thanks to the National Key Research and Development Program of China (Grant no. 2016YFC1100100) and the National Natural Science Foundation of China (Grant nos. 81572203 and 91649204); all the authors want to show their special thanks to their families, as well as for their support and love.

References

[1] K. Luoma, H. Riihimaki, R. Luukkonen, R. Raininko, E. Viikari-Juntura, and A. Lamminen, "Low back pain in relation to lumbar disc degeneration," *Spine*, vol. 25, no. 4, pp. 487–492, 2000.

[2] Y. R. Rampersaud, A. Bidos, C. Fanti, and A. V. Perruccio, "The need for multidimensional stratification of chronic low back pain (LBP)," *Spine*, vol. 42, no. 22, pp. E1318–E1325, 2017.

[3] W. Tong, Z. Lu, L. Qin et al., "Cell therapy for the degenerating intervertebral disc," *Translational Research*, vol. 181, pp. 49–58, 2017.

[4] D. Oehme, T. Goldschlager, P. Ghosh, J. V. Rosenfeld, and G. Jenkin, "Cell-based therapies used to treat lumbar degenerative disc disease: a systematic review of animal studies and human clinical trials," *Stem Cells International*, vol. 2015, Article ID 946031, 16 pages, 2015.

[5] D. Sakai, "Stem cell regeneration of the intervertebral disk," *Orthopedic Clinics of North America*, vol. 42, no. 4, pp. 555–562, 2011.

[6] D. Sakai and S. Grad, "Advancing the cellular and molecular therapy for intervertebral disc disease," *Advanced Drug Delivery Reviews*, vol. 84, pp. 159–171, 2015.

[7] H. Yang, C. Cao, C. Wu et al., "TGF-βl suppresses inflammation in cell therapy for intervertebral disc degeneration," *Scientific Reports*, vol. 5, no. 1, article 13254, 2015.

[8] L. Orozco, R. Soler, C. Morera, M. Alberca, A. Sánchez, and J. García-Sancho, "Intervertebral disc repair by autologous mesenchymal bone marrow cells: a pilot study," *Transplantation*, vol. 92, no. 7, pp. 822–828, 2011.

[9] D. Sakai and G. B. J. Andersson, "Stem cell therapy for intervertebral disc regeneration: obstacles and solutions," *Nature Reviews Rheumatology*, vol. 11, no. 4, pp. 243–256, 2015.

[10] Q. Shen, L. Zhang, B. Chai, and X. Ma, "Isolation and characterization of mesenchymal stem-like cells from human nucleus pulposus tissue," *Science China Life Sciences*, vol. 58, no. 5, pp. 509–511, 2015.

[11] J. F. Blanco, I. F. Graciani, F. M. Sanchez-Guijo et al., "Isolation and characterization of mesenchymal stromal cells from human degenerated nucleus pulposus: comparison with bone marrow mesenchymal stromal cells from the same subjects," *Spine*, vol. 35, no. 26, pp. 2259–2265, 2010.

[12] F. Wang, R. Shi, F. Cai, Y.-T. Wang, and X.-T. Wu, "Stem cell approaches to intervertebral disc regeneration: obstacles from the disc microenvironment," *Stem Cells and Development*, vol. 24, no. 21, pp. 2479–2495, 2015.

[13] H. Li, Y. Tao, C. Liang et al., "Influence of hypoxia in the intervertebral disc on the biological behaviors of rat adipose- and nucleus pulposus-derived mesenchymal stem cells," *Cells, Tissues, Organs*, vol. 198, no. 4, pp. 266–277, 2013.

[14] J. Liu, H. Tao, H. Wang et al., "Biological behavior of human nucleus pulposus mesenchymal stem cells in response to changes in the acidic environment during intervertebral disc degeneration," *Stem Cells and Development*, vol. 26, no. 12, pp. 901–911, 2017.

[15] C. Neidlinger-Wilke, F. Galbusera, H. Pratsinis et al., "Mechanical loading of the intervertebral disc: from the macroscopic to the cellular level," *European Spine Journal*, vol. 23, no. S3, pp. 333–343, 2014.

[16] R. D. Bowles and L. A. Setton, "Biomaterials for intervertebral disc regeneration and repair," *Biomaterials*, vol. 129, pp. 54–67, 2017.

[17] K.-G. Ma, Z.-W. Shao, S.-H. Yang et al., "Autophagy is activated in compression-induced cell degeneration and is mediated by reactive oxygen species in nucleus pulposus cells exposed to compression," *Osteoarthritis and Cartilage*, vol. 21, no. 12, pp. 2030–2038, 2013.

[18] S. Chen, X. Lv, B. Hu et al., "RIPK1/RIPK3/MLKL-mediated necroptosis contributes to compression-induced rat nucleus pulposus cells death," *Apoptosis*, vol. 22, no. 5, pp. 626–638, 2017.

[19] M. Dominici, K. Le Blanc, I. Mueller et al., "Minimal criteria for defining multipotent mesenchymal stromal cells. The International Society for Cellular Therapy position statement," *Cytotherapy*, vol. 8, no. 4, pp. 315–317, 2006.

[20] F. Ding, Z.-W. Shao, S.-H. Yang, Q. Wu, F. Gao, and L.-M. Xiong, "Role of mitochondrial pathway in compression-induced apoptosis of nucleus pulposus cells," *Apoptosis*, vol. 17, no. 6, pp. 579–590, 2012.

[21] M. V. Risbud, A. Guttapalli, T. T. Tsai et al., "Evidence for skeletal progenitor cells in the degenerate human intervertebral disc," *Spine*, vol. 32, no. 23, pp. 2537–2544, 2007.

[22] H. B. Henriksson, M. Thornemo, C. Karlsson et al., "Identification of cell proliferation zones, progenitor cells and a potential stem cell niche in the intervertebral disc region: a study in four species," *Spine*, vol. 34, no. 21, pp. 2278–2287, 2009.

[23] C. Sang, X. Cao, F. Chen, X. Yang, and Y. Zhang, "Differential characterization of two kinds of stem cells isolated from rabbit nucleus pulposus and annulus fibrosus," *Stem Cells International*, vol. 2016, Article ID 8283257, 14 pages, 2016.

[24] L. T. Liu, B. Huang, C. Q. Li, Y. Zhuang, J. Wang, and Y. Zhou, "Characteristics of stem cells derived from the degenerated human intervertebral disc cartilage endplate," *PLoS One*, vol. 6, no. 10, article e26285, 2011.

[25] C. Liu, Q. Guo, J. Li et al., "Identification of rabbit annulus fibrosus-derived stem cells," *PLoS One*, vol. 9, no. 9, article e108239, 2014.

[26] B. Huang, L.-T. Liu, C.-Q. Li et al., "Study to determine the presence of progenitor cells in the degenerated human cartilage endplates," *European Spine Journal*, vol. 21, no. 4, pp. 613–622, 2012.

[27] H. Wang, Y. Zhou, T.-W. Chu et al., "Distinguishing characteristics of stem cells derived from different anatomical regions of human degenerated intervertebral discs," *European Spine Journal*, vol. 25, no. 9, pp. 2691–2704, 2016.

[28] R. Shi, F. Wang, X. Hong et al., "The presence of stem cells in potential stem cell niches of the intervertebral disc region: an in vitro study on rats," *European Spine Journal*, vol. 24, no. 11, pp. 2411–2424, 2015.

[29] W. M. Erwin, D. Islam, E. Eftekarpour, R. D. Inman, M. Z. Karim, and M. G. Fehlings, "Intervertebral disc-derived stem cells," *Spine*, vol. 38, no. 3, pp. 211–216, 2013.

[30] S. Liu, H. Liang, S. M. Lee, Z. Li, J. Zhang, and Q. Fei, "Isolation and identification of stem cells from degenerated human intervertebral discs and their migration characteristics," *Acta Biochimica et Biophysica Sinica*, vol. 49, no. 2, pp. 101–109, 2016.

[31] H. Clevers, K. M. Loh, and R. Nusse, "An integral program for tissue renewal and regeneration: Wnt signaling and stem cell control," *Science*, vol. 346, no. 6205, article 1248012, 2014.

[32] J. Dai, H. Wang, G. Liu, Z. Xu, F. Li, and H. Fang, "Dynamic compression and co-culture with nucleus pulposus cells promotes proliferation and differentiation of adipose-derived mesenchymal stem cells," *Journal of Biomechanics*, vol. 47, no. 5, pp. 966–972, 2014.

[33] D. H. Kim, S. H. Kim, S. J. Heo et al., "Enhanced differentiation of mesenchymal stem cells into NP-like cells via 3D co-culturing with mechanical stimulation," *Journal of Bioscience and Bioengineering*, vol. 108, no. 1, pp. 63–67, 2009.

[34] H.-J. Wilke, A. Rohlmann, S. Neller, F. Graichen, L. Claes, and G. Bergmann, "ISSLS prize winner: a novel approach to determine trunk muscle forces during flexion and extension: a comparison of data from an in vitro experiment and in vivo measurements," *Spine*, vol. 28, no. 23, pp. 2585–2593, 2003.

[35] R. Pochampally, "Colony forming unit assays for MSCs," *Methods in Molecular Biology*, vol. 449, pp. 83–91, 2008.

[36] G. Chamberlain, J. Fox, B. Ashton, and J. Middleton, "Concise review: mesenchymal stem cells: their phenotype, differentiation capacity, immunological features, and potential for homing," *Stem Cells*, vol. 25, no. 11, pp. 2739–2749, 2007.

[37] C. C. Tsai, P. F. Su, Y. F. Huang, T. L. Yew, and S. C. Hung, "Oct4 and Nanog directly regulate Dnmt1 to maintain self-renewal and undifferentiated state in mesenchymal stem cells," *Molecular Cell*, vol. 47, no. 2, pp. 169–182, 2012.

[38] R. Feng and J. Wen, "Overview of the roles of Sox2 in stem cell and development," *Biological Chemistry*, vol. 396, no. 8, pp. 883–891, 2015.

[39] P. Colombier, J. Clouet, C. Boyer et al., "TGF-β1 and GDF5 act synergistically to drive the differentiation of human adipose stromal cells toward *nucleus pulposus*-like cells," *Stem Cells*, vol. 34, no. 3, pp. 653–667, 2016.

[40] R. Tsaryk, A. Gloria, T. Russo et al., "Collagen-low molecular weight hyaluronic acid semi-interpenetrating network loaded with gelatin microspheres for cell and growth factor delivery for nucleus pulposus regeneration," *Acta Biomaterialia*, vol. 20, pp. 10–21, 2015.

The Differential Effects of Leukocyte-Containing and Pure Platelet-Rich Plasma on Nucleus Pulposus-Derived Mesenchymal Stem Cells: Implications for the Clinical Treatment of Intervertebral Disc Degeneration

Jun Jia,[1] Shan-zheng Wang,[2,3] Liang-yu Ma,[1] Jia-bin Yu,[1] Yu-dong Guo,[2] and Chen Wang ⓘ[1]

[1]*School of Medicine, Southeast University, 87 Ding Jia Qiao Road, Nanjing, Jiangsu 210009, China*
[2]*Department of Orthopaedics, Zhongda Hospital, School of Medicine, Southeast University, 87 Ding Jia Qiao Road, Nanjing, Jiangsu 210009, China*
[3]*The First Clinical Medical School, Nanjing Medical University, 300 Guangzhou Road, Nanjing, Jiangsu 210029, China*

Correspondence should be addressed to Chen Wang; wangchen_seu_edu@163.com

Academic Editor: Stefania Cantore

Background. Platelet-rich plasma (PRP) is a promising strategy for intervertebral disc degeneration. However, the potential harmful effects of leukocytes in PRP on nucleus pulposus-derived mesenchymal stem cells (NPMSCs) have seldom been studied. This study aimed at comparatively evaluating effects of pure platelet-rich plasma (P-PRP) and leukocyte-containing platelet-rich plasma (L-PRP) on rabbit NPMSCs in vitro. *Methods.* NPMSCs isolated from rabbit NP tissues were treated with L-PRP or P-PRP in vitro, and then cell proliferation and expression of stem cell markers, proinflammatory cytokines (TNF-α, IL-1β), production of ECM (extracellular matrix-related protein), and NF-κB p65 protein were validated by CCK-8 assay, real-time polymerase chain reaction, enzyme-linked immunosorbent assay, immunofluorescence, and western blot respectively. *Results.* NPMSCs differentiate into nucleus pulposus-like cells after treatment of PRPs (P-PRP and L-PRP), and NPMSCs exhibited maximum proliferation at a 10% PRP dose. L-PRP had observably higher concentration of leukocytes, TNF-α, and IL-1β than P-PRP. Furthermore, compared to P-PRP, L-PRP induced the differentiated NPMSCs to upregulate the expression of TNF-α and IL-1β, enhanced activation of the NF-κB pathway, increased the expression of MMP-1 and MMP-13, and produced less ECM in differentiated NPMSCs. *Conclusions.* Both P-PRP and L-PRP can induce the proliferation and NP-differentiation of NPMSCs. Compared to L-PRP, P-PRP can avoid the activation of the NF-κB pathway, thus reducing the inflammatory and catabolic responses.

1. Introduction

As a major cause of low back pain, intervertebral disc degeneration (IDD) is drawing increasing attention for substantial financial and health care burdens worldwide [1]. Although the etiology of IDD is currently unknown, mounting evidence has shown that the mechanical and biological degradation of the discs is considered as one of the common major causes of IDD [2]. Intervertebral disc consists of three distinct structural compositions, the outer annulus fibrosis, the inner NP (nucleus pulposus), and the upper and lower layers of endplates [3]. As the core portion of the intervertebral disc, NP plays a critical role in transmitting the load [4]. The failure of the load transmission is often considered the initiation of the disc degeneration [2]. Thus, the preservation and regeneration of the NP are often the concerns for the therapeutic strategies [5]. Currently, conservative treatments, including oral analgesics and NSAIDs, are clinically applied to alleviate the symptoms [6]. Spinal surgeries, especially those with minimal invasive techniques, can efficiently relieve the symptoms of neural compression. However, the degradation of the intervened or the adjacent discs may undergo an increasing degeneration course [7].

Currently, stem cell transplantation therapy is becoming a promising strategy when transplanted into the degenerated discs [8]. The convincing outcomes were well illustrated in many clinical and basic studies [9–11]. The microenvironment of IVD has the characteristics of low nutrition, acidity, hypertonicity, hypoxia, and high mechanical load [12]. This microenvironment not only has negative influence on original cells of the disc but also promotes apoptosis of transplanted cells [13]. It should be noted that the mesenchymal stem cells (MSCs) reside in the degenerated nucleus pulposus tissues for their regenerative potential. A recent study confirmed that the endogenic MSCs in the nucleus pulposus tissues (NPMSCs) were more resistant to hyperosmotic, acidic, and anoxic environment than the MSCs of fat sources [14]. Thus, in the degenerative disc microenvironment, the activation or transplantation of NPMSCs may have more advantages over MSCs from other tissues. As a useful MSC activator, PRP is widely investigated in tissue engineering strategy for its potential in cell proliferation and extracellular matrix [15–17]. When activated, a variety of growth factors, including PDGF, TGF, EGF, and VEGF, are secreted from the platelets, contributing to a joint regenerative effect on the damaged tissues [18]. Direct injection of PRP has been proven effective in IDD treatment by comprehensive researches [19, 20].

Although PRP is widely used for its regenerative potential, the efficacy was often in debate for its indeterminate therapeutic effect. Some studies revealed that PRP was effective in the repair of tendon injury [21–23], while others did not confirm the functional recovery of the repaired tendon and pain relief of the patients [24–26]. The inconsistency might be caused by the individual difference in patients and different preparations of PRP in each study [27]. Different preparations for PPR bring out various components, and leukocyte is one of the critical elements. Exclusion of leukocytes in PRP has been proven more beneficial for osteoarthritis [28] and bone defects [29]. In addition, PRP rich in leukocytes (L-PRP) can release high concentrations of inflammatory cytokines, which result in the activation of NF-κB pathway [28, 29]. However, the potential harmful effects of leukocytes in PRP on nucleus pulposus-derived mesenchymal stem cells (NPMSCs) have seldom been studied.

The objective of this study is to comparatively evaluate effects of P-PRP and L-PRP on rabbit NPMSCs in vitro, and a new insight is provided to improve the efficiency of PRP treatment in disc regeneration.

2. Methods

2.1. Preparation of L-PRP, P-PRP, NPMSCs, Spleen Cells, and NPCs. The use of rabbits was approved and supervised by the Animal Care and Use Committee of Southeast University. Autologous whole blood and NPMSCs were harvested from 24 New Zealand white rabbits (8 months old, 3.0–4.0 kg, female) respectively. About 27 ml of autologous whole blood was collected from each New Zealand white rabbit through the carotid artery and mixed with 3 ml acid-citrate dextrose solution A (Santa Cruz, catalog no. SC-214744) to make 30 ml of anticoagulated whole blood. 2 ml whole blood was

used in quantifying the platelet and leukocyte concentrations in whole blood, and the rest 28 ml blood was left for preparation of PRP (P-PRP, L-PRP). The method of two-step centrifugation process [30] was applied to prepare the P-PRP and L-PRP. Briefly, 14 ml whole blood was centrifuged at 250g for 10 minutes at room temperature to separate the blood into three layers, platelet-containing plasma at the top, buffy coat (rich in leukocytes and platelets) in the middle, and erythrocytes at the bottom. The top two layers were transferred into a new tube and spun again at 250g for 10 minutes; most of the leukocytes, platelets, and fibrinogen precipitated. Then, most of the supernatant (poor in platelet) was discarded. The left plasma and precipitate, which were almost 2 ml, were resuspended to form the L-PRP. The other 14 ml whole blood was centrifuged at 160g for 10 minutes to separate platelet-containing plasma from buffy coat (rich in leukocytes) and erythrocytes. Then plasma layer was aspirated carefully to avoid the buffy coat and erythrocyte pollution. The plasma layer was centrifuged again at 250g for 15 minutes. Then, most of the supernatant (poor in platelet) was discarded. The left plasma and precipitate, which were almost 1.5 ml, were resuspended to form the P-PRP.

Nucleus pulposus tissue was isolated from IVDs of the New Zealand white rabbits above, minced into 1mm^3 tissue block, and digested using 0.2 mg/ml type II collagenase (Thermo Fisher, catalog no. DS56580) in DMEM-LG (GIBCO, catalog no. AB10104399) medium for 4–6 h. After centrifugation at 1500 r/min for 10 minutes (DragonLab, D3024R), the cell pellet from the discs (lumbar 3-5) of the same rabbit was cultured in 25 cm^2 cell culture dish at a density of 10^4 cells/cm^2. The cells were cultured in DMEM-LG medium supplemented with 10% fetal bovine serum (FBS) (Sigma, catalog no. BK20170120), 100 U/ml penicillin G (Hyclone, lot: J150019) and 0.1 mg/mL streptomycin (Hyclone, catalog no. K270109) under a humidified atmosphere of 95% air and 5% CO$_2$ at 37°C. The medium was changed every 3 days until the cells reached 80%–90% subconfluence, then cells were harvested using 0.25% trypsin and 0.02% EDTA (Hyclone, lot: J160004) and re-suspended in the same medium. Then the cell suspension was inoculated into tissue culture dishes at a density of 50 cells/cm^2 for further culture. The images of cell morphology were performed using microscope attaching camera (OLYMPU, IX51). The NPMSCs of passage 2 were selected for further experiments.

NPCs were isolated and harvested as previously reported [31]. Nucleus pulposus tissue were obtained from the rabbits above and immediately minced into 1 mm3 tissue block and digested using 0.25% trypsin (Thermo Fisher, catalog no. 25200056) for 5 to10 minutes and 0.25% type I collagenase (Thermo Fisher, catalog no. 17100017) for 20 to 25 minutes. After centrifugation (1500 r/min, 10 min), the cell pellets were re-suspended in monolayer culture supplemented with DMEM medium containing 10% fetal bovine serum (Sigma, catalog no. BK20170120), 100 U/ml penicillin G (Hyclone, lot: J150019), and 0.1 mg/ml streptomycin (Hyclone, catalog no. K270109) under standard conditions (37°C, 21% O$_2$, and 5% CO$_2$). The medium was changed every 3 days after the primary started to grow by static adherence. The NPCs were collected and subcultured at a ratio of 1:3 until the cells

TABLE 1: Sequences of primers used for RT-PCR.

Gene	Forward primers (5′-3′)	Reverse primers (5′-3′)
GAPDH	ACTTTGTGAAGCTCATTTCCTGGTA	GTGGTTTGAGGGCTCTTACTCCTT
CD29	GTCACCAACCGTAGCAA	CTCCTCATCTCATTCATCAG
CD44	CGATTTGAATATAACCTGCCGC	CGTGCCCTTCTATGAACCCA
CD166	GGACAGCCCGAAGGAATACGAA	GACACAGGCAGGGAATCACCAA
CD4	GATGGAGGTGGAACTGC	GGAAAGCCCAACACTATG
CD8	GGGTGGAAAAGGAGAAGC	AGGTGAGTGCGGGAGAC
CD14	CAGGTGCCTAAGGGACT	AATAAAGTGGGAAGCGG
IL-1β	CGGTCAAGGAGAGGAGCTTAC	GGACTAGCCCTCGCTTATCTTT
TNF-α	GGAGAAGCCGGTAGTGGAGAT	GGTCTGGTCACGGTTTGGAA
MMP-1	CGACTCGCTATCTCCAAGTGA	GTTGAACCAGTCTCCGACCA
MMP-13	GGAGGCGAGAACATCAAGCC	CGGCCTTCCCTCGTAGTGA
Oct-4	ACCTTCATCGGAAACTCCAAAG	ACTGTTAGGCTCAGGTGAACT
Nanog	CTGTGGGTTTCTGTGCTGG	CCGGCTTCAAGGCTTTCAG
Collagen II	CAGGATGTCCAGGAGGCT	GCAGTGGCGAGGTCAGTAG
Aggrecan	GGAGCCCGAGCCTATACTATTT	CCCAAGGACCAATCA

reached 80%–90% subconfluence. The P2 NPCs were used for total RNA extraction.

Spleen cells were isolated according to the method described previously [32]. Briefly, the harvested spleen tissue from the rabbits above was minced and filtrated with 70 μm cell strainer (Corning, catalog no. 431751) to obtain single-cell solution. The cell solution was subsequently centrifuged at 1000 r/min for 10 minutes. The cell pellet was subsequently treated with blood cell lysis buffer (Solarbio, catalog no. R1010-500 ml) to remove red blood cells. The precipitate of mixture of cells was used for total RNA extraction.

2.2. Component Analysis of P-PRP, L-PRP, and Whole Blood. The concentrations of leukocyte and platelet in PRP and whole blood were measured by an automatic hematology analyzer (XP-300, Sysmex, Houston, America). The P-PRP and L-PRP were activated with 10% calcium chloride solution and then incubated at 37°C for 7 d. Moreover, the supernatants were extracted from PRP which had been centrifugated at 2800g for 15 minutes. The concentrations of TNF-α and IL-1β were explored using ELISA kit (Xitang, Shanghai, China) according to the manufacturer's instructions.

2.3. Identification of Nucleus Pulposus Mesenchymal Stem Cells. The NPMSCs of passage 2 were subjected to induced differentiation by culturing them in chondrogenic, adipogenic, and osteogenic media, respectively. The cells were evaluated using Alcian blue (Sigma, catalog no. B8438), Oil Red O (Sigma, catalog no. O8010), and alizarin red (Solabio, catalog no. G8550-25), staining respectively. The outcomes were examined by an inverted microscope. RT-PCR was used to determine the expression of MSC (mesenchymal stem cell) mark genes (CD166, CD44, CD29, CD14, CD8, and CD4) from the NPMSCs, NPCs (nucleus pulposus cells), and spleen cells. Briefly, total RNA was extracted from NPMSCs, NPCs, and spleen tissue using TRIzol reagent (Thermo Fisher, catalog no. 10296010) according to the manufacturer's

instructions. Reverse transcription was gained by a reverse transcription kit (Thermo Fisher, catalog no.AM334) according to the instruction sequences of the manufacturer. The sequences of primers which were used in the reactions are listed in Table 1.

2.4. Proliferation of NPMSCs in Different Concentrations of PRPs (P-PRP, L-PRP). To determine the cell viability and cell proliferation capacity, cells were examined with CCK-8 assay. The P2 NPMSCs obtained as described above were seeded in a 24-well plate (Yu can Corning/Costar, catalog no. 3415) at 10000 cells per well and maintained in a culture medium containing 2% FBS and P-PRP or L-PRP at various volume percent fractions: 0%, 5%, 10%, 15%, and 20% for 7 days. 100 μl of fresh medium containing 0.5% FBS and 10 μl CCK-8 were added to each plate and incubated for 4 h at 37°C. The optical density was detected at 450 nm, and the experiment was independently performed for three times.

2.5. Coculture of NPMSCs In Vitro. The transwell system (Costar, catalog no.JM-3450) was used for coculture of NPMSCs in this study. This transwell consists microporous membrane (0.4um) between upper and lower compartments so that there is free flow of culture medium in the two compartments. The P2 NPMSCs in the basal medium (DMEM + 2% FBS) were seeded into the bottom of the transwell system allocated to three groups (P-PRP, L-PRP, and control). The experimental groups (P-PRP or L-PRP group) were put into 10%P-PRP or 10%L-PRP, respectively, in the top compartment of the transwell system, and the top compartment containing basal medium only was set as the control group. The NPMSCs from all groups were cocultured for 14 days, and the culture medium was changed every 3 days. Concentration of PRPs in this study was adjusted to 10% (vol/vol) using basal medium (DMEM + 2% FBS) according to the proliferation of NPMSC assay above.

2.6. Measuring Expression of MMP-1, MMP-13, IL-1β, and TNF-α in Coculture NPMSCs. Cells from all groups mentioned above were harvested on day 14 by trypsinization and centrifugation. The cell pellet was used to measure cell count by an auto cellometer (Cellometer Auto 2000, Nexcelom, America), and the supernatant was used to estimate the concentrations of MMP-1, MMP-13, TNF-α, and IL-1β by respective ELISA kits according to the manufacturer's instructions (Xitang, Shanghai, China). Each experiment was repeated in triplicate.

2.7. qRT-PCR Analysis. The NPMSCs which were cultured in the transwell described above were harvested on day 14 by 2.5% trypsin and 0.02% EDTA. The gene nucleus pulposus cell-related genes (collagen II and aggrecan), mesenchymal stem cell-related genes (Oct-4, Nanog), inflammatory marker genes (TNF-α, IL-1β), and catabolic genes (MMP-1, MMP-13) were determined by qRT-PCR. In brief, TRIzol reagent (Invitrogen, CA, USA) was used to extract the total RNA from cells according to the manufacturer's instructions. Real-time PCR was performed using SYBR Premix Ex Taq II (TaKaRa, Dalian, China) and measured on an iQ5 Real-Time PCR Detection System (Bio-Rad, Hercules, CA). The PCR conditions were performed by denaturing the cDNA at 94°C for 4 min, followed by 40 cycles of amplification: 94°C for 40 s, 52°C for 40 s, and 72°C for 40 s for data collection. All samples were normalized to control and calculated using the $2^{-\Delta\Delta CT}$ analysis method. We used GAPDH expression as the endogenous control, and the sequences of primers which are used in the reactions are listed in Table 1.

2.8. Immunofluorescence. The NPMSCs were collected from the experimental groups and control groups as described above. And then, the cells were fixed with PBS containing 4% paraformaldehyde (Sigma, catalog no. D56988) for 20 minutes and washed with PBS including 1% Triton for 5 minutes. Immunostaining for nucleus pulposus cell-related proteins (collagen II and aggrecan) was implemented by blocking the cells in 2% mouse serum (Novus Biologicals, catalog no. NB600-504) and then incubated with mouse anti-rabbit collagen II antibody (Aridobio, catalog no. ARG62450) or anti-rabbit aggrecan (Novus Biologicals, catalog no. NB600-504) at 4°C overnight. The cells were washed 3 times with PBS for 5 minutes each and incubated with Alexa Fluor 594-conjugated goat anti-mouse IgG secondary antibody (Bastet, catalog no. BK0027) for 90 minutes at room temperature. The cell nucleus was counterstained by Hoechst 33342 (Thermo Fisher, catalog no. 62249). The inverted fluorescence microscope (BX53, Olympus, Japan) was used to observe the stained cells.

2.9. Western Blot Analysis. The cells from all groups mentioned above were harvested after culturing for two weeks. Extraction of total proteins in the cells was performed by using M-PER (mammalian protein extraction reagent) (Fermenta, catalog no. 26616) supplementing 1.5% (vol/vol) protease inhibitors (Bio-Rad catalog no. 161-0156). Concentration of proteins in the supernatant was measured by using the BCA Protein Assay Kit (Thermo Fisher catalog no.

EC60980) according to manufacturer's instruction after centrifugation at 10000 r/min for 10 minutes. 20 μg of total cell protein extracts from each group was separated by 25% SDS polyacrylamide gel electrophoresis (Thermo Fisher, catalog no. DF65896) at 100 V for 60 minutes, then transferred onto PVDF membranes (Millipore catalog no. IPVH00010) at 100 V for 30 minutes which was blocked with 3% fat-free milk in Tris-buffered saline at room temperature for 30 minutes. The blots were incubated with anti-P65 antibody (Abcam, catalog no. ab154036), anti-aggrecan antibody (Novus Biologicals, catalog no. NB600-504), anti-collagen II antibody (Aridobio, catalog no. ARG62450), and anti-GAPDH antibody at a dilution of 1 : 1000 at 4°C overnight, followed by incubation with IgG-HRP (goat anti-mouse peroxidase-conjugated secondary antibody) (Bastet, catalog no. BK0027) at a dilution of 1 : 5000 for 1 h at room temperature. The expression of protein was detected by ECL kit (Biyuntian, catalog no. ce7827) according to the manufacturer's suggested protocols. GAPDH was used as an internal control.

2.10. Statistical Analysis. The difference between different two groups of three independent experiments was analyzed by Student's *t*-test. One-way analysis of variance (ANOVA) was used to analyze the difference among more than two groups. The data are presented as means ± S.D. $P < 0.05$ was considered to be statistically significant.

3. Results

3.1. NPMSCs Possessed the Typical Characteristics of MSCs for Self-Renewing, Clonogenicity, Stem Cell Markers, and Multidifferentiation Potential. After inoculation, the cells isolated from the nucleus pulposus of the disc started to grow by static adherence after 10–14 days, and the primary cells showed various shapes. They mainly comprise round macrophage-like cells and spindle-shaped fibroblast-like cells (Figure 1(a)). After low-density (50/cm^2) cell passage, the cells formed typical sunflower-like cell colonies (Figure 1(b)). In addition, the cells displayed a uniform cobblestone-like morphology at passage 2 (Figure 1(c)); RT-PCR was performed to determine the gene expression of typical MSC surface marks. As shown in Figure 1(d), the results indicated that the expression of markers in passage 2 including CD166, CD44, and CD29 which frequently exist in MSCs was significantly higher than that in NPCs. In addition, the markers containing CD14, CD8, and CD4 were seldom expressed which are negative in MSCs. Meanwhile, the cells were induced to differentiation of chondrogenesis, osteogenesis, and adipogenesis respectively (Figures 1(e)–1(g)). When the cells were cultivated in the osteogenic medium, the morphology of the cells changed on the fifth day. The calcium deposits in the cells were highly visible after 3 weeks, and then they were fixed and stained by "alizarin red." In contrast, the cells in the control group did not produce any calcium deposits which were cultivated in basic medium (Figure 1(e)). After culturing in adipogenic induction medium for 1 week, the cells gradually developed lipid droplets. The cells were stained with "Oil Red O" on day 21.

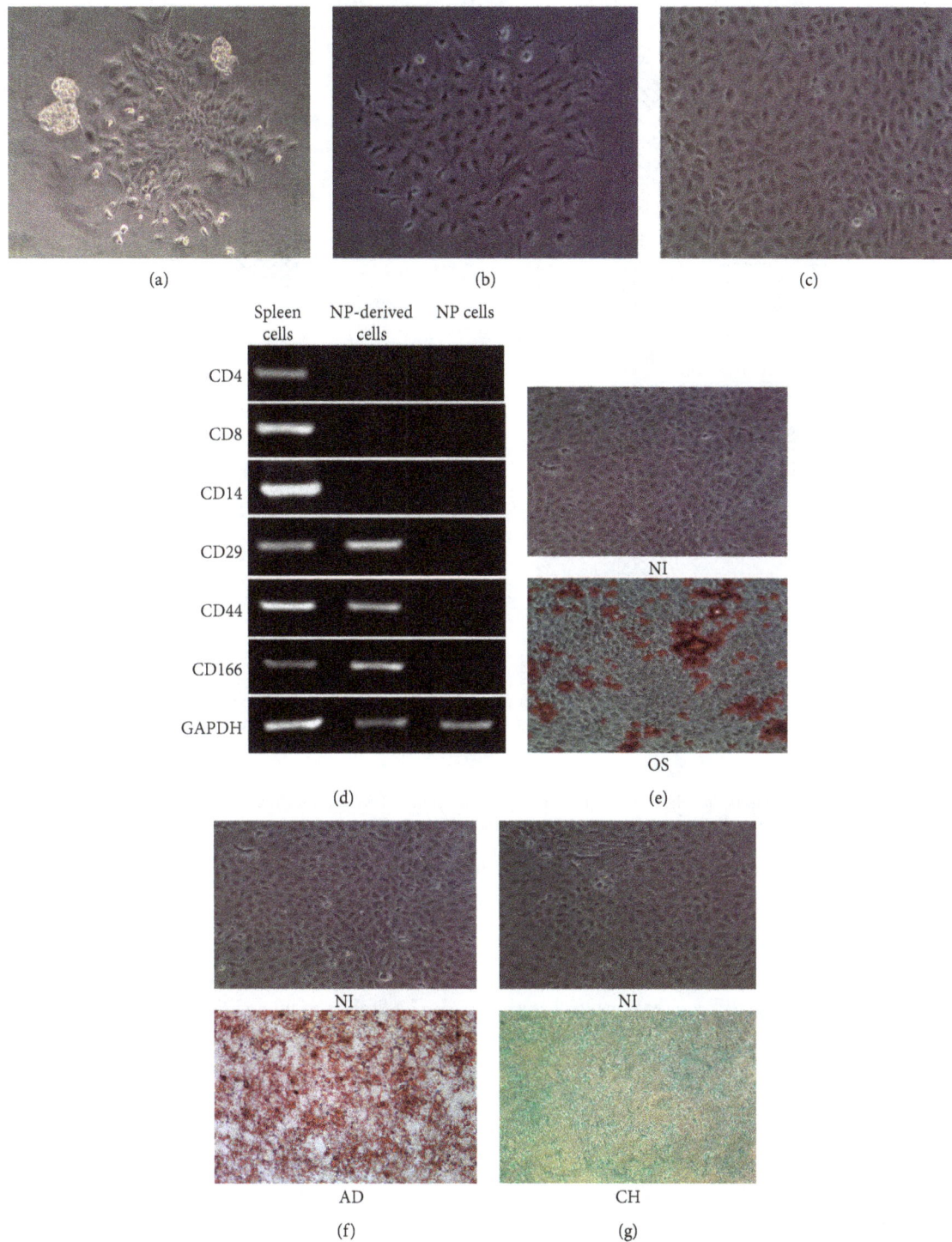

FIGURE 1: NPMSCs possessed the typical characteristics of MSCs for self-renewing, clonogenicity, stem cell markers, and multidifferentiation potential. (a) The morphology of primary cells (100x). (b) A typical sunflower-like cell colony at passage 1 (100x). (c) Cells displayed a uniform cobblestone-like morphology (100x). (d) The genes of CD29, CD44, and CD166 expressed strongly in cells of passage 2 but not in NP cells and seldom expressed CD14, CD8, and CD4; The spleen cells expressed all genes above as positive controls; the NP cells did not express these genes as a negative control. (e) Micrographs showing accumulation of mineralized calcium deposition in noninduced cells (NI) and osteoinduced cells (OS), as determined by alizarin red staining (100x). (f) Micrographs showing degree of lipid droplets in noninduced cells (NI) and adipoinduced cells (AD) as assessed by Oil red O staining (NI100x, AD400x). (g) Micrographs showing the levels of chondrogenesis in noninduced cells (NI) and chondrogenic induction cell (CH), as measured by Alcian blue staining.

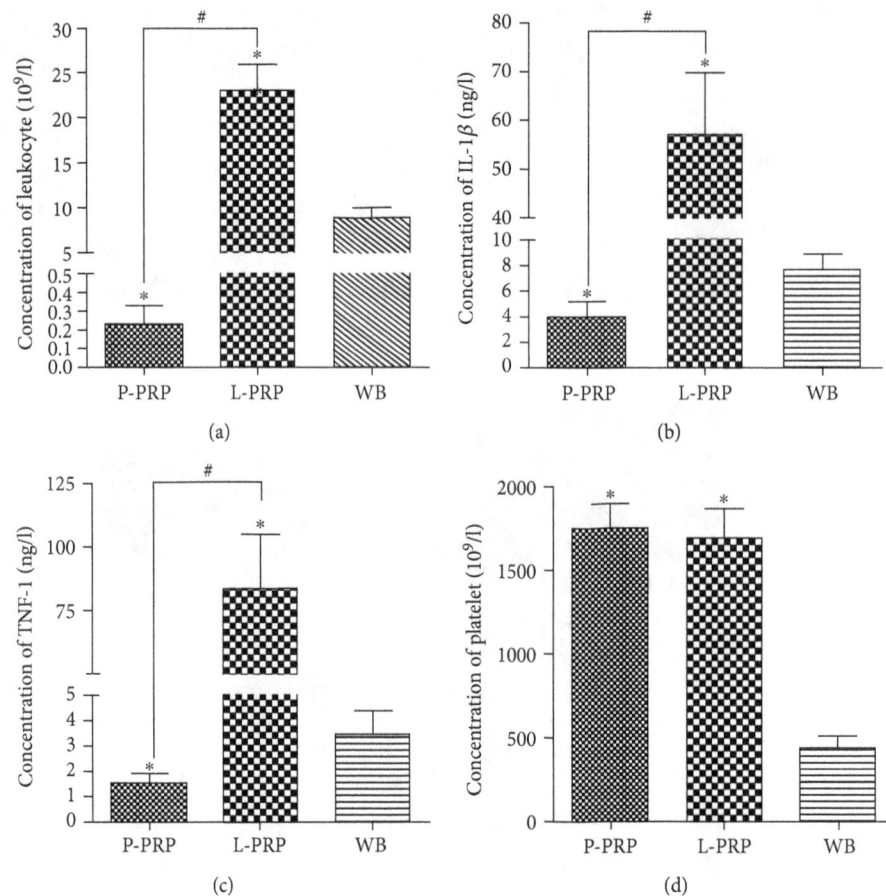

FIGURE 2: The concentrations of leukocytes, inflammatory cytokines (IL-1β and TNF-α), and platelet in whole blood, L-PRP and P-PRP. (a–c) The leukocytes, inflammatory cytokines, IL-1β, and TNF-α in P-PRP, L-PRP, and whole blood. (d) Platelet concentrations of P-PRP, L-PRP, and whole blood. "*" indicates that the difference between P-PRP or L-PRP and whole blood was statistically significant ($P < 0.05$). "#" indicates that the difference between L-PRP and P-PRP was statistically significant ($P < 0.05$). Statistical analysis using ANOVA, $n = 8$.

The cells of the control group did not have any change (Figure 1(f)). The cells differentiated into chondrocyte-like cells and emerged a much higher level of "Alcian blue" staining after culturing in a chondrogenic differentiation medium compared with control cells (Figure 1(g)).

3.2. The Concentrations of Leukocytes, Inflammatory Cytokines (IL-1β and TNF-α), and Platelet in Whole Blood, L-PRP, and P-PRP. We found that the leukocyte concentration in L-PRP was markedly higher than that in whole blood while the concentration of leukocyte in P-PRP was significantly lower than that in whole blood (Figure 2(a), $P < 0.05$). The levels of IL-1β and TNF-α in L-PRP were elevated. As shown in Figures 2(b) and 2(c), the levels of IL-1β and TNF-α in L-PRP were significantly higher than those in whole blood and P-PRP, while the levels of IL-1β and TNF-α in P-PRP were evidently lower than those in whole blood ($P < 0.05$). The concentration of platelet was similar between P-PRP and L-PRP. In addition, concentrations of platelet in P-PRP and L-PRP were 3.8-fold higher than those in whole blood (Figure 2(d)).

3.3. The Proliferation of Cells Is Dose-Dependent to PRPs. To ascertain whether PRP could functionally regulate proliferation, we performed CCK-8 assays to evaluate the role of PRPs in the progression of cells. When the cells cultured in the medium comprising different concentrations of PRPs as described above, the results displayed that cell proliferation rate showed dose-dependent response on P-PRP and L-PRP (Figure 3). The cell proliferation rate had no significant difference at the presence of 5%, 15%, and 20% P-PRP or L-PRP and increased by 60% compared with the control groups (0% PRPs). The presence of 10% P-PRP or 10% L-PRP obtained the maximum proliferation rate. There was no significant difference between L-PRP and P-PRP in each concentration ($P > 0.05$).

3.4. PRPs Promote the Differentiation of NPMSCS into Nucleus Pulposus-like Cells. To observe the effects of P-PRP and L-PRP on differentiation of NPMSCS, we first investigate the cell morphology. The results showed that controls were mainly cobblestone-like without any change (Figure 4(a)), while cell morphology of experimental groups gradually

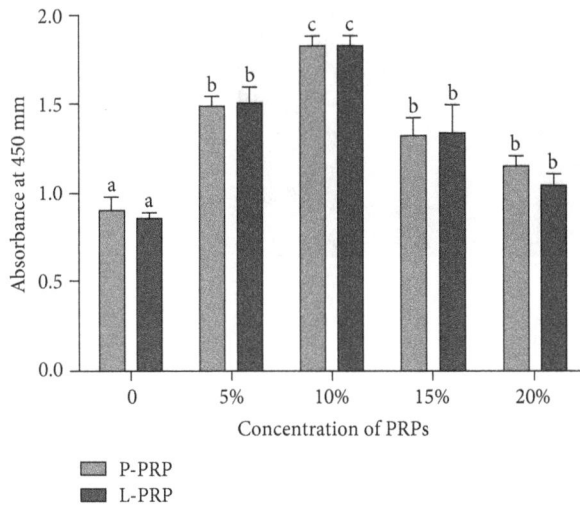

FIGURE 3: The proliferation of cells derived from nucleus pulposus in different concentrations of P-PRP or L-PRP. Cell proliferation was evaluated on day 7 by CCK-8 assay. The cell proliferation showed a maximum effect on 10% P-PRP and 10% L-PRP. Differences for the date from each group (P-PRP or L-PRP) performed by using one-way analysis of variance. A t test was used for determining the statistical significant difference between P-PRP and L-PRP in each concentration of PRPs. Different letters above bars indicate that the difference is statistically significant ($P < 0.05$).

changed from cobblestone-like cells to elongated spindle-shaped nucleus pulposus-like cells (Figure 4(b)). Furthermore, the results of qRT-PCR suggested that the expression of stem cell marker gene including "Oct-4 and Nanog" in the experimental groups decreased 30% compared with that in the control (Figures 4(c)). In contrast, the expression of nucleus pulposus cell-related genes (collagen II and aggrecan) in the experimental groups was 3- to 4-folds higher than that in the control group (Figure 4(d)) Moreover, there was no significant difference between P-PRP groups and L-PRP groups (Figures 4(b)–4(d)). These results indicate that both L-PRP and P-PRP induced the differentiation of NPMSCs towards the mature NP-like cells.

3.5. L-PRP Activates NF-κB Pathway in Differentiated Nucleus Pulposus-like Cells. To explore the effects of L-PRP and P-PRP on the activation of NF-κB pathway in the newly nucleus pulposus-like cells, the expression of proinflammatory genes (IL-1β, TNF-α) and catabolic genes (MMP-1, MMP-13) was determined by qRT-PCR. We observed that the expression of these genes in the L-PRP group was significantly higher than that in the P-PRP and control group (Figures 5(a) and 5(b)). In addition, we used ELISA assay to further investigate these cytokine productions in all groups. The results indicated that the L-PRP group was also significantly higher than P-PRP and control groups (Figures 5(c) and 5(d)). As shown in Figure 5(e), western blot analysis revealed that production of NF-κB/p65 in the L-PRP group was highest in all groups. Moreover, there were no significant differences about all results in the P-PRP and control group.

3.6. P-PRP Induces Differentiated Nucleus Pulposus-like Cells to Produce More Extracellular Matrix-Related Proteins. In order to evaluate the effect of P-PRP and L-PRP on productions of extracellular matrix-related proteins in nucleus pulposus-like cells, we measured the levels of collagen II and aggrecan by immunofluorescence staining and western blot analysis, respectively. Immunofluorescence staining showed that PRP treatment upregulated the productions of collagen II and aggrecan when compared with control and the cells obtained the highest staining after P-PRP treatment (Figure 6(a)). We further performed western blot analysis to determine the levels of these factors; the results also identified the result, indicating that P-PRP induced the maximum production of collagen II and aggrecan in cells (Figure 6(b)).

4. Discussion

This study determined the significance of leukocyte exclusion in PRP for the culture of NPMSCs in vitro. The isolated NPMSCs possessed the typical characteristics of MSCs for self-renewing, clonogenicity, and multidifferentiation potential. The platelet concentration was over 3 times higher in either P-PRP or L-PRP compared to the whole blood. Concentrations of leukocytes, TNF-α, and IL-1β were significantly lower in P-PRP compared with those in L-PRP. Both L-PRP and P-PRP induced the differentiation of NPMSCs towards the mature NP cells. P-PRP which induced lower concentrations of MMP-1, MMP-13, TNF-α, and IL-1β had superior efficacy on the production of ECM (collagen II and aggrecan). In addition, western blot results confirmed the high expression of NF-κB/P65 protein in the L-PRP group.

In the characterization of NPMSCs, we did not test the classic surface markers of MSCs for the lack of specific rabbit antigens by flow cytometry. To solve this problem, we conducted RT-PCT to determine the expression of these markers from the gene level. The colony-forming cells isolated from the NP highly expressed MSC-specific markers (CD29, CD44, and CD166) while minimally expressed the hematopoietic markers (CD8, CD8, and CD14). Spleen cells were used as the positive control for this study, because spleen cells, mainly including lymphocytes and monocytes, are positive for the expression of both MSC-specific and hematopoietic markers [33, 34].

Given the value of endogenic MSCs to the metabolic homeostasis of the disc, an ideal therapy is to activate and proliferate the resident MSC population. PRP, prepared by autologous blood, has been proven effective in the restoration of the degenerated discs [19, 20]. When activated, a variety of growth factors (PDGF, TGF, EGF, and VEGF) released from platelet α-granules in PRP are able to increase cell proliferation and cartilaginous matrix secretion in vitro [18]. In this study, both P-PRP and L-PRP had over 3 times higher platelet concentration compared to the whole blood. After 7 days of coculture with PRPs, NPMSCs proliferated faster than the control group. Moreover, NPMSCs exhibited active NPC shape with increased expression of nucleus pulposus cell-related genes (collagen II and aggrecan) and their protein production after treatment of PRPs for 14 days. Therefore, PRPs not only improved cell proliferation but also induced

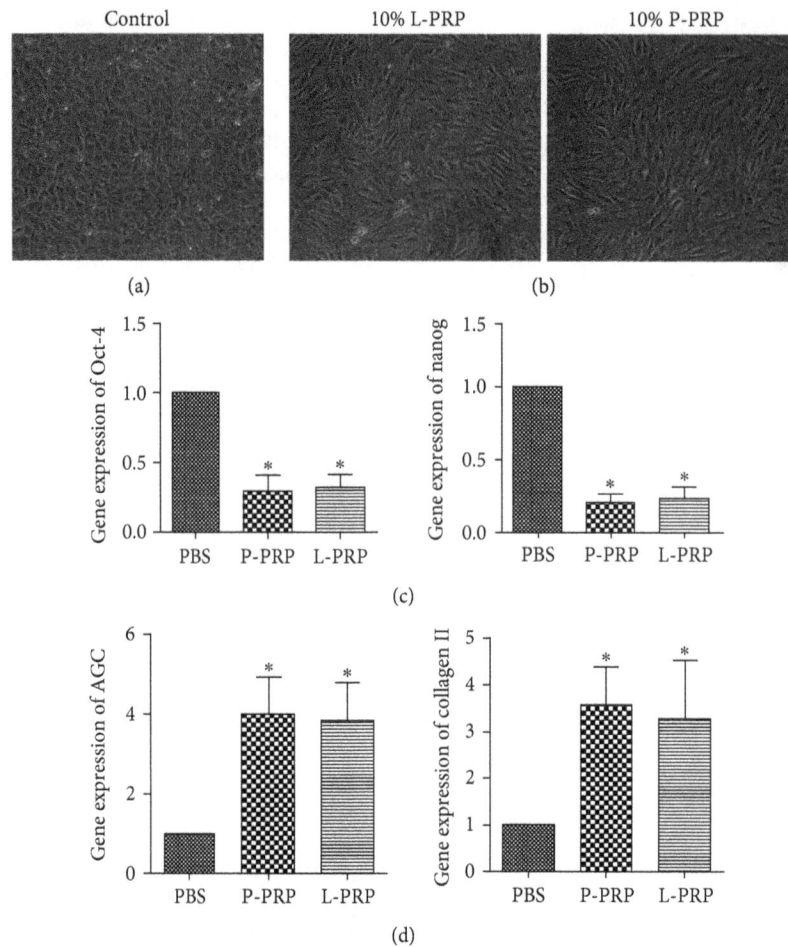

(a)

(b)

(c)

(d)

FIGURE 4: Effects of P-PRP and L-PRP on differentiation in the NPMSCS. (a) Cells morphology in the control. (b) Morphology of the cells treated with 10% L-PRP and 10% P-PRP. (c) mRNA expression of stem cell markers Oct-4 and Nanog, as determined by qRT-PCR. (d) mRNA expression of NP cell-related genes, aggrecan (AGC) and collagen II. "∗" indicates that the difference between P-PRP or L-PRP and control is statistically significant ($P < 0.05$). Note that cell morphology was observed under an inverted microscope (×100).

the active differentiation of NPMSCs for upregulating the extracellular matrix-related protein production.

Variations in the composition of the PRP may contribute to distinct results [21]. The exclusion of leukocytes has been proven more effective when applied in the treatment of bone defect [29], osteoarthritis [35], and acute tendon injury [36]. In this study, similar platelet concentrations of P-PRP and L-PRP resulted in significantly different ECM production in each individual group. P-PRP presents better ECM production function, which could be attributed to the exclusion of leukocytes compared to L-PRP. As typical proinflammatory cytokines, IL-1β and TNF-α are efficient activators of NF-κB signaling pathway [37–39]. In the present study, the proinflammatory genes (TNF-α and IL-1β) as well as their respective protein expression of differentiated NPMSCs in the L-PRP group were significantly higher than those in the P-PRP group. Western blot results showed the higher expression of NF-κB/P65 protein in the L-PRP group compared with P-PRP. These results are consistent with previous 132#studies showing that the NF-κB pathway is activated by the high concentration of leukocytes in L-PRP [28, 29, 40].

NF-κB signaling pathway is intimately involved in the impaired anabolism and enhanced catabolism by upregulating catabolic cytokines, MMP-1 and MMP-13 in intervertebral disc cells [41]. The anti-inflammatory effect of PRP is well confirmed by previous studies [42, 43]. In addition, PRP cleavage products were reported to be able to terminate the NF-κB pathway and downregulate the production of COX-2 [44]. However, the high concentration of leukocytes in L-PRP may counteract the anti-inflammatory potential of growth factors released from platelets [45]. In our study, L-PRP highly induced the inflammation compared to PRP with negligible leukocytes (P-PRP). In addition, NPMSCs treated with L-PRP upregulated catabolism-related genes (MMP-1, MMP-13) and their proteins compared with P-PRP. Thus, the activation of NF-κB pathway can be largely attributed to the inclusion of leukocytes in PRP. The exclusion of leukocytes from PRP resulted in less production of IL-1β and TNF-α, thus prohibiting the activation of NF-κB signaling pathway.

Our study has several limitations. First, we preliminarily confirmed the superiority of P-PRP over L-PRP

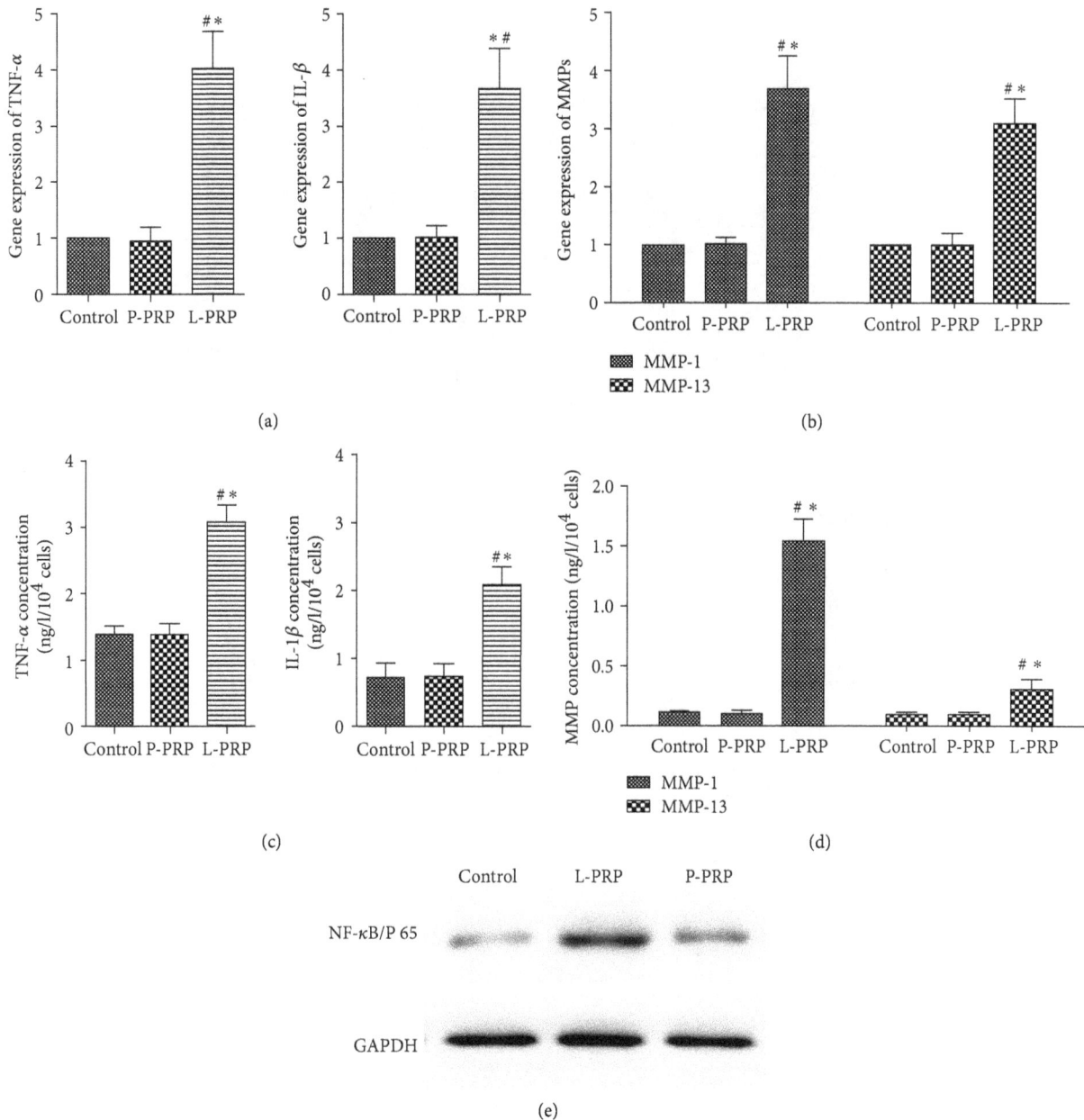

(a)

(b)

(c)

(d)

(e)

Figure 5: Effects of P-PRP and L-PRP on activation of NF-κB pathway. (a, b) mRNA expression of proinflammatory genes (IL-1β, TNF-α) and catabolic marker genes (MMP-1, MMP-13), as measured by qRT-PCR. (c, d) Production of proinflammatory cytokines (IL-1β, TNF-α) and catabolic cytokines (MMP-1, MMP-13), as determined by ELISA assay. (e) Production of NF-κB/p65 in the nucleus, as assessed by western blot. "*" indicates that the difference between the P-PRP or L-PRP and control was statistically significant ($P < 0.05$). "#" indicates that the difference between L-PRP and P-PRP was statistically significant ($P < 0.05$).

in the extracellular matrix-related protein accumulation of NPMSCs. However, the precise mechanism, especially the activation of NF-κB pathway, should be investigated in depth for further studies. Second, in this study, we only tested the in vitro effects of PRPs on NPMSCs. Cell culture system cannot necessarily guarantee the effect of P-PRP on NPMSCs when injected into animal models. Third, we did not investigate the effect of PRPs on the NPMSCs from the degenerated discs. When applied in a clinic, how PRPs can influence the already degenerated NPMSCs should be determined in further studies.

5. Conclusion

We demonstrated that both L-PRP and P-PRP induced the differentiation of NPMSCs towards the mature NP-like cells and exhibited similar proliferation effects on NPMSCs. However, different leukocyte levels contributed to distinct effects on the activation of NF-κB signaling pathway. Concentrated leukocytes in the L-PRP released high levels of proinflammatory cytokines, resulting in the strong activation of NF-κB signaling pathway. Although P-PRP and L-PRP exerted similar proliferation effects on NPMSCs, P-PRP showed superior

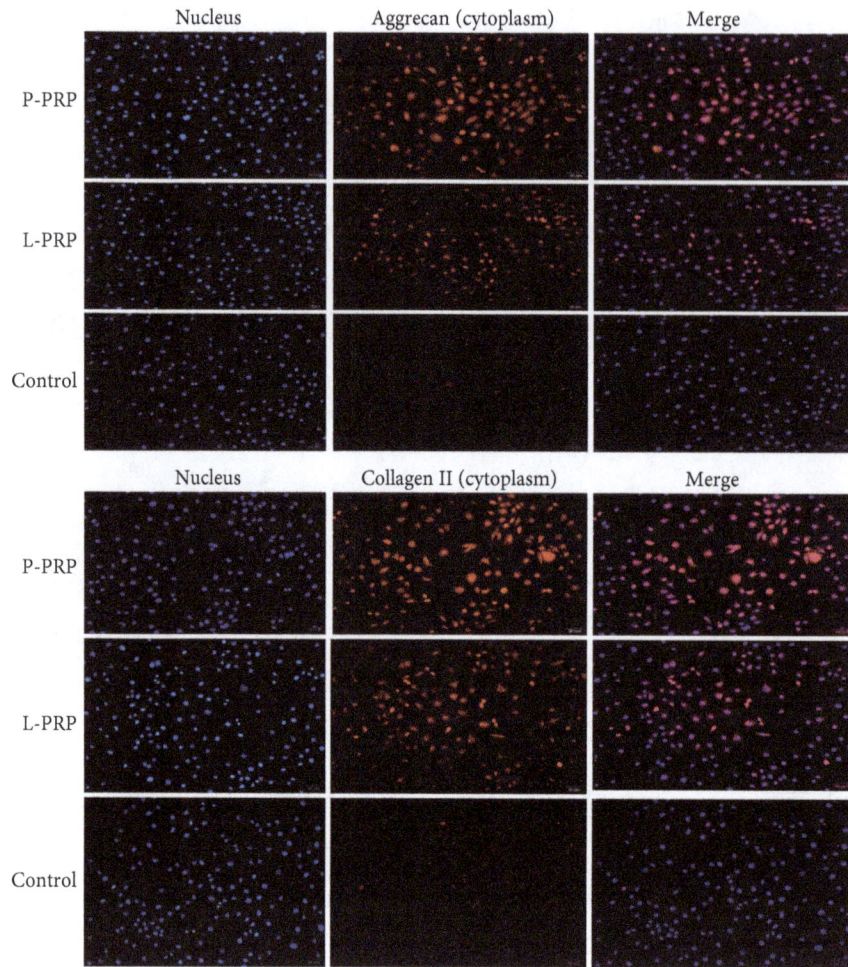

(a)

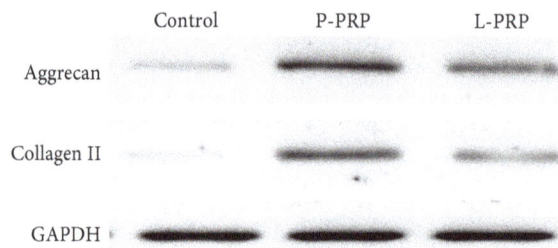

(b)

FIGURE 6: P-PRP induces more extracellular matrix-related proteins. (a) Collagen II and aggrecan in the cytoplasm of the coculture cells imaged by fluorescence microscopy. (b) Production of collagen II and aggrecan, as measured by western blot.

efficacy on the production of extracellular matrix-related protein. Therefore, when applied in IDD therapy, P-PRP exhibited a superior agent, which could better restore the degenerated ECM accumulation and function by activation of NPMSCs.

Acknowledgments

The funding support from the National Natural Science Foundation of China (Grant no. 81572188) for this work is gratefully acknowledged (CW).

References

[1] A. C. Schwarzer, C. N. Aprill, R. Derby, J. Fortin, G. Kine, and N. Bogduk, "The prevalence and clinical features of internal disc disruption in patients with chronic low back pain," *Spine*, vol. 20, no. 17, pp. 1878–1883, 1995.

[2] M. A. Adams and P. J. Roughley, "What is intervertebral disc degeneration, and what causes it?," *Spine*, vol. 31, no. 18, pp. 2151–2161, 2006.

[3] S. Roberts, H. Evans, J. Trivedi, and J. Menage, "Histology and pathology of the human intervertebral disc," *The Journal of Bone and Joint Surgery*, vol. 88, Supplement 2, pp. 10–14, 2006.

[4] H. A. Horner, S. Roberts, R. C. Bielby, J. Menage, H. Evans, and J. P. G. Urban, "Cells from different regions of the intervertebral disc: effect of culture system on matrix expression and cell phenotype," *Spine*, vol. 27, no. 10, pp. 1018–1028, 2002.

[5] D. Sakai, "Future perspectives of cell-based therapy for intervertebral disc disease," *European Spine Journal*, vol. 17, Supplement 4, pp. 452–458, 2008.

[6] S. K. Mirza and R. A. Deyo, "Systematic review of randomized trials comparing lumbar fusion surgery to nonoperative care for treatment of chronic back pain," *Spine*, vol. 32, no. 7, pp. 816–823, 2007.

[7] J. Karppinen, F. H. Shen, K. D. K. Luk, G. B. J. Andersson, K. M. C. Cheung, and D. Samartzis, "Management of degenerative disk disease and chronic low back pain," *The Orthopedic Clinics of North America*, vol. 42, no. 4, pp. 513–528, 2011.

[8] D. Sakai and G. B. J. Andersson, "Stem cell therapy for intervertebral disc regeneration: obstacles and solutions," *Nature Reviews Rheumatology*, vol. 11, no. 4, pp. 243–256, 2015.

[9] Y. C. Huang, V. Y. L. Leung, W. W. Lu, and K. D. K. Luk, "The effects of microenvironment in mesenchymal stem cell-based regeneration of intervertebral disc," *The Spine Journal*, vol. 13, no. 3, pp. 352–362, 2013.

[10] L. M. Benneker, G. Andersson, J. C. Iatridis et al., "Cell therapy for intervertebral disc repair: advancing cell therapy from bench to clinics," *European Cells & Materials*, vol. 27, pp. 5–11, 2014.

[11] S. Ikehara and M. Li, "Stem cell transplantation improves aging-related diseases," *Frontiers in Cell and Development Biology*, vol. 2, p. 16, 2014.

[12] J. P. G. Urban, "The role of the physicochemical environment in determining disc cell behaviour," *Biochemical Society Transactions*, vol. 30, no. 6, pp. 858–863, 2002.

[13] K. Wuertz, K. Godburn, C. Neidlinger-Wilke, J. Urban, and J. C. Iatridis, "Behavior of mesenchymal stem cells in the chemical microenvironment of the intervertebral disc," *Spine*, vol. 33, no. 17, pp. 1843–1849, 2008.

[14] B. Han, H. C. Wang, H. Li et al., "Nucleus pulposus mesenchymal stem cells in acidic conditions mimicking degenerative intervertebral discs give better performance than adipose tissue-derived mesenchymal stem cells," *Cells, Tissues, Organs*, vol. 199, no. 5-6, pp. 342–352, 2015.

[15] W. H. Chen, H. Y. Liu, W. C. Lo et al., "Intervertebral disc regeneration in an *ex vivo* culture system using mesenchymal stem cells and platelet-rich plasma," *Biomaterials*, vol. 30, no. 29, pp. 5523–5533, 2009.

[16] M. Nagae, T. Ikeda, Y. Mikami et al., "Intervertebral disc regeneration using platelet-rich plasma and biodegradable gelatin hydrogel microspheres," *Tissue Engineering*, vol. 13, no. 1, pp. 147–158, 2007.

[17] S. Z. Wang, J. Y. Jin, Y. D. Guo et al., "Intervertebral disc regeneration using platelet-rich plasma-containing bone marrow-derived mesenchymal stem cells: a preliminary investigation," *Molecular Medicine Reports*, vol. 13, no. 4, pp. 3475–3481, 2016.

[18] M. Leslie, "Cell biology. Beyond clotting: the powers of platelets," *Science*, vol. 328, no. 5978, pp. 562–564, 2010.

[19] S. Obata, K. Akeda, T. Imanishi et al., "Effect of autologous platelet-rich plasma-releasate on intervertebral disc degeneration in the rabbit anular puncture model: a preclinical study," *Arthritis Research & Therapy*, vol. 14, no. 6, p. R241, 2012.

[20] G. B. Gullung, J. W. Woodall, M. A. Tucci, J. James, D. A. Black, and R. McGuire, "Platelet-rich plasma effects on degenerative disc disease: analysis of histology and imaging in an animal model," *Evidence-Based Spine-Care Journal*, vol. 2, no. 4, pp. 13–18, 2011.

[21] M. Sanchez, E. Anitua, and I. Andia, "Poor standardization in platelet-rich therapies hampers advancement," *Arthroscopy*, vol. 26, no. 6, pp. 725–726, 2010.

[22] J. C. Peerbooms, J. Sluimer, D. J. Bruijn, and T. Gosens, "Positive effect of an autologous platelet concentrate in lateral epicondylitis in a double-blind randomized controlled trial," *American Journal of Sports Medicine*, vol. 38, no. 2, pp. 255–262, 2010.

[23] R. R. Monto, "Platelet rich plasma treatment for chronic Achilles tendinosis," *Foot & Ankle International*, vol. 33, no. 5, pp. 379–385, 2012.

[24] S. de Jonge, R. J. de Vos, A. Weir et al., "One-year follow-up of platelet-rich plasma treatment in chronic Achilles tendinopathy: a double-blind randomized placebo-controlled trial," *The American Journal of Sports Medicine*, vol. 39, no. 8, pp. 1623–1630, 2011.

[25] R. J. de Vos, A. Weir, H. T. M. van Schie et al., "Platelet-rich plasma injection for chronic Achilles tendinopathy: a randomized controlled trial," *JAMA*, vol. 303, no. 2, pp. 144–149, 2010.

[26] T. Schepull, J. Kvist, H. Norrman, M. Trinks, G. Berlin, and P. Aspenberg, "Autologous platelets have no effect on the healing of human Achilles tendon ruptures: a randomized single-blind study," *The American Journal of Sports Medicine*, vol. 39, no. 1, pp. 38–47, 2011.

[27] J. H. Wang, "Can PRP effectively treat injured tendons?," *Muscles, Ligaments and Tendons Journal*, vol. 4, no. 1, pp. 35–37, 2014.

[28] W. J. Yin, H. T. Xu, J. G. Sheng et al., "Advantages of pure platelet-rich plasma compared with leukocyte- and platelet-rich plasma in treating rabbit knee osteoarthritis," *Medical Science Monitor*, vol. 22, pp. 1280–1290, 2016.

[29] W. Yin, X. Qi, Y. Zhang et al., "Advantages of pure platelet-rich plasma compared with leukocyte- and platelet-rich plasma in promoting repair of bone defects," *Journal of Translational Medicine*, vol. 14, no. 1, p. 73, 2016.

[30] W. Yin, H. Xu, J. Sheng et al., "Optimization of pure platelet-rich plasma preparation: a comparative study of pure platelet-rich plasma obtained using different centrifugal conditions in a single-donor model," *Experimental and Therapeutic Medicine*, vol. 14, no. 3, pp. 2060–2070, 2017.

[31] P. Li, Y. Gan, Y. Xu et al., "17beta-estradiol attenuates TNF-α-induced premature senescence of nucleus pulposus cells through regulating the ROS/NF-κB pathway," *International Journal of Biological Sciences*, vol. 13, no. 2, pp. 145–156, 2017.

[32] C. Liu, Q. Guo, J. Li et al., "Identification of rabbit annulus fibrosus-derived stem cells," *PLoS One*, vol. 9, no. 9, article e108239, 2014.

[33] D. Gibbings and A. D. Befus, "CD4 and CD8: an inside-out coreceptor model for innate immune cells," *Journal of Leukocyte Biology*, vol. 86, no. 2, pp. 251–259, 2009.

[34] M. C. Levesque, C. S. Heinly, L. P. Whichard, and D. D. Patel, "Cytokine-regulated expression of activated leukocyte cell adhesion molecule (CD166) on monocyte-lineage cells and in rheumatoid arthritis synovium," *Arthritis and Rheumatism*, vol. 41, no. 12, pp. 2221–2229, 1998.

[35] E. Assirelli, G. Filardo, E. Mariani et al., "Effect of two different preparations of platelet-rich plasma on synoviocytes," *Knee Surgery, Sports Traumatology, Arthroscopy*, vol. 23, no. 9, pp. 2690–2703, 2015.

[36] Y. Zhou, J. Zhang, H. Wu, M. V. Hogan, and J. H-C. Wang, "The differential effects of leukocyte-containing and pure platelet-rich plasma (PRP) on tendon stem/progenitor cells - implications of PRP application for the clinical treatment of tendon injuries," *Stem Cell Research & Therapy*, vol. 6, 173 pages, 2015.

[37] K. Wuertz, N. Vo, D. Kletsas, and N. Boos, "Inflammatory and catabolic signalling in intervertebral discs: the roles of NF-κB and MAP kinases," *European Cells & Materials*, vol. 23, pp. 102–120, 2012.

[38] M. Klawitter, L. Quero, J. Klasen et al., "Triptolide exhibits anti-inflammatory, anti-catabolic as well as anabolic effects and suppresses TLR expression and MAPK activity in IL-1β treated human intervertebral disc cells," *European Spine Journal*, vol. 21, no. S6, Supplement 6, pp. 850–859, 2012.

[39] L. Quero, M. Klawitter, A. Schmaus et al., "Hyaluronic acid fragments enhance the inflammatory and catabolic response in human intervertebral disc cells through modulation of toll-like receptor 2 signalling pathways," *Arthritis Research & Therapy*, vol. 15, no. 4, p. R94, 2013.

[40] Z. Xu, W. Yin, Y. Zhang et al., "Comparative evaluation of leukocyte- and platelet-rich plasma and pure platelet-rich plasma for cartilage regeneration," *Scientific Reports*, vol. 7, article 43301, 2017.

[41] K. Wuertz, N. Vo, D. Kletsas, and N. Boos, "Inflammatory and catabolic signalling in intervertebral discs: the roles of NF-κB and MAP kinases," *European Cells & Materials*, vol. 23, pp. 103–119, 2012.

[42] M. Moussa, D. Lajeunesse, G. Hilal et al., "Platelet rich plasma (PRP) induces chondroprotection via increasing autophagy, anti-inflammatory markers, and decreasing apoptosis in human osteoarthritic cartilage," *Experimental Cell Research*, vol. 352, no. 1, pp. 146–156, 2017.

[43] J. Zhang, K. K. Middleton, F. H. Fu, H. J. Im, and J. H. C. Wang, "HGF mediates the anti-inflammatory effects of PRP on injured tendons," *PLoS One*, vol. 8, no. 6, article e67303, 2013.

[44] R. C. Pereira, M. Scaranari, R. Benelli et al., "Dual effect of platelet lysate on human articular cartilage: a maintenance of chondrogenic potential and a transient proinflammatory activity followed by an inflammation resolution," *Tissue Engineering. Part A*, vol. 19, no. 11-12, pp. 1476–1488, 2013.

[45] F. Réadini, A. Mauviel, S. Pronost, G. Loyau, and J. P. Pujol, "Transforming growth factor β exerts opposite effects from interleukin-1β on cultured rabbit articular chondrocytes through reduction of interleukin-1 receptor expression," *Arthritis and Rheumatism*, vol. 36, no. 1, pp. 44–50, 1993.

Differentiation of Human Embryonic Stem Cells to Sympathetic Neurons: A Potential Model for Understanding Neuroblastoma Pathogenesis

Jane Carr-Wilkinson,[1,2,3] Nilendran Prathalingam,[2,4] Deepali Pal,[1,2] Mohammad Moad,[5] Natalie Lee,[1] Aishwarya Sundaresh,[1] Helen Forgham,[3] Peter James,[6] Mary Herbert,[2,4,7] Majlinda Lako,[2,4] and Deborah A. Tweddle (iD)[1,2,8]

[1]Wolfson Childhood Cancer Research Centre, Northern Institute for Cancer Research, Newcastle University, UK
[2]North East Stem Cell Institute, Newcastle University, UK
[3]Faculty of Health Sciences and Wellbeing, University of Sunderland, UK
[4]Institute of Genetic Medicine, Newcastle University, UK
[5]Northern Institute for Cancer Research, Paul O-Gorman Building, Newcastle University, UK
[6]Institute of Health & Society, Newcastle University, UK
[7]Newcastle Fertility Centre, Newcastle University, UK
[8]Great North Children's Hospital, Newcastle upon Tyne Hospitals NHS Trust, UK

Correspondence should be addressed to Deborah A. Tweddle; deborah.tweddle@newcastle.ac.uk

Guest Editor: Hui Li

Background and Aims. Previous studies modelling human neural crest differentiation from stem cells have resulted in a low yield of sympathetic neurons. Our aim was to optimise a method for the differentiation of human embryonic stem cells (hESCs) to sympathetic neuron-like cells (SN) to model normal human SNS development. *Results.* Using stromal-derived inducing activity (SDIA) of PA6 cells plus BMP4 and B27 supplements, the H9 hESC line was differentiated to neural crest stem-like cells and SN-like cells. After 7 days of PA6 cell coculture, mRNA expression of *SNAIL* and *SOX-9* neural crest specifier genes and the neural marker *peripherin* (*PRPH*) increased. Expression of the pluripotency marker *OCT 4* decreased, whereas *TP53* and *LIN28B* expression remained high at levels similar to SHSY5Y and IMR32 neuroblastoma cell lines. A 5-fold increase in the expression of the catecholaminergic marker *tyrosine hydroxylase (TH)* and the noradrenergic marker *dopamine betahydroxylase (DBH)* was observed by day 7 of differentiation. Fluorescence-activated cell sorting for the neural crest marker p75, enriched for cells expressing *p75, DBH, TH,* and *PRPH*, was more specific than p75 neural crest stem cell (NCSC) microbeads. On day 28 post p75 sorting, dual immunofluorescence identified sympathetic neurons by PRPH and TH copositivity cells in 20% of the cell population. Noradrenergic sympathetic neurons, identified by copositivity for both PHOX2B and DBH, were present in $9.4\% \pm 5.5\%$ of cells. *Conclusions.* We have optimised a method for noradrenergic SNS development using the H9 hESC line to improve our understanding of normal human SNS development and, in a future work, the pathogenesis of neuroblastoma.

1. Introduction

The neural crest is a transient embryonic cell population which undergoes extensive migration and differentiation to give rise to a diverse range of cell populations in the embryo, ranging from the peripheral nervous system (sensory, enteric, and autonomic (sympathetic and parasympathetic)) to the craniofacial skeleton and pigment cells (reviewed by [1]). Neural crest cells are multipotent stem cells which can self-renew and in humans undergo extensive migration around the third to fourth weeks of gestation [2].

Sympathetic neurons originate from trunk neural crest cells that arrest their migration upon arrival at the dorsal aorta and begin to express the catecholaminergic and noradrenergic biosynthetic enzymes tyrosine hydroxylase (TH) and dopamine betahydroxylase (DBH), respectively (Figures 1(a) and 1(b)). Bone morphogenetic proteins (BMPs), multifunctional secreted proteins of the transforming growth factor β superfamily, are secreted in the dorsal aorta and the gut [3] and are important for noradrenergic autonomic specification from the neural crest [4, 5].

Neuroblastoma is an embryonal malignancy originating from neural crest cells which give rise to the sympathetic nervous system (SNS) [3]. It is the most common childhood solid tumour outside the central nervous system, and in contrast to many other paediatric malignancies, high-risk neuroblastoma is fatal in around 50% of patients despite intensive multimodal therapy [6]. *In vivo* and *in vitro* observations have shown that neuroblastic tumours appear to recapitulate the development of differentiating, predominantly noradrenergic, sympathetic neurons, and chromaffin cells of the adrenal medulla, suggesting that neuroblastoma arises from aberrant or blocked differentiation in normal SNS development (reviewed in [7]). By modelling the normal development of the neural crest and SNS, it may be possible to understand the pathogenesis of neuroblastoma and other abnormalities of the neural crest, e.g., neurocristopathies.

Human embryonic stem cells (hESCs) and induced pluripotent stem cells (IPSC) have the potential to provide an unlimited source of cells for both disease modelling and cell replacement therapy. The ability to differentiate hESC to neural crest-derived stem-like cells (NCDSC) and autonomic progenitors provides an important tool for modelling human neural crest development.

Kawasaki and colleagues were the first to demonstrate efficient induction of peripheral autonomic neuronal lineages from murine and primate hESC by coculture with PA6 cells, which possess stromal-derived inducing activity (SDIA) [8, 9]. Mizuseki et al. showed that early exposure of cocultured cells to BMP4 inhibited neural differentiation, whereas late exposure to high concentrations of BMP4 (days 5–9) induced differentiation to neural crest cells and autonomic progenitors [9]. Recently, other studies differentiating hESC have used BMP4 [10] or a feeder layer [11] to help induce SN differentiation.

The aim of this study was to develop an *in vitro* model using both BMP4 and a stromal feeder layer for efficient differentiation of hESC to noradrenergic sympathetic neurons (Figures 1(a) and 1(b)). We sought to determine the optimum conditions for the differentiation of hESC to SN by comparing different neural differentiation media, sorting methods for neural crest-like cells, and plating conditions for sorted cells.

Understanding normal SNS development in hESC models will enable us to learn more about the SNS as well as neural crest-derived malignancies such as neuroblastoma.

2. Materials and Methods

2.1. Cell Culture. H9 cells were obtained from the WiCell Bank (Wisconsin) following approval from the UK Medical Research Council (MRC) Stem Cell Steering Committee.

Undifferentiated H9 hESCs [12] were cultured on either the human foreskin fibroblast cell line (NclFed(R)1A) [13], inactivated with 35Gy ionising radiation, or irradiated MEF-CF1 standard density cells (AMSBIO, UK). hESCs were cultured in stem cell media (20% KnockOut Serum Replacement (Invitrogen, USA), 0.1% nonessential amino acids (NEAA) (Invitrogen, USA), 0.1 mM β-mercaptoethanol (Invitrogen, USA), 2 mM Glutamax (Invitrogen, USA), and 8 ng/ml FGF2 (Invitrogen, USA) in KO-DMEM (Invitrogen, USA)). Cells were passaged weekly and replated on 6-well plates coated with irradiated feeder cells at a density of 6.5×10^3 cells per well. The mouse stromal PA6 cell line was obtained from the Riken Cell Bank (Japan).

All cell lines were checked regularly and found to be free from contamination with Mycoplasma. Karyotypic analysis of H9 cells was also undertaken to confirm their identity using standard Giemsa banding techniques.

SKNAS (S-substrate adherent type, non-*MYCN* amplified) [14], IMR32 (N-neuronal type, *MYCN* amplified [15]), and SHSY5Y (N type, non-*MYCN* amplified) [16] human neuroblastoma cell lines were used as controls.

2.2. Differentiation to Neural Crest-Like Cells and Sympathetic Progenitors. Neural crest differentiation was induced by coculture of hESC with PA6 cells in neural differentiation media as outlined in Figure 1(c). Cells were detached from Fed1A feeders using 1 mg/ml collagenase IV and incubated for 10 minutes at 37°C to detach hESC colonies. 500–800 cells were transferred to 12- or 24-well plates, each well containing 1 or 0.5×10^4 PA6 cells, respectively, and cultured for up to 28 days.

To optimise differentiation to p75+ve neural crest-like cells, two neural differentiation media were compared: (1) neural BHK media (90% BHK-21 medium/Glasgow modified Eagle medium (MEM) with 10% KO-SR, 1% L-Glutamax, 0.5% NEAA, 1% pyruvate, 1% penicillin/streptomycin, and $2 \times N2$ neuronal supplement) and (2) 90% MACS® neuronal media plus 2% MACS B27 supplement, 1% L-Glutamax, 0.5% NEAA, and 1% penicillin/streptomycin. Conditions required for optimal development of noradrenergic sympathetic neurons were established by comparing the addition or withdrawal of 10 ng/ml BMP4 and 10 ng/ml BMP2 and 4 with 10 ng/ml BMP4 alone, on days 5 to 9 of differentiation. N2 supplement (Life Technologies) and 10 ng/ml nerve growth factor (NGF) (R&D systems) were added to the media from day 4 of differentiation and 0.1 mM dibutyryl cyclic AMP (dbcAMP) was added on day 8 and withdrawn from the media after 10 days of differentiation. Cells were further differentiated for 3–4 weeks, and media were changed every two days. Differentiation experiments were carried out to $n = 3$.

2.3. p75 (CD271) Fluorescence-Activated Cell Sorting (FACS) of Differentiating Cells. Two methods of cell sorting for p75-positive cells were used to compare the yield of p75-positive cells obtained.

H9 cells were harvested on day 8 of PA6 coculture, which was found to yield the optimal number of p75-positive cells (data not shown) using 1 mg/ml collagenase, incubated for

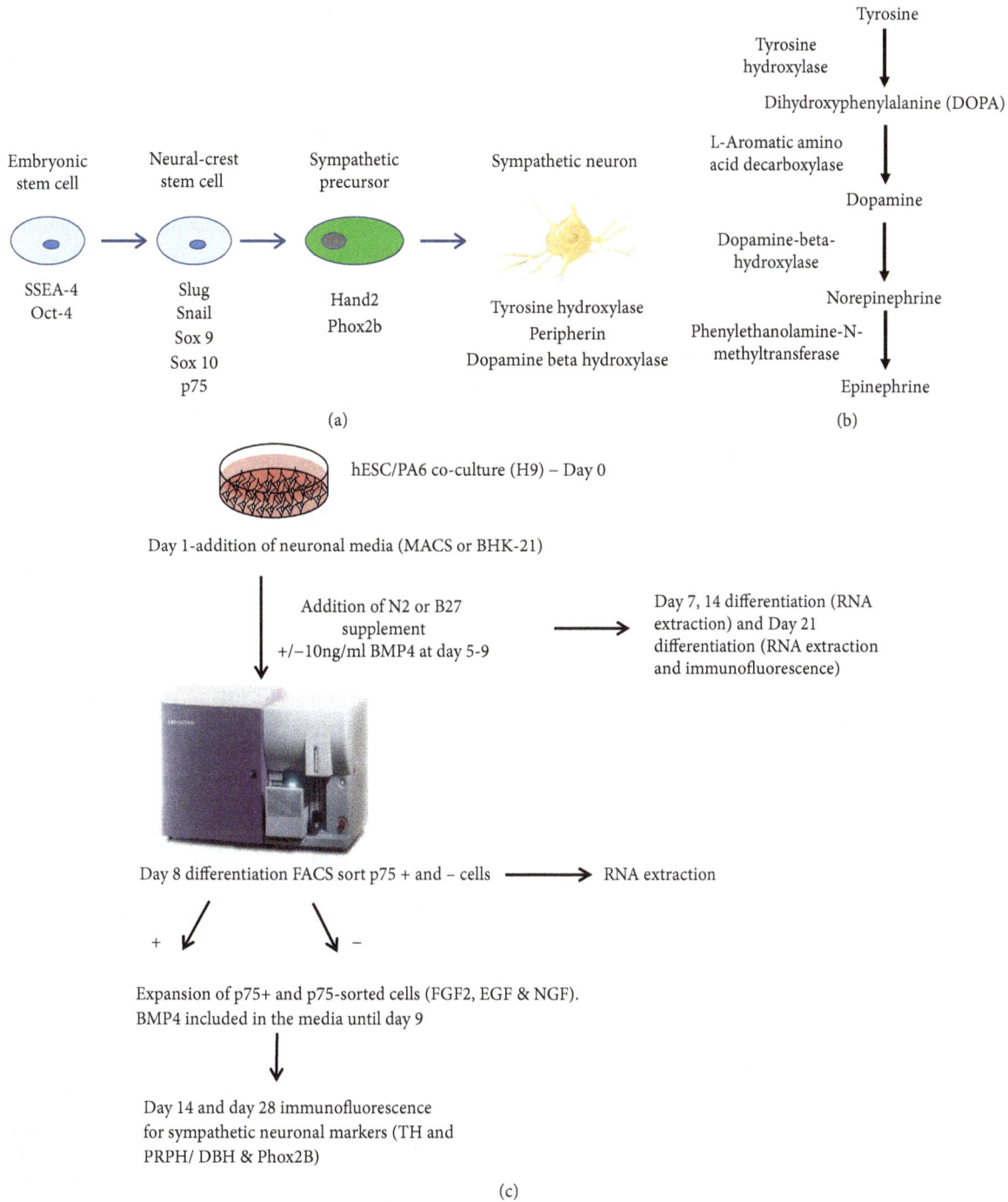

Figure 1: (a) Markers used to identify cell populations in this study. (b) The catecholamine biosynthesis pathway. (c) Flow chart detailing experimental outline of neural differentiation.

10 minutes at 37°C, followed by incubation in Accumax (Stemgent) for 10 minutes with gentle agitation to obtain a single cell suspension. Cells were washed once in FACS wash buffer (1 in 20 dilution of bovine serum albumin (Miltenyi Biotec, UK) in MACs rinsing solution (Miltenyi Biotec) and centrifuged at 150 g for 4 minutes. 10% Fc block in FACS wash buffer was added to the cell suspension and incubated for 10 minutes at room temperature. Anti-p75 (CD 271) primary antibody directly conjugated with phycoerythrin (PE)

(Miltenyi Biotec) was added to cells at 1 in 33 dilution. Multiple cell sorts were performed ($n = 3$) using a FACS Aria II Cell Sorter (BD Bioscience™) and a minimum of 5.5×10^4 p75+ ve and p75– ve cells plated onto either PA6-coated 24 well plates or BD BioCoat™ poly-l-ornithine/laminin-coated 24 well plates (BD Biosciences). All sorted cells were cultured in MACS neuronal medium containing B27 supplement, 10 ng/ml NGF, 10 ng/ml fibroblast growth factor (FGF2), and 10 ng/ml epidermal growth factor (EGF).

2.4. Neural Crest Stem Cell (NCSC) Microbead Sorting. Differentiating H9 cells were harvested using Trypsin/EDTA and dissociated to a cell suspension. Positive cell enrichment was performed using anti-p75- (CD271) coated NCSC MicroBeads, according to the manufacturer's instructions (Miltenyi Biotec). Sorted cells were cultured in either 24-well PA6-coated plates or BD BioCoat™ poly-l-ornithine/laminin-coated 24-well plates.

2.5. Live Cell Immunofluorescence of Undifferentiated H9 Cells. Undifferentiated H9 hESC colonies were immunostained with 1 : 100 dilutions of TRA-1-60-FITC conjugate (Millipore) and anti-SSEA-4/clone MC-813-70-PE conjugate (Millipore). HESC colonies were incubated with primary antibodies at 37°C for 2 hours followed by a 10-minute incubation with 0.5 μg/ml Hoechst-hESC media solution and twice washed with hESC media to ensure all Hoechst dye was removed. The colonies were then imaged in hESC media under a Nikon eclipse TE2000U inverted microscope after which the media was replaced with fresh hESC media containing 10 μM Rho-associated kinase (ROCK) inhibitor Stemolecule™ Y27632 [17] (Stemgent, MA, USA).

2.6. Immunofluorescence of Differentiating Cells. H9 cells were immunostained for stem cell and neuronal markers. Cells were washed in PBS and fixed in 4% paraformaldehyde for 10 minutes. After washing in PBS (3 × 5-minute washes), the samples were incubated in blocking solution containing 1% BSA and 10% goat serum. The following antibodies were used at the dilutions indicated: OCT4 1 : 400 (Abcam), NANOG (R&D systems) 1 : 200, neural cell adhesion molecule (NCAM) 1 : 200 (Millipore), peripherin (PRPH) 7C5 and C-19 1 : 200 (Santa Cruz Biotechnology), TH 1 : 450 (Millipore), DBH, 1 : 450 (Abcam), and paired like homeobox2B (PHOX2B) 1 : 450 (Santa Cruz Biotechnology). Cells were incubated with primary antibodies overnight at either 4°C or room temperature for 1.5 hours. Secondary antibodies coupled to Alexa Fluor 488 or 568 (Molecular Probes, USA) were used for detection and were used alone as controls for two-colour costaining as well as comparison with single markers alone. Cells were washed with 3 × 10-minute washes and nuclei stained using 4′,6-diamidino-2-phenylindole, dihydrochloride DAPI (Vectashield) diluted 1 : 10 in PBS in 24-well plates, and coverslips were stained with DAPI. 24-well plates and 4-well chamber slides (Millipore, UK) were viewed and photographed using a Nikon A1r confocal microscope. Percentages of positively immunostained cells were obtained by counting 100 cells each in 3 different areas of the slide and then scoring the number of positive cells. This scoring process was applied to all experimental replicates.

2.7. Time Lapse Photography. Live cell analysis and imaging of p75+ and p75− H9 cells were performed over 4 days using a Nikon Biostation Cell Tracker. Cells were imaged on both PA6-coated 24-well plates and poly-l-ornithine/laminin 24-well plates. The migration rates, including velocity and meandering index, were measured using the Volocity™ software programme (Perkin Elmer, UK).

2.8. RNA Analysis-RT-PCR. RNA was extracted using the RNeasy mini kit (Qiagen) and 0.5 μg reverse transcribed using the iscript cDNA synthesis kit (BioRAD™). RNA was isolated from differentiated H9 cells on day 7, 14, and 21 of differentiation. Undifferentiated stem cells and SKNAS, SHSY5Y, and IMR-32 neuroblastoma cell lines were used as controls. In addition, normal human adrenal cortex, medulla, and dorsal root ganglion tissue from a 14-week gestation fetus were supplied by the Human Developmental Biology Resource (http://www.hdbr.org).

RT-PCR reactions were set up in a total volume of 20 μl, containing 10% PCR buffer, 10% magnesium chloride (MgCl₂), 10% dNTPs, 1 μl of 10 μM forward and reverse primers, and 1% Amplitaq Gold™ (Applied Biosystems). RT-PCR was performed for neural crest specifiers (*SNAIL*, and *SOX9*), SNS precursors, (*PHOX2b* and *TH*), noradrenergic sympathetic neurons (*DBH*), and other neuronal markers (*NCAM*, *PRPH*) on days 7, 14, and 21 of coculture of unsorted cells, as well as on day 8 for p75+ ve FACS sorting (see Supplementary Information 1 for primer sequences). Densitometry was performed using ImageJ software (NIH, USA). Total intensity was calculated from PCR bands and first normalised to *GAPDH*; mRNA expression for each target was then calculated as fold change relative to undifferentiated H9 stem cells.

2.9. Quantitative Reverse Transcriptase PCR (QRT-PCR). Taqman® gene expression assay primers and probes were used to amplify *OCT4*, *TP53*, *DBH*, and *GAPDH*. RT-PCR was performed in a total reaction volume of 10 μl containing 5 μl of Taqman universal PCR master mix, 0.5 μl of primers and probes mix (Applied Biosystems), 2.5 μl cDNA, and 2 μl H₂O. Reactions were performed in triplicate then quantified using the ABI Prism 7900HT sequence detection system (Applied Biosystems) relative to *GAPDH*.

2.10. Statistics. A chi-squared test was used to compare the percentages of p75+ and p75− ve cells obtained using MACS® neuronal media and neural BHK media ($n = 3$).

Continuous velocity data for p75+ cells grown on PA6 cells v poly-l-ornithine/laminin plates was summarised using the mean and standard deviation for normally distributed data and medians with quartiles for skewed data. Log transformations were performed to reduce skewness, and two sample *t*-tests were used to compare normally distributed data. The statistical package STATA version 14.1 (StataCorp 2015, Stata Statistical Software: Release 14; College Station, TX: StataCorp LP) was used for statistical analyses.

3. Results

3.1. Confirmation of Phenotype and Karyotype of H9-Undifferentiated hESC. Live cell staining using antibodies specific to the pluripotency markers SSEA4 and TRA-1-60 showed intense staining of undifferentiated H9 ES cell colonies (Figures 2(a-iii) and 2(b-iii)). Hoechst staining of H9 cells was less intense than in the Fed1A feeder cell layer, indicative of a "Hoechst dim" phenotype due to efflux of Hoechst dye by stem cells, in contrast to brighter staining

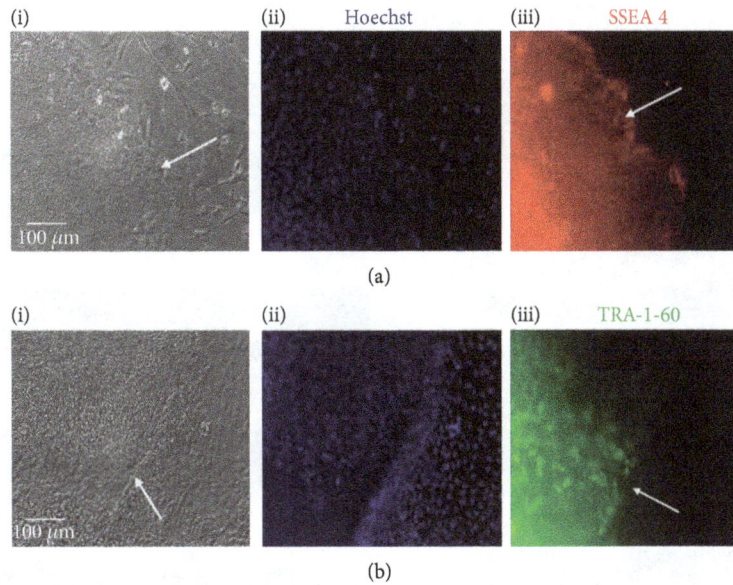

FIGURE 2: H9 hESC live cell staining for pluripotency markers SSEA4 and TRA-1-60. (a-i, b-i) Phase contrast microscopy. (a-ii, b-ii) Hoechst staining showing efflux of Hoechst from stem cells but not feeder layer. (a-iii) SSEA-4 (red) and (b-iii) TRA-1-60 (green) showing specific staining for human ES cell colonies compared with control feeder cells. White arrows highlight the stem cell colony borders.

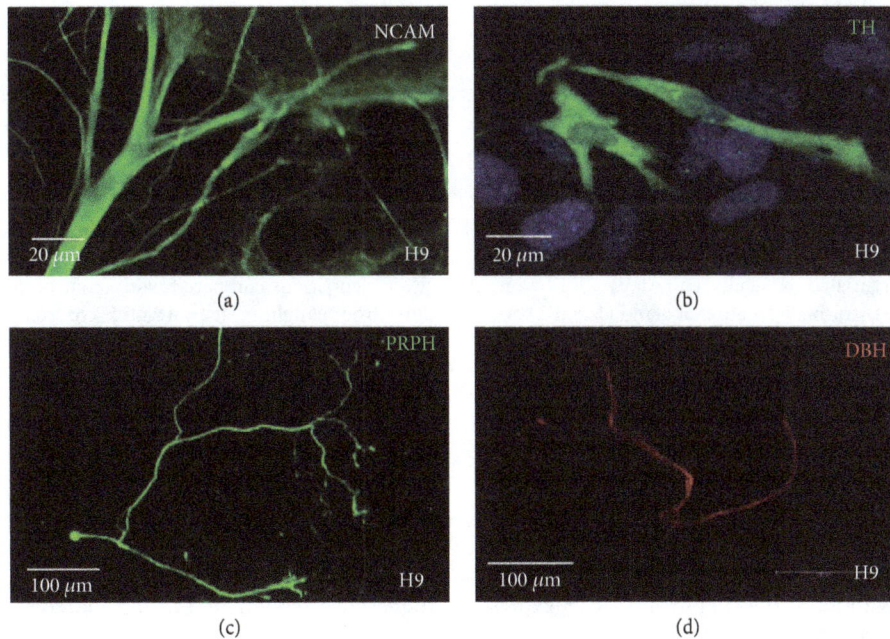

FIGURE 3: Immunofluorescence of unsorted H9 hESCs on day 21 of neuronal differentiation demonstrating expression of (a) neural cell adhesion molecule (NCAM), (b) tyrosine hydroxylase (TH), (c) peripherin (PRPH), and (d) dopamine betahydroxylase (DBH).

observed on the feeder layer (Figures 2(a-ii) and 2(b-ii)). Karyotyping of H9 cells confirmed a normal female karyotype (Figure S1).

3.2. Sympathetic Neuronal Differentiation of H9 Cells Detected by Immunofluorescence and RT-PCR. Following 7 days of PA6 coculture, morphological changes towards a neuronal phenotype were observed in H9 cells using phase contrast microscopy. Immunofluorescence of H9 cells on day 21 of differentiation for neuronal markers showed >90% of cocultured cells immunostained positive for NCAM (Figure 3(a)) with PRPH positivity in 20% (Figure 3(c)). TH-positive cells were observed in around 10% of the cell population (Figure 3(b)). DBH was detected in approximately 5% of differentiated cells (Figure 3(d)). This cell population included around 10% PA6 cells, and thus, the percentage of cells differentiating towards a sympathetic neuronal lineage is likely to be slightly higher than this.

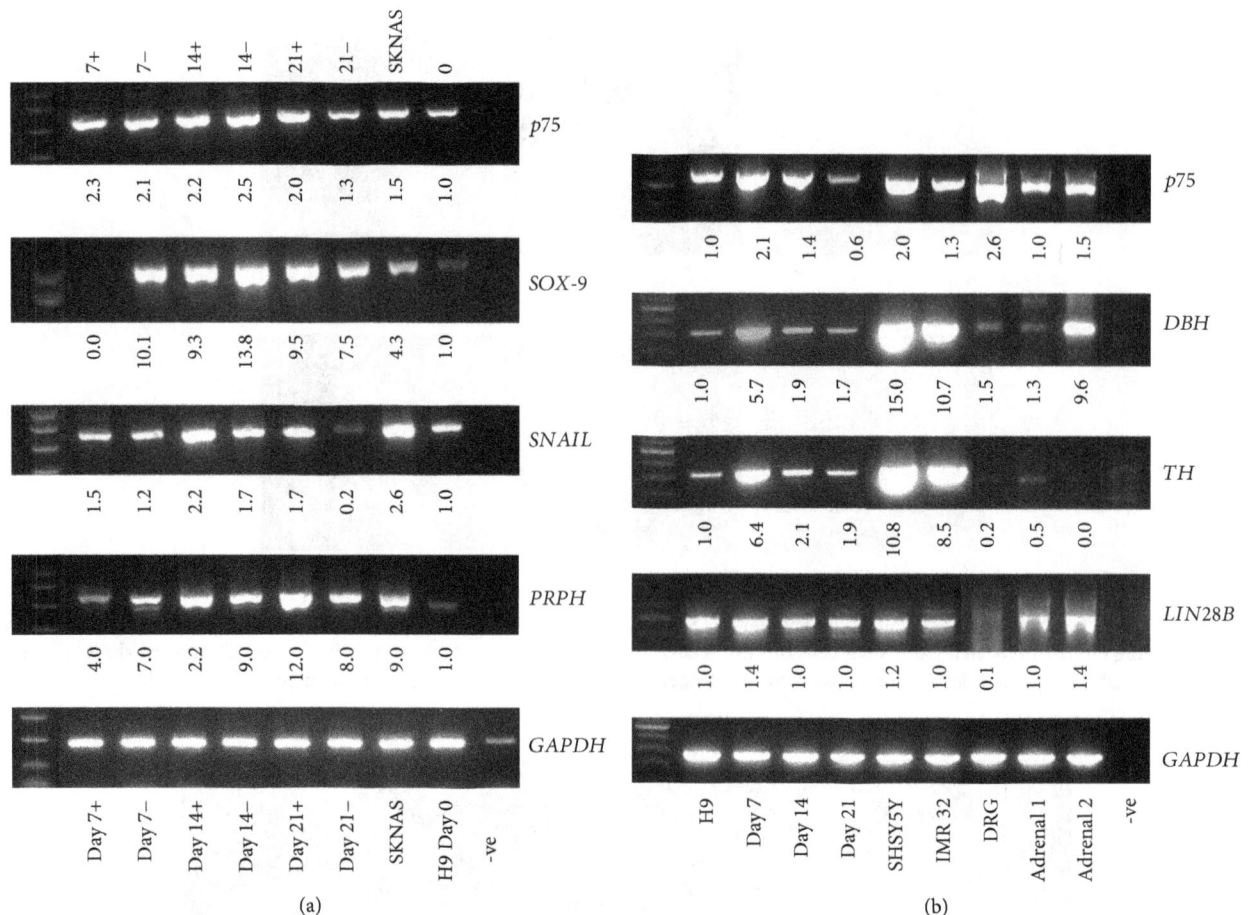

(a)   (b)

FIGURE 4: Neuronal differentiation in H9 cells. (a) Semiquantitative RT-PCR showing mRNA expression of neural crest specifiers *p75*, *SOX-9*, and *SNAIL* and the neuronal marker *PRPH* on days 0, 7, 14, and 21 of differentiation in the presence (+) or absence (−) of 10 ng/ml BMP4 on days 5–9 of differentiation with the SKNAS neuroblastoma cell line as a + control. (b) RT-PCR expression of *p75*, *DBH*, *TH*, and *LIN28B* expression in undifferentiated H9 cells and days 7, 14, and 21 of differentiation compared with control SHSY5Y and IMR-32 neuroblastoma cell lines, normal fetal adrenal gland (1 and 2) and fetal dorsal root ganglion. −ve = negative control.

mRNA expression by RT-PCR of early neural crest specifier genes including *SNAIL* showed a twofold increase between day 0 and day 14, and *SOX-9* expression increased 14-fold by day 14 (Figure 4(a)). The addition of BMP4 (10 ng/ml) on days 5–9 of coculture led to a 12-fold increase in *PRPH* expression from day 7 to day 21 of differentiation compared to 8-fold without BMP4 (Figure 4(a)). *p75* expression was highest between day 7 and day 14 of differentiation and increased upon addition of BMP4 (Figures 4(a) and 4(b)). Low basal expression of *p75*, *DBH*, and *TH* was detected, possibly due to spontaneous differentiation into neuronal cells as has previously been reported for H9 hESC [18]. High expression of *p75* was observed in the neural crest-derived control tissues, fetal adrenal gland comprising adrenal cortex and medulla and control dorsal root ganglion (sensory neurons). There was a 5-fold increase in *DBH* expression and a 6-fold increase in *TH* expression by day 7 of differentiation compared to control H9 cells. High expression of *TH* and *DBH* was observed in the positive controls (IMR32 and SHSY5Y cells). *DBH* expression on day 7 was comparable with one of the fetal adrenal glands, and as

expected, the fetal dorsal root ganglion showed low expression of *DBH* (Figure 4(b)). The highest expression of the pluripotency gene *LIN28B* expression was observed in H9 cells on day 7 of differentiation (Figure 4(b)).

3.3. Quantitative RT-PCR of Differentiating H9 Cells. The highest expression of the pluripotency marker *OCT4* was observed in undifferentiated H9 cells, decreasing by day 7 through day 21 of differentiation (Figure 5(a)). SHSY5Y and IMR-32 neuroblastoma cell lines expressed low levels of *OCT4* compared with undifferentiated H9 cells (Figure 5(a)). *TP53* was expressed in pluripotent H9 cells and expression maintained throughout differentiation at levels comparable with the neuroblastoma cell lines (Figure 5(b)). *DBH* expression was very low in undifferentiated H9 cells and increased to a maximum on day 7 of differentiation before declining during the later stages of differentiation (Figure 5(c)), consistent with the data obtained by RT-PCR where the highest expression of *DBH* was also on day 7 of differentiation (Figure 4(b)). As expected, control neuroblastoma cell lines expressed very high levels of *DBH* (Figure 5(c)).

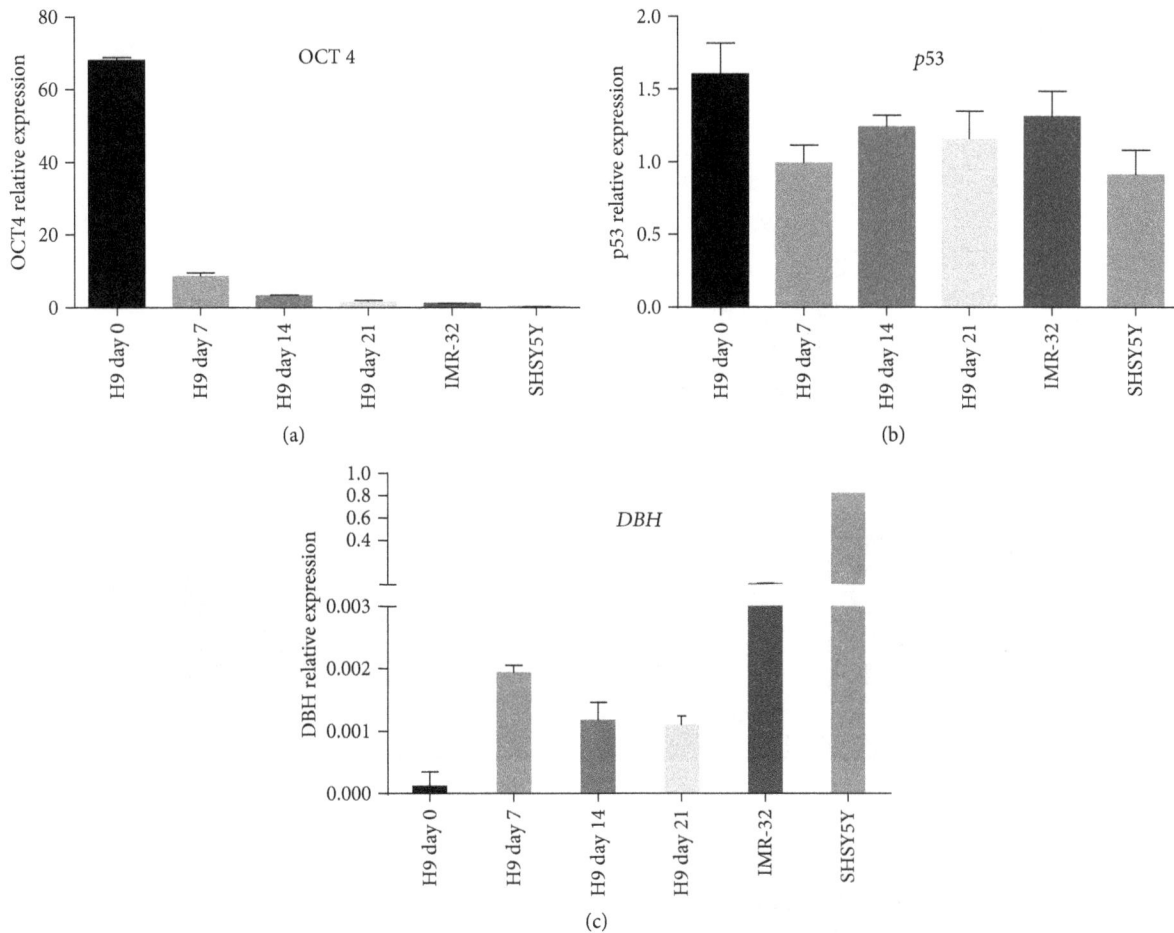

FIGURE 5: Quantitative RT-PCR of H9 cells. (a) High mRNA expression of *OCT4* in pluripotent H9 cells decreases throughout neuronal differentiation with low expression in SHSY5Y and IMR-32 neuroblastoma cell lines. (b) Sustained *TP53* expression throughout differentiation at levels similar to SHSY5Y and IMR-32 neuroblastoma cell lines. (c) Low *DBH* expression in undifferentiated H9 cells increases to a maximum on day 7 of differentiation but is less than SHSY5Y and IMR32 neuroblastoma cell lines ($n = 3$ in triplicate, values relative to *GAPDH*).

3.4. Enrichment of Sympathetic Progenitor-Like Cells by p75 Sorting.

To enrich for NCDSC and sympathetic neuron-like cells, cells were sorted using FACS for the NCSC marker p75 (CD271) on day 8 of coculture (Figure 4(b)). To optimise neural crest stem cell differentiation further, two different neuronal media types were compared: (a) MACS® neuronal media + B27 and (b) neural BHK media + N2 supplement. On day 8 of differentiation, an increased proportion of p75 + ve cells were observed using MACS® neuronal media 45.0% ± 0.8 (95% confidence interval) compared with 32.7 ± 0.8 (95% confidence interval) using neural BHK media ($n = 3$, $p < 0.0001$, chi-squared test) (Figure 6(a)). Preliminary results undertaking FACS for both p75 and DBH on day 8 of differentiation showed that 5.5 and 5.7% of cells were p75 and DBH+, by FACS following culture in BHK and MACS media, respectively (data not shown).

Following p75 sorting, autonomic neuronal populations were enriched when cells were grown in preconditioned media from cultured hESC in the presence of N2 supplement, NGF, and dbcAMP (data not shown). On day 28 post p75 sorting, dual immunofluorescence identified sympathetic neurons by PRPH and TH copositivity cells in H9 cells (Figure 6(b-i)) in up to 20% cells. Noradrenergic sympathetic neurons identified by copositivity for both PHOX2B and DBH were present in 9.4% ± 5.5% H9 cells (Figure 6(b-ii)). mRNA expression by RT-PCR of p75+ ve H9 cells showed enrichment for *p75* and the sympathetic neuronal markers, *TH* and *DBH*, together with *PRPH* where expression was observed exclusively in p75+ ve cells (Figure 6(c)). This was in contrast to the early neural crest specifier *SNAIL* which was expressed in both p75+ ve and p75– ve cells. Following selection of p75+ ve cells using neural crest stem cell microbeads in differentiating H9 cells, *p75* mRNA expression was highly enriched in the p75+ ve cell fraction and *DBH* was expressed exclusively in p75+ ve cells whereas *TH* was expressed in both the p75-enriched and the p75-depleted cell populations (Figure 6(d)). This indicates possible contamination of p75+ ve cells in the p75-depleted population.

3.5. Live Cell Imaging (Biostation).

p75+ ve-sorted cells plated onto PA6-coated plates cells survived better compared to those on poly-l-ornithine/laminin-coated plates (data not

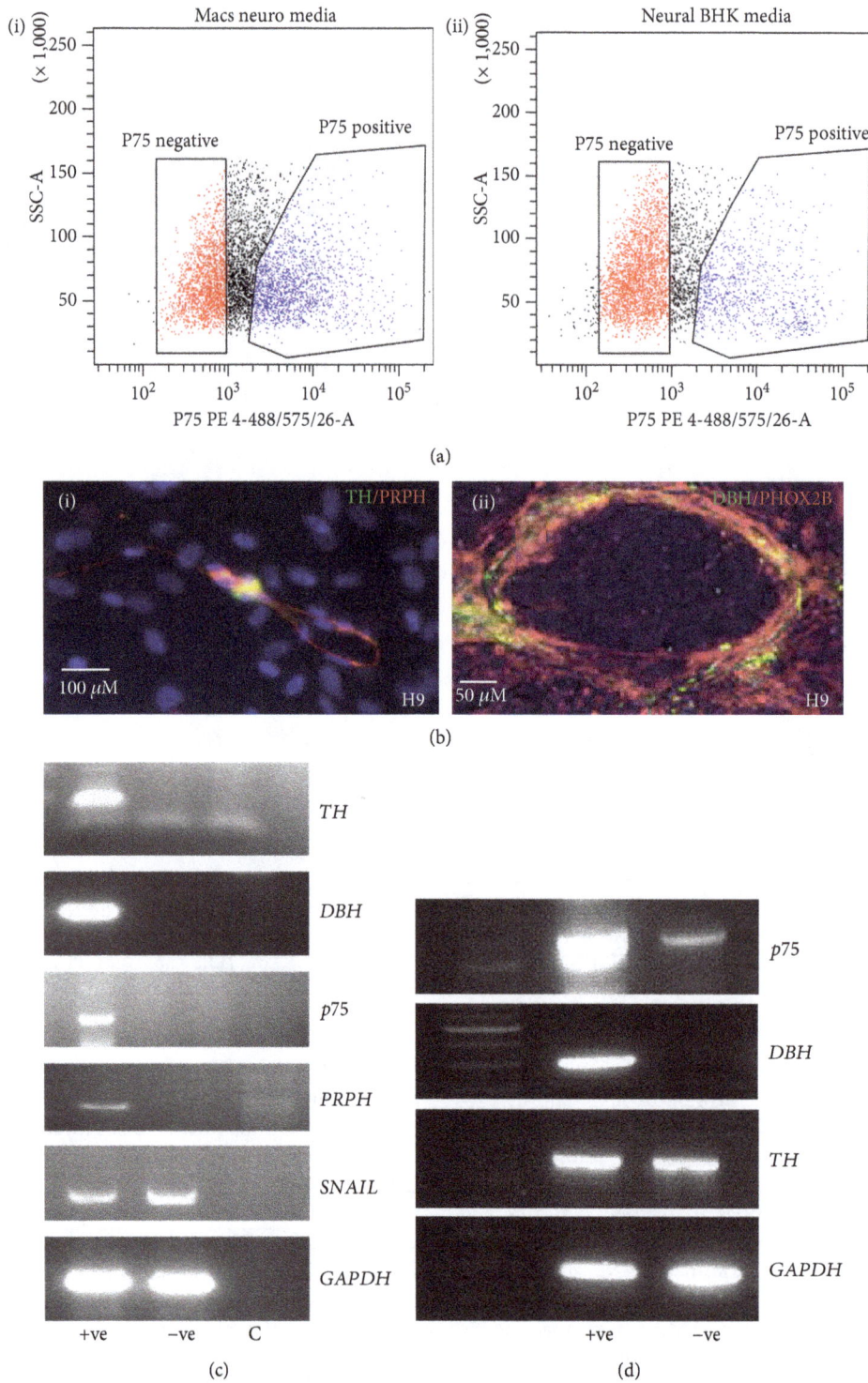

FIGURE 6: (a–c) Fluorescence-activated cell sorting (FACS) for p75 (neural crest stem cell marker). (a) FACS plots for H9 cells sorted on day 8 of differentiation. (a-i) 44.7% ± 6.1 p75+ viable cells in MACS® neuronal media. (a-ii) 32.5% ± 1.4 p75+ viable cells in neural BHK media. (b) Immunofluorescence of p75+ FACS-sorted H9 cells at different stages of differentiation. (b-i) PRPH and TH copositive H9 cells at 14 days post cell sort. (b-ii) PHOX2B and DBH copositive H9 cells at 14 days post cell sort. (c) mRNA expression by RT-PCR of FACS sorted H9 p75+ and p75− ve fractions showing high expression of *TH*, *DBH*, and *PERIPHERIN* in p75+ cells and undetectable expression in p75− cells and equivalent *SNAIL* expression in both populations. (d) RT-PCR of p75-enriched H9 cells isolated using anti-human p75 antibody-coated magnetic MicroBeads showing *TH* and *p75* expression in p75-depleted population. +ve = p75 positive fraction, −ve = p75 negative fraction, and c = negative control.

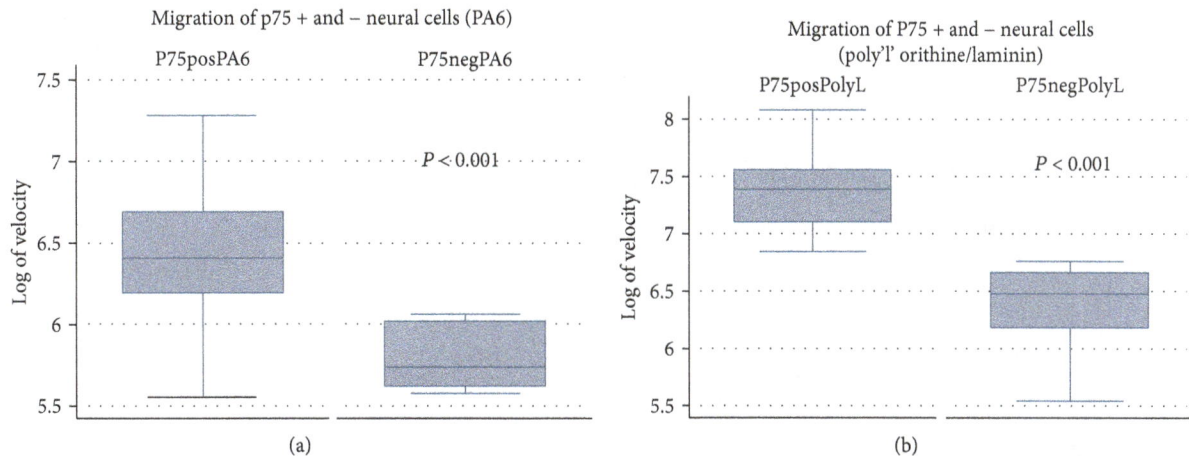

FIGURE 7: Migration of p75+ and p75– H9 cells sorted by FACS on (a) PA6 coated wells showing a higher mean logged velocity of p75+ cells compared with p75– cells ($p < 0.001$), and (b) poly 'L'ornithine/Laminin coated plates again showing a higher mean logged velocity in p75+ cells ($p < 0.001$).

shown). H9 cells appeared to track and follow PA6 cells adhering to them which in turn led to enhanced survival. Time-lapse microscopy revealed that p75+ ve cells showed increased migration compared with p75– ve cells. A t-test for independent groups with correction for unequal variances showed that the mean logged velocity for p75+ ve cells grown on PA6 cells was higher than that for p75– ve cells ($p < 0.001$). A similar analysis showed that the mean logged velocity for p75+ ve cells grown on poly-l-ornithine /laminin cells was higher than that for p75– ve cells ($p < 0.001$) (Figures 7(a) and 7(b); Supplementary online video 1).

4. Discussion

The aim of the current study was to optimise a model of normal human sympathetic neuronal development using hESC, which could be used to understand the normal development of the SNS and in the future the pathogenesis of neuroblastoma and other neural crest-derived malignancies.

In this study, we optimised derivation of neural crest-like cells and noradrenergic sympathetic neuron-like cells using a variety of methods. Initially, we tested conditions for neural crest-derived stem line cell differentiation by comparison of two media types: (1) MACS® neuronal media and (2) neural BHK media, where the former was found to be superior for the generation of p75+ ve cells. We also optimised BMP exposure and showed that BMP4 exposure alone was superior, in agreement with previous studies showing that although early exposure to BMP4 can promote dorsal neural differentiation, when applied at later stages, BMP4 enhances the production of NCSC and autonomic neurons in primate and murine cells [9, 19]. BMP signalling is essential for the initiation of differentiation of neural crest cells into sympathetic neurons in the developing embryo [20, 21]. To our knowledge, there is only one other study differentiating hESC to autonomic neurons which has employed the use of BMP4 during differentiation [10], but this study did not use SDIA

which is likely to be at least partly responsible for the higher yields of sympathetic neurons we observed (Table 1).

p75 is the low affinity NGF receptor and a well-characterised marker for neural crest-derived stem-like cells [22]. Using a murine in vivo model, NGF was shown to bind the high-affinity NGF receptor (TRKA) which regulates the expression of both TH and DBH in developing and maturing sympathetic neurons [23]. p75 cell sorting has been used previously to purify neural crest stem cells from hESCs [24, 25], and our work has extended this field by showing that day 8 of differentiation induced by SDIA is the optimal time for p75 cell sorting.

The presence of TH and PRPH costaining or DBH and PHOX2B was used to identify catecholaminergic and noradrenergic sympathetic neurons, respectively. TH is the rate-limiting enzyme in the biosynthesis of dopamine and noradrenaline and is a useful marker for catecholaminergic neurons (Figure 1(b)) [26]. PRPH is expressed in neurons of the developing peripheral nervous system [27].

PHOX2B regulates the expression of PHOX2A and heart and neural crest-derived expressed protein 2 (HAND2). Hand2 is induced by BMPs and is first observed after the onset of Phox2B and Asc-1 expression. Overexpression of Hand2 has been shown to induce the generation of catecholaminergic neurons from neural precursor cells both in vitro and in vivo [4, 5]. Furthermore, germline mutations in *PHOX2B* have been identified in hereditary neuroblastoma [28, 29]. DBH, a specific marker of noradrenergic sympathetic neurons, is expressed in some neuroblastoma cell lines [30]; it catalyses the conversion of dopamine to noradrenaline in the catecholamine synthesis pathway leading to noradrenergic neurons [31]. In the current study, noradrenergic sympathetic neurons were identified by *DBH* mRNA expression and immunostaining for DBH alone and DBH/ PHOX2B copositivity.

Time-lapse analysis of p75+ ve and p75– ve cells showed that p75+ ve cells had increased migration compared with p75– ve cells, consistent with migratory properties of neural

TABLE 1: Comparison of the current study with previously published studies reporting the differentiation of pluripotent stem cells to sympathetic neurons.

Reference	Methods	Cell type	Markers used to identify SNS progenitors	Yield
Mizuseki et al. [9]	PA6 stromal cells/BMP4	mESCs, primate ESCs	TH+/PRPH+/Phox2b	Not quantified—very low
Pomp et al. [33]	PA6 coculture BHK-21 medium/Glasgow MEM + N2 supplement	HES1, HUES1, HUES7	TH+/PRPH+	<1%
Lee et al. [25]	MS5 stromal cell line 28 days, FGF2/EGF exposure	H9	TH+/PRPH+	1-2%
Jiang et al. [24]	PA6 stromal cell line—7 days BHK-21 medium/Glasgow modified Eagle's medium + N2 supplement	H1, H9	TH+/PRPH+	18%
Acevedo et al. [34]	Embryoid bodies (EBs)—onto collagen plates	H9	Dopa decarboxylase (DDC), TH+, Mash 1	Not determined
Huang et al. [10]	Exposure to retinoic acid, BMP2, BMP4, BMP7	H1, WTC iPSC	TH+/DBH+	Not determined
This study	PA6 stromal cells, MACS® neuronal media + BMP4	H9	TH+/PRPH+, DBH+/PHOX2B+	20% and 9.4% ± 5.5%, respectively

crest cells [1]. These results mirror findings observed in vivo using live cell imaging during embryogenesis [32].

QRT-PCR gene expression analysis showed high expression of the pluripotency markers OCT4 and LIN28B in pluripotent H9 cells decreasing with the onset of neural differentiation as expected [35].

TP53 expression was observed throughout differentiation at levels similar to those in neuroblastoma cell lines consistent with evidence that p53 regulates the proliferation and differentiation of neural progenitor cells independently of its role in the induction of apoptosis. In vivo studies using transgenic mouse models have demonstrated a fundamental role for p53 during neural stem cell self-renewal and differentiation [36, 37].

Previous studies have used murine neural crest systems to investigate neuroblastoma development by MYCN transformation of primary neural crest cells derived from day 9.5 mouse embryos [38]. Further studies also reported that MYCN and common ALK mutations exert a role in neuroblastoma tumour initiation using neural crest progenitor cell lines MONC-1 and JoMa1 [39, 40]. Very recently, human NCSC derived from hESC have been transformed by MYCN to form neuroblastoma in vivo [11]. The use of human stem cell models of sympathoadrenal development such as ours will develop this field further.

In conclusion, our study describes advancement in the generation of noradrenergic sympathetic neuron-like cells from hESC to improve our understanding of the normal development of the human SNS and abnormalities thereof including neural crest-derived malignancies such as neuroblastoma. This model could later be perturbed by oncogenic transformation of these cells with genes known to be important in the development of neuroblastoma including MYCN and/or ALK as has been reported for NCDSC, to better understand events leading to the development of neuroblastoma, its cell of origin, and new potential treatment targets.

Abbreviations

BMP: Bone morphogenetic protein
hESC: Human embryonic stem cells
DBH: Dopamine betahydroxylase
NCAM: Neural cell adhesion molecule
SDIA: Stromal-derived inducing activity
PRPH: Peripherin
SNS: Sympathetic nervous system
TH: Tyrosine hydroxylase.

Acknowledgments

We would like to thank the following for neuroblastoma cell lines: Dr. Jean Bernard (SKNAS) and Prof. Penny Lovat (IMR32 and SHSY5Y). We acknowledge the Newcastle University Flow Cytometry Core Facility (FCCF) for the assistance with the generation of flow cytometry data and in particular are very grateful to Mr. Ian Dimmick, Mr. Ian Harvey, and Dr. Owen Hughes. We thank Dr. Alex Laude for the assistance with the use of the Biostation and confocal microscopy and Mr. Jerome Evans for karyotyping the H9 cell line. We are also grateful to Professor Alison Murdoch and staff at the Newcastle Fertility Centre for an additional hESC line (NCL-14) which was used to replicate some of the experimental data obtained with H9 cells (not shown). The human embryonic and fetal material was provided by the Joint MRC/Wellcome Trust Human Developmental Biology Resource (http://www.hdbr.org). This study was supported by Neuroblastoma UK, Children with Cancer UK, Newcastle Healthcare Charity, Wellcome Trust (grant # 099175/Z/12/Z), JGW Patterson Foundation, and the North of England Children's Cancer Research Fund.

References

[1] T. Sauka-Spengler and M. Bronner-Fraser, "A gene regulatory network orchestrates neural crest formation," *Nature Reviews. Molecular Cell Biology*, vol. 9, no. 7, pp. 557–568, 2008.

[2] S. Thomas, M. Thomas, P. Wincker et al., "Human neural crest cells display molecular and phenotypic hallmarks of stem cells," *Human Molecular Genetics*, vol. 17, no. 21, pp. 3411–3425, 2008.

[3] S. A. Mohlin, C. Wigerup, and S. Pahlman, "Neuroblastoma aggressiveness in relation to sympathetic neuronal differentiation stage," *Seminars in Cancer Biology*, vol. 21, no. 4, pp. 276–282, 2011.

[4] M. J. Howard, M. Stanke, C. Schneider, X. Wu, and H. Rohrer, "The transcription factor dHAND is a downstream effector of BMPs in sympathetic neuron specification," *Development*, vol. 127, no. 18, pp. 4073–4081, 2000.

[5] C. Schneider, H. Wicht, J. Enderich, M. Wegner, and H. Rohrer, "Bone morphogenetic proteins are required in vivo for the generation of sympathetic neurons," *Neuron*, vol. 24, no. 4, pp. 861–870, 1999.

[6] J. M. Maris, "Recent advances in neuroblastoma," *The New England Journal of Medicine*, vol. 362, no. 23, pp. 2202–2211, 2010.

[7] N. K. Cheung and M. A. Dyer, "Neuroblastoma: developmental biology, cancer genomics and immunotherapy," *Nature Reviews Cancer*, vol. 13, no. 6, pp. 397–411, 2013.

[8] H. Kawasaki, K. Mizuseki, S. Nishikawa et al., "Induction of midbrain dopaminergic neurons from ES cells by stromal cell-derived inducing activity," *Neuron*, vol. 28, no. 1, pp. 31–40, 2000.

[9] K. Mizuseki, T. Sakamoto, K. Watanabe et al., "Generation of neural crest-derived peripheral neurons and floor plate cells from mouse and primate embryonic stem cells," *Proceedings of the National Academy of Sciences of the United States of America*, vol. 100, no. 10, pp. 5828–5833, 2003.

[10] M. Huang, M. L. Miller, L. K. McHenry et al., "Generating trunk neural crest from human pluripotent stem cells," *Scientific Reports*, vol. 6, no. 1, article 19727, 2016.

[11] E. A. Newman, S. Chukkapalli, D. Bashllari et al., "Alternative NHEJ pathway proteins as components of MYCN oncogenic activity in human neural crest stem cell differentiation: implications for neuroblastoma initiation," *Cell Death & Disease*, vol. 8, no. 12, p. 3208, 2017.

[12] J. A. Thomson, J. Itskovitz-Eldor, S. S. Shapiro et al., "Embryonic stem cell lines derived from human blastocysts," *Science*, vol. 282, no. 5391, pp. 1145–1147, 1998.

[13] N. Prathalingam, L. Ferguson, L. Young et al., "Production and validation of a good manufacturing practice grade human fibroblast line for supporting human embryonic stem cell derivation and culture," *Stem Cell Research & Therapy*, vol. 3, no. 2, p. 12, 2012.

[14] D. Goldschneider, E. Horvilleur, L. F. Plassa et al., "Expression of C-terminal deleted p 53 isoforms in neuroblastoma," *Nucleic Acids Research*, vol. 34, no. 19, pp. 5603–5612, 2006.

[15] J. J. Tumilowicz, W. W. Nichols, J. J. Cholon, and A. E. Greene, "Definition of a continuous human cell line derived from neuroblastoma," *Cancer Research*, vol. 30, no. 8, pp. 2110–2118, 1970.

[16] J. L. Biedler, L. Helson, and B. A. Spengler, "Morphology and growth, tumorigenicity, and cytogenetics of human neuroblastoma cells in continuous culture," *Cancer Research*, vol. 33, no. 11, pp. 2643–2652, 1973.

[17] K. Watanabe, M. Ueno, D. Kamiya et al., "A ROCK inhibitor permits survival of dissociated human embryonic stem cells," *Nature Biotechnology*, vol. 25, no. 6, pp. 681–686, 2007.

[18] O. A. Kozhich, R. S. Hamilton, and B. S. Mallon, "Standardized generation and differentiation of neural precursor cells from human pluripotent stem cells," *Stem Cell Reviews*, vol. 9, no. 4, pp. 531–536, 2013.

[19] Y. Sasai, "Directed differentiation of neural and sensory tissues from embryonic stem cells in vitro," *Ernst Schering Research Foundation Workshop*, vol. 54, pp. 101–109, 2005.

[20] H. Liu, J. F. Margiotta, and M. J. Howard, "BMP4 supports noradrenergic differentiation by a PKA-dependent mechanism," *Developmental Biology*, vol. 286, no. 2, pp. 521–536, 2005.

[21] E. Reissmann, U. Ernsberger, P. H. Francis-West, D. Rueger, P. M. Brickell, and H. Rohrer, "Involvement of bone morphogenetic protein-4 and bone morphogenetic protein-7 in the differentiation of the adrenergic phenotype in developing sympathetic neurons," *Development*, vol. 122, no. 7, pp. 2079–2088, 1996.

[22] D. J. Anderson and R. Axel, "A bipotential neuroendocrine precursor whose choice of cell fate is determined by NGF and glucocorticoids," *Cell*, vol. 47, no. 6, pp. 1079–1090, 1986.

[23] R. Andres, L. A. Herraez-Baranda, J. Thompson, S. Wyatt, and A. M. Davies, "Regulation of sympathetic neuron differentiation by endogenous nerve growth factor and neurotrophin-3," *Neuroscience Letters*, vol. 431, no. 3, pp. 241–246, 2008.

[24] X. Jiang, Y. Gwye, S. J. McKeown, M. Bronner-Fraser, C. Lutzko, and E. R. Lawlor, "Isolation and characterization of neural crest stem cells derived from in vitro–differentiated human embryonic stem cells," *Stem Cells and Development*, vol. 18, no. 7, pp. 1059–1071, 2009.

[25] G. Lee, H. Kim, Y. Elkabetz et al., "Isolation and directed differentiation of neural crest stem cells derived from human embryonic stem cells," *Nature Biotechnology*, vol. 25, no. 12, pp. 1468–1475, 2007.

[26] S. C. Daubner, T. Le, and S. Wang, "Tyrosine hydroxylase and regulation of dopamine synthesis," *Archives of Biochemistry and Biophysics*, vol. 508, no. 1, pp. 1–12, 2011.

[27] S. Z. Krister S Eriksson, L. Lin, R. C. Larivière, J.-P. Julie2, and E. Mignot, "The type III neurofilament peripherin is expressed in the tuberomammillary neurons of the mouse," *BMC Neuroscience*, vol. 9, no. 1, p. 26, 2008.

[28] D. Trochet, F. Bourdeaut, I. Janoueix-Lerosey et al., "Germline mutations of the paired-like homeobox 2B (*PHOX2B*) gene in neuroblastoma," *American Journal of Human Genetics*, vol. 74, no. 4, pp. 761–764, 2004.

[29] V. van Limpt, A. Schramm, A. van Lakeman et al., "The Phox2B homeobox gene is mutated in sporadic neuroblastomas," *Oncogene*, vol. 23, no. 57, pp. 9280–9288, 2004.

[30] A. M. F. P. Oyarce, "Multiple forms of human dopamine β-hydroxylase in SH-SY5Y neuroblastoma cells," *Archives of Biochemistry and Biophysics*, vol. 290, no. 2, pp. 503–510, 1991.

[31] J. H. Yan Fan, N. Kieran, and M.-Y. Zhu, "Effects of transcription factors Phox2 on expression of norepinephrine transporter and dopamine β-hydroxylase in SK-N-BE(2)C cells," *Journal of Neurochemistry*, vol. 110, no. 5, pp. 1502–1513, 2009.

[32] M. R. Clay and M. C. Halloran, "Control of neural crest cell

behavior and migration: insights from live imaging," *Cell Adhesion & Migration*, vol. 4, no. 4, pp. 586–594, 2010.

[33] O. Pomp, I. Brokhman, I. Ben-Dor, B. Reubinoff, and R. S. Goldstein, "Generation of peripheral sensory and sympathetic neurons and neural crest cells from human embryonic stem cells," *Stem Cells*, vol. 23, no. 7, pp. 923–930, 2005.

[34] L. M. Acevedo, J. N. Lindquist, B. M. Walsh et al., "hESC differentiation toward an autonomic neuronal cell fate depends on distinct cues from the co-patterning vasculature," *Stem Cell Reports*, vol. 4, no. 6, pp. 1075–1088, 2015.

[35] M. Patterson, D. N. Chan, I. Ha et al., "Defining the nature of human pluripotent stem cell progeny," *Cell Research*, vol. 22, no. 1, pp. 178–193, 2012.

[36] E. Gottlieb, R. Haffner, A. King et al., "Transgenic mouse model for studying the transcriptional activity of the p53 protein: age- and tissue-dependent changes in radiation-induced activation during embryogenesis," *The EMBO Journal*, vol. 16, no. 6, pp. 1381–1390, 1997.

[37] E. A. Komarova, M. V. Chernov, R. Franks et al., "Transgenic mice with p53-responsive lacZ: p53 activity varies dramatically during normal development and determines radiation and drug sensitivity in vivo," *The EMBO Journal*, vol. 16, no. 6, pp. 1391–1400, 1997.

[38] R. R. Olsen, J. H. Otero, J. Garcia-Lopez et al., "MYCN induces neuroblastoma in primary neural crest cells," *Oncogene*, vol. 36, no. 35, pp. 5075–5082, 2017.

[39] G. Montavon, N. Jauquier, A. Coulon et al., "Wild-type ALK and activating ALK-R1275Q and ALK-F1174L mutations upregulate Myc and initiate tumor formation in murine neural crest progenitor cells," *Oncotarget*, vol. 5, no. 12, pp. 4452–4466, 2014.

[40] J. H. Schulte, S. Lindner, A. Bohrer et al., "MYCN and ALKF1174L are sufficient to drive neuroblastoma development from neural crest progenitor cells," *Oncogene*, vol. 32, no. 8, pp. 1059–1065, 2013.

4

Characterization of Human Mesenchymal Stem Cells Isolated from the Testis

Letizia De Chiara (ID),[1,2] **Elvira Smeralda Famulari,**[2] **Sharmila Fagoonee,**[2,3]
Saskia K. M. van Daalen,[4] **Stefano Buttiglieri,**[2] **Alberto Revelli,**[5] **Emanuela Tolosano,**[2]
Lorenzo Silengo,[2] **Ans M. M. van Pelt,**[4] **and Fiorella Altruda** (ID)[2]

[1]*Centro di Eccellenza DeNothe, Department of Biomedical, Experimental and Clinical Sciences, University of Florence,
Viale Pieraccini 6, 50139 Firenze, Italy*
[2]*Molecular Biotechnology Center, Department of Molecular Biotechnology and Health Sciences, University of Turin, Via Nizza 52,
10126 Turin, Italy*
[3]*The Institute of Biostructure and Bioimaging (CNR) c/o Molecular Biotechnology Center, Turin, Italy*
[4]*Center for Reproductive Medicine, Women's and Children's Hospital, Academic Medical Center, University of Amsterdam,
Meibergdreef 9, 1105 AZ Amsterdam, Netherlands*
[5]*Obstetrics and Gynecology 1U, Physiopathology of Reproduction and IVF Unit, Department of Surgical Sciences,
Sant'Anna Hospital, University of Turin, Corso Spezia 60, 10126 Turin, Italy*

Correspondence should be addressed to Letizia De Chiara; letizia.dechiara@gmail.com
and Fiorella Altruda; fiorella.altruda@unito.it

Academic Editor: Peter J. Quesenberry

Mesenchymal stem cells hold great promise for regenerative medicine as they can be easily isolated from different sources such as adipose tissue, bone marrow, and umbilical cord blood. Spontaneously arising pluripotent stem cells can be obtained in culture from murine spermatogonial stem cells (SSCs), while the pluripotency of the human counterpart remains a matter of debate. Recent gene expression profiling studies have demonstrated that embryonic stem cell- (ESC-) like cells obtained from the human testis are indeed closer to mesenchymal stem cells (MSCs) than to pluripotent stem cells. Here, we confirm that colonies derived from human testicular cultures, with our isolation protocol, are of mesenchymal origin and do not arise from spermatogonial stem cells (SSCs). The testis, thus, provides an important and accessible source of MSCs (tMSCs) that can be potentially used for nephrotoxicity testing *in vitro*. We further demonstrate, for the first time, that tMSCs are able to secrete microvesicles that could possibly be applied to the treatment of various chronic diseases, such as those affecting the kidney.

1. Introduction

Mesenchymal stem cells (MSCs) are multipotent stem cells first postulated by Owen et al. to be derived from bone marrow [1]. Since then, this stromal cell type has been found in a myriad of different tissues [2–4]. As MSCs are able to home to sites of inflammation and differentiate into various cell types and are immunomodulatory, they are ideal candidates for clinical applications. Unlike multipotent stem cells, SSCs are unipotent stem cells that reside on the basal membrane of the testis and can give rise only to spermatozoa. SSCs are defined by their ability to balance between self-renewal and differentiation, a feature which is supported by Sertoli and stromal cells that represent the main components of the SSC niche [5]. The study of SSCs has always been challenging as they are very limited in number [6, 7], and specific markers have not yet been identified [8].

Intriguingly, murine SSCs, under specific culture conditions, are able to spontaneously convert into pluripotent embryonic-like stem cells, known as germline cell-derived pluripotent stem cells (GPSCs) [9–12]. Recently, a number of groups have claimed that pluripotent stem cells can be derived from unipotent human SSCs [13, 14]. Nevertheless, these findings have been subsequently challenged [15], demonstrating that these "embryonic-like colonies" have an expression profile more similar to that of fibroblasts than to that of embryonic stem cells (ESCs) [16] and are, in fact, of mesenchymal origin [17, 18].

Here, we confirm that a mesenchymal population can be easily established from small human biopsies without employing any particular separation protocol. Interestingly, we demonstrate that these testicular MSCs (tMSCs) can be established from very small testis biopsies making them an attractive and novel source of MSC for cell therapy. Furthermore, we evaluate the microvesicle profile of these tMSCs derived from the human testis, which was never shown before. The therapeutic potential of extracellular vesicles is very broad, with applications including as a drug delivery route and as biomarkers for diagnosis [19, 20]. Extracellular vesicles extracted from stem cells may be used for treatment of many diseases including those affecting the kidney [21–23].

2. Materials and Methods

2.1. Culture Conditions and Isolation Protocol. tMSC colonies were derived from primary testicular cultures, starting with 1×10^6 to 1×10^7 cells and are based on previously published protocols [24, 25], from frozen-thawed testis material of TESE (testicular sperm extraction) pellets of 10 individuals that underwent IVF (*in vitro* fertilization). The protocol was approved by the LIVET Srl local Ethical Committee (approval date 14 March 2015). After obtaining the written informed consent, the testis material was donated for research. Testicular cells were isolated with a cocktail of enzymes, trypsin (Sigma), collagenase type I (Worthington), and hyaluronidase (Sigma), in MEM1x (Invitrogen) containing DNase (Sigma) and cultured in supplemented StemPro-34 (Invitrogen) medium as previously described for mouse testicular cells [26], with the omission of feeder cells. After their initial appearance, colonies morphologically resembling ESC colonies were picked and subcultured as described previously [27] with some modifications. Briefly, individual colonies were subcultured in ESC medium composed of DMEM-KO medium (Invitrogen), 20% ES qualified fetal calf serum (FCS, Gibco), 0.01 mM nonessential amino acid (NEAA, Gibco), 100 U/ml penicillin (Gibco), 100 μg/ml streptomycin (Gibco), 0.05 mM β-mercaptoethanol (Sigma), a cocktail of insulin, transferrin, and sodium selenite (10 μg/ml, 5.5 μg/ml, and 5 ng/ml, resp.; ITS 100X, Sigma), and 25 ng/ml bFGF (basic fibroblast growth factor, Voden). Testicular somatic cells (TSCs) were isolated using the same protocol and maintained in MEM1x (Invitrogen) with 10% FCS.

2.2. Culture of IMCD3. IMCD3 (inner medullary collecting duct cells) were maintained in DMEM-F12 (Invitrogen) added with calf serum (Gibco), 100 U/ml penicillin (Gibco), and 100 μg/ml streptomycin (Gibco).

2.3. Analysis of mRNA Expression. Total RNA was extracted from tMSCs at passage 6, according to the manufacturer's instruction (TRI Reagent®, Ambion). cDNA was synthesized starting from 500 ng of RNA as previously described [28]. Quantitative real-time PCR was performed using the following sets of primers: VASA (forward: 5′-CGCCAAACCCT TATGTTCAG-3′ and reverse: 5′-AAAAACTCTGCAGC CAACCTT-3′), VIMENTIN (forward: 5′-TACAGGAAG CTGCTGGAAGG-3′ and reverse: 5′-ACCAGAGGGAG TGAATCCAG-3′), CD90 (forward: 5′-AGGACGAGGGC ACCTACAC-3′ and reverse: 5′-GCCCTCACTTGACCAG TT-3′), NANOG (forward: 5′-AGATGCCTCACACGGA GAC-3′ and reverse: 5′-TTTGCGACACTCTTCTCTGC-3′), SOX2 (forward: 5′-TGCTGCCTCTTTAAGACTA-3′ and reverse: 5′-CCTGGGGCTCAAACTTCTCT-3′), and OCT4 (forward: 5′-CTTCGCAAGCCCTCATTTC-3′ and reverse: 5′-GAGAAGGCGAAATCCGAAG-3′).

2.4. Immunofluorescence Staining. tMSCs were fixed with 4% paraformaldehyde for 10 minutes, and the primary antibody was diluted in 1% bovine serum albumin (BSA, Sigma) and incubated for 1 h at room temperature. The goat polyclonal anti-vimentin (Santa Cruz) antibody was used. Nuclei were counterstained with DAPI (4,6 diamidino-2-phenylindole, Sigma).

2.5. Flow Cytometry Analysis. Flow cytometry was performed using a FACSCalibur Cytometer (BD Biosciences); a phenotyping kit (MSC phenotyping kit, Miltenyi) was used to characterize the tMSCs. The following antibodies were used: anti-CD34PerCP, anti-CD45PerCP, anti-CD20PerCP, anti-CD14PerCP, anti-CD73APC, anti-CD9FITC, and anti-CD105PE (BD Pharmingen). Matched isotype controls were applied to determine background fluorescence levels.

2.6. Adipogenic Differentiation and Oil Red Staining. tMSCs were plated at a density of 3×10^5 in a 6-well culture dish and incubated O/N in a humidified incubator. Adipogenic induction medium was prepared in DMEM-low glucose (Invitrogen) with the addition of 10% fetal bovine serum (FBS), 10 mM dexamethasone (Sigma), 10 mg/mL insulin (Sigma), 100 U/ml penicillin (Gibco), and 100 μg/ml streptomycin (Gibco). Adipogenic maintenance medium was prepared as the induction medium with the exception of dexamethasone. The medium was added following the differentiation schedule: 4 days in the induction medium and 2 days in the maintenance medium (repeated 3 times).

For the red oil staining, cells were fixed for 10′ in 4% paraformaldehyde (PFA) and then incubated for 10′ in 60% isopropanol. The staining for the lipid droplets was accomplished through the incubation of cells with oil red O solution (Sigma) for 5′, and then the cells were washed with phosphate-buffered saline (PBS) and mounted. Nuclei were counterstained with hematoxylin (Bioptica).

2.7. Osteogenic Differentiation and Alizarin Red Staining. tMSCs were plated at a density of 1×10^5 in a 6-well culture dish and incubated O/N in a humidified incubator. Cells

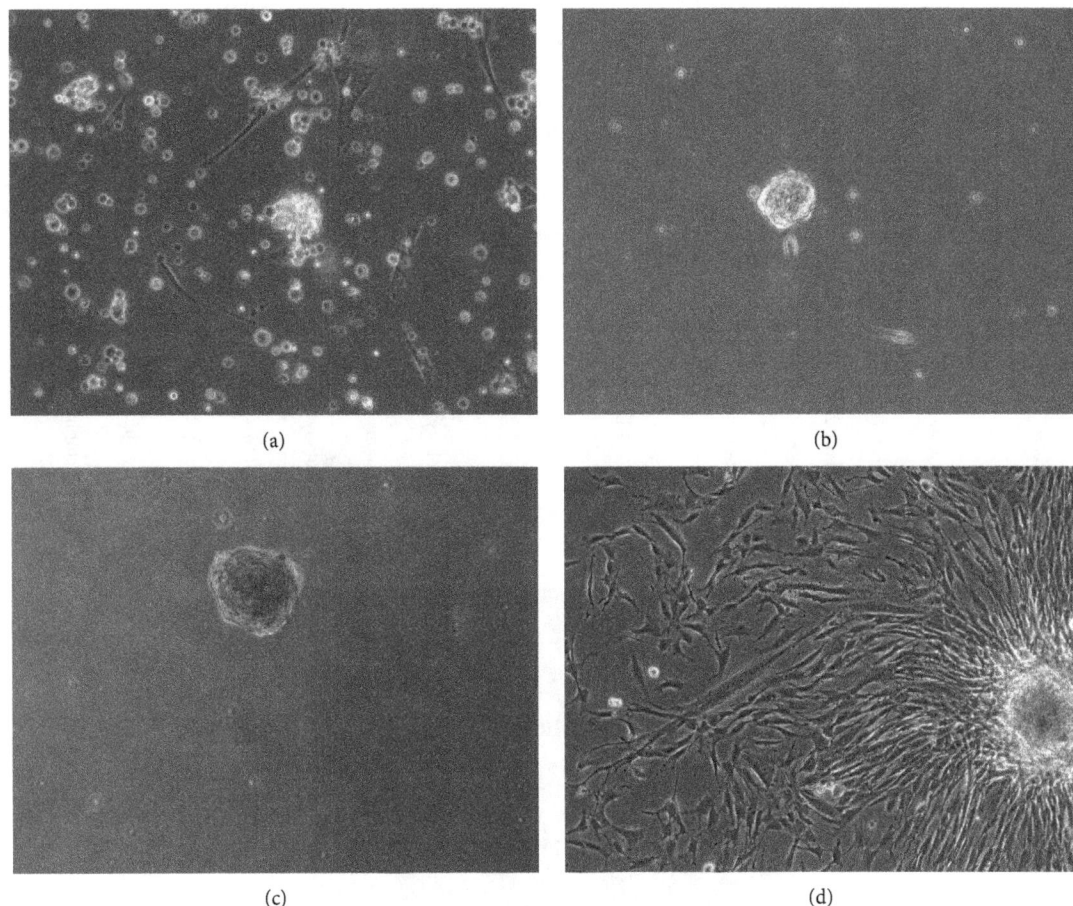

(a)

(b)

(c)

(d)

FIGURE 1: Appearance of tMSC colonies. The day after cell purification from testis biopsies, a mixed population of cells was present in the culture (a). Floating clusters started to appear between 1 week and 3 weeks postseparation (b, c). Once isolated and cultured on plastic, these colonies start to expand and proliferate (d). Original magnification: ×200.

were treated for 3 weeks with a commercial medium for osteogenic differentiation (Euroclone). For alizarin red S staining, cells were fixed for 10′ in 4% PFA and stained with the alizarin red solution (Sigma) for 30″ to 5′, while observing the reaction microscopically. Cells were dehydrated in acetone and mounted. Nuclei were counterstained with hematoxylin (Bioptica).

2.8. Alkaline Phosphatase Staining. For the alkaline phosphatase assay, cells at passage 6 were seeded onto a chamber slide (Thermo Scientific) and allowed to reach 80% confluence. They were then fixed with 4% PFA for 2′ and stained with a commercial kit, according to the manufacturer's instruction (Millipore).

2.9. Microvesicle (MV) Isolation from tMSCs and TSCs. MVs were isolated according to previously published protocols [21]. Briefly, MVs were obtained from supernatants of tMSCs at early passages (p6) and from testicular somatic cells as a control. tMSCs were cultured in DMEM-KO (Invitrogen), and testicular somatic cells in MEM1x (Invitrogen) both deprived of FCS for 24 h. After centrifugation at 3000 RPM for 10′ to remove debris, cell-free supernatants

were centrifuged at 100,000g (Beckman Coulter Optima L-100K ultracentrifuge) for 2 h at 4°C. MV concentration was determined by protein quantification (Bradford assay, Bio-Rad).

2.10. Labelling of MVs Derived from tMSCs. 50 μg/ml of MVs was labelled with PKH67 dye (Sigma) according to the manufacturer's protocol. The MVs were then incubated on IMCD3 for 4 h, 12 h, and 24 h at 37°C. Following incubation, the cells were fixed, counterstained with DAPI, and analyzed by fluorescence microscopy.

2.11. Statistical Analysis. Values are reported as the mean ± standard error of mean. Statistical analysis was performed by using two-tailed Student's t-tests ($^*P < 0.05$, $^{**}P < 0.01$, and $^{***}P < 0.001$) for the graphs comparing only two variables. For the analysis of more than two categories, the statistical significance was calculated with one-way ANOVA and Bonferroni posttest ($^*P < 0.05$, $^{**}P < 0.01$, and $^{***}P < 0.001$). All the analyses were performed with PRISM5 (GraphPad Software Inc., La Jolla CA, USA).

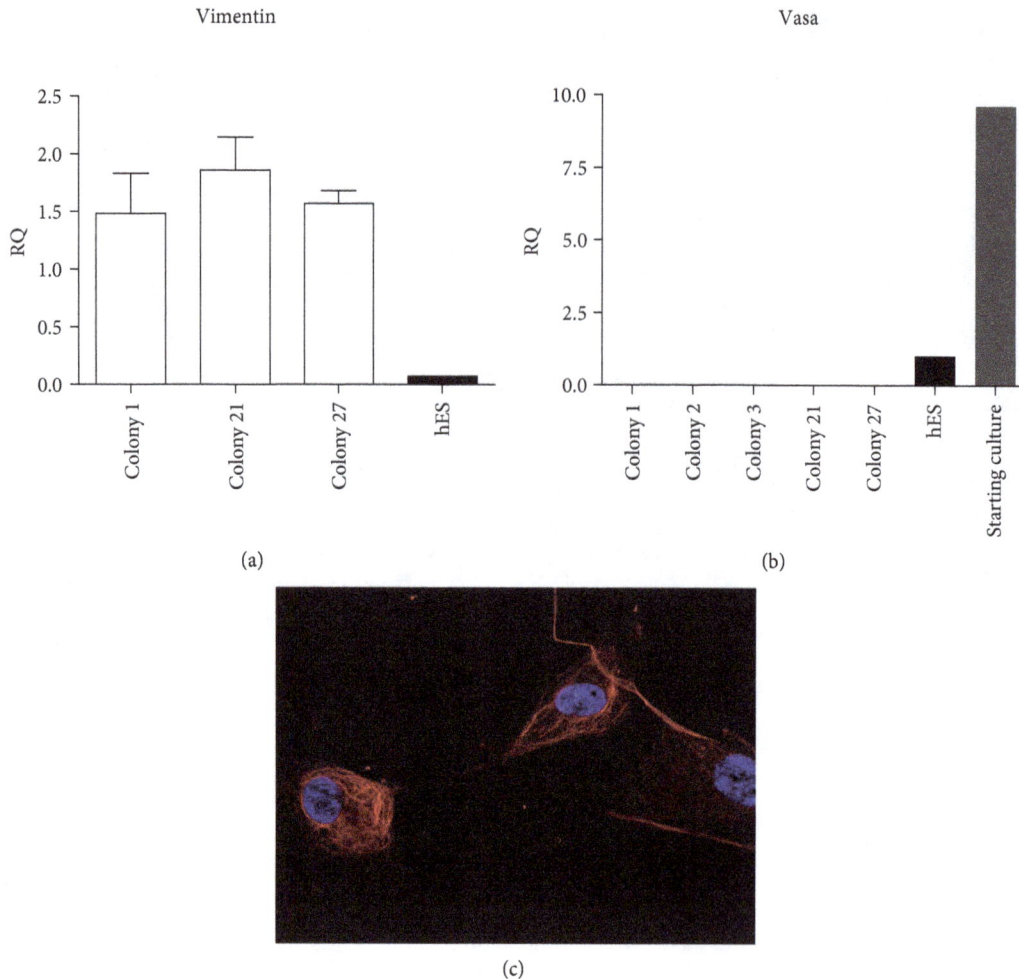

(a)

(b)

(c)

FIGURE 2: Mesenchymal phenotype of isolated tMSCs. Cells expanded from tMSC colony strongly express vimentin both at mRNA level (a) and at protein level (c). Moreover, they do not express VASA (b), a marker of cells originating from the germ lineage. Original magnification: (c) ×630.

3. Results

3.1. Mesenchymal Stem Cells from Testis Biopsies. Due to a lack of specific markers for SSCs [8], we chose not to sort our mixed population, composed of somatic cells, Sertoli cells, and SSCs (Sup. Figure S1A, B, and C), isolated from testicular biopsies. One week postisolation, some cells formed aggregated floating colonies (Figure 1(a)) and became granulated with time (Figures 1(b) and 1(c)). Two days after picking, colonies attached to the plates and started to proliferate (Figure 1(d)), but despite their resemblance to ESC colonies, further analysis revealed the nongermline origin of these cells (referred to as testicular mesenchymal stem cells (tMSCs) from now on) (Figure 2). We successfully isolated 27 colonies from up to 10 different biopsies, and we were able to maintain them in culture for at least 20 passages with comparable proliferation rates. All colonies analyzed gave equivalent results and showed the same mesenchymal characteristics. RNA was extracted at different passages. The expression of VASA was not detected in any colony (Figure 2(b)). VASA is a specific protein expressed by mammalian germ cells [29], and it is essential for germ cell

development [30]. Furthermore, cells derived from these colonies expressed high levels of vimentin, a typical mesenchymal marker, at both mRNA (Figure 2(a)) and protein level (Figure 2(c)). When we analyzed the expression of pluripotent markers in numerous tMSC colonies, none were found to be positive for any of the classical pluripotent markers (Sup. Figure S2A, B, and C). Moreover, they were unable to give rise to any of the three embryonic germ layers (data not show). The ability to grow on plastic and differentiate toward three mesodermal lineages (adipo-, osteo-, and chondrogenic) and the relevant presence and absence of specific antigens are the defining criteria of MSCs [31]. These colony-derived tMSCs were capable of growing on plastic (Figure 3(a)) and were positive for CD105, CD73, and CD90 (Figure 3(g)) and negative for CD14 and CD34 (Figure 3(h)). Finally, under appropriate conditions, tMSC differentiated toward mesodermal lineages. In the case of osteogenic differentiation, calcium deposition was observed (Figure 3(e)), while lipid accumulation (Figure 3(f)) was observed in the case of adipogenic differentiation of tMSCs. Intriguingly, some of the tMSC colonies showed positive staining for alkaline phosphatase (AP) (Figure 3(c)). Once

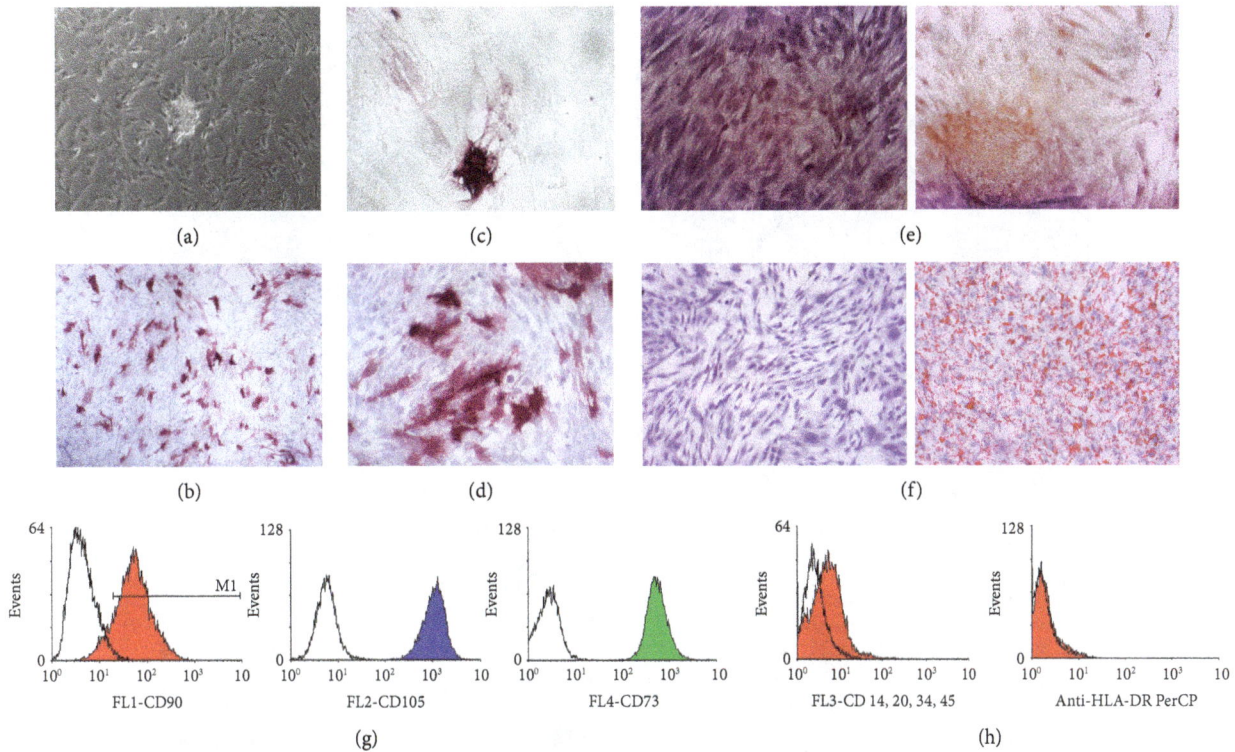

FIGURE 3: Characterization of the mesenchymal phenotype of tMSCs. (a–d) A representative picture of a tMSC colony (a) positive for AP staining and the correspondent colony in brightfield (c). Once picked and expanded, the colonies gave rise to a heterogeneous population expressing alkaline phosphatase (b–d). (e–f) Representative pictures of alizarin red staining (e) and oil red staining (f) of tMSCs, indicating osteogenic and adipogenic differentiation. Negative staining is represented on the left side, and positive staining on the right side. Original magnification: (a–c) ×100, (d) ×200, and (e, f) ×100. (g, h) A flow cytometry analysis of one of the tMSC colonies (colony #27). The analysis demonstrates that the cells are positive for CD73, CD105, and CD90 (g). As expected, the cells are negative for CD14, CD34, and HLA-DR (h). This analysis is representative of three independent experiments performed on various colonies.

isolated and cultured, these colonies, regardless of their initial positive staining for AP, gave rise to a mixed population of cells, in which about 50% of tMSCs were positive for AP (Figures 3(b) and 3(d)), reflecting the heterogeneous nature of other types of MSCs [32]. AP is demonstrated to be identical to the mesenchymal stem cell antigen MSCA-1 [33], and it can be used as a selective marker for MSC isolation [34]. Taken together, this data confirms the mesenchymal nature of these colonies and demonstrates for the first time the expression of AP in MSCs isolated from the human testis.

3.2. Characterization of MVs Derived from tMSCs. MVs were isolated from tMSCs following ultracentrifugation of the serum-starved culture supernatant. tMSC-derived microvesicles were labelled with PKH26 dye. IMCD3 (inner medullary collecting duct cells) were treated with the MV suspension for 4 h, 12 h, and 24 h. Uptake of MVs by the renal cells was evident at 4 h postincubation and continued in a time-dependent manner reaching the maximum uptake 24 h postincubation (Figure 4(a)). Intriguingly, we found that the testicular somatic cells used as a control were able to secrete MVs incorporated by the IMCD3, though to a lesser extent (data not shown). Real-time PCR analysis of these MVs was performed in order to evaluate their

mRNA composition and verify their mesenchymal origin. We demonstrated that tMSC-MVs of mesenchymal origin express higher level of both vimentin and CD90 mRNA than MVs isolated from testicular somatic cells (Figure 4(b)). Taken together, this data demonstrates for the first time that tMSCs are able to secrete MVs that are easily taken up by renal cells.

4. Discussion

Mesenchymal stem cells can be obtained from a number of different tissues, including bone marrow [4], umbilical cord [2], and adipose tissue [3]. It has been previously suggested that testicular tissue contains a mesenchymal population [35] of cells, and a study from 2014 identified these mesenchymal progenitors as the source of the ESC-like colonies isolated from the human testis [17]. In the present study, we confirmed independently that the "ESC-like" colonies arising from human testicular culture are indeed of mesenchymal origin and do not possess any pluripotent characteristics. Furthermore, we demonstrated the feasibility of isolating tMSC-derived MVs, highlighting the utility of this novel source of mesenchymal stem cells as an avenue to derive MVs for regenerative medicine applications.

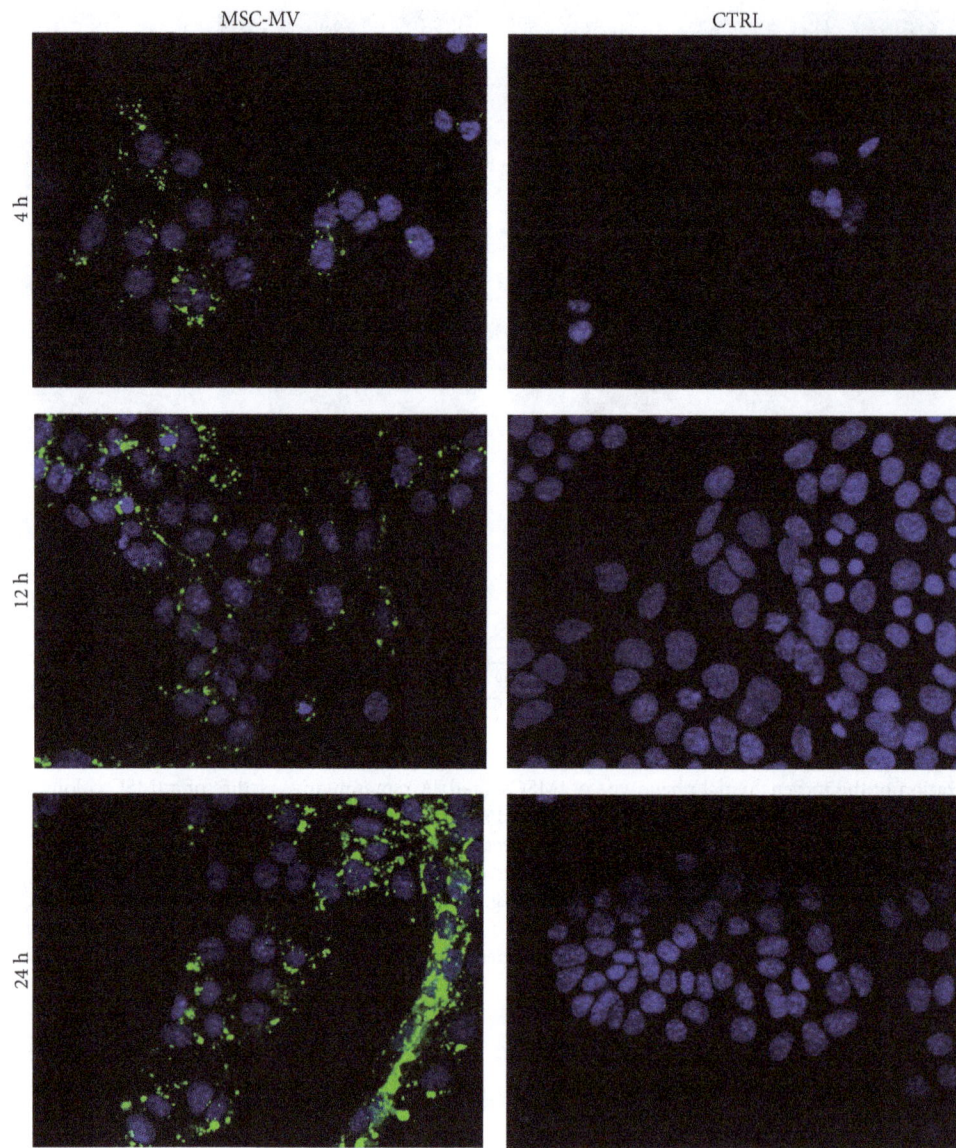

(a)

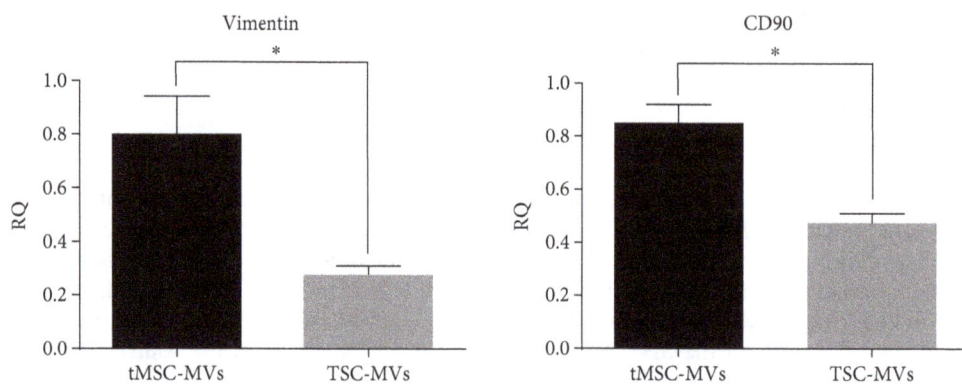

(b)

FIGURE 4: GFP$^+$ MVs derived from tMSCs are incorporated by IMCD3. (a) Representative pictures of IMDC3 incubated with GFP-labelled MVs at 4, 12, and 24 hours and the control (CTRL) cells incubated only with the labelling reagent. The MVs are progressively fused with the cells as demonstrated by the increased amount of fluorescence. Original magnification: ×400. (b) Finally, real-time analysis shows that MVs derived from tMSCs are positively enriched in vimentin and CD90 when compared to the MVs obtained from testicular somatic cells isolated from the same biopsy (TSC-MVs) ($N = 3$, $^*P < 0.05$).

Different lines of tMSCs were established from up to 10 testis biopsies, all with consistent features. The isolated colonies started to appear after differential passaging around 7–14 days postisolation. Although the shape of the colonies closely resembled that of ESC colonies, once isolated, they became granulated, giving rise to a population of "spindle"-like cells able to grow on plastic as a single layer. This population of cells was positive for the expression of the mesenchymal marker vimentin at both RNA and protein levels. It is interesting to note that none of the populations arising from the various colonies showed any indication of pluripotency. When cultured in suspension, these tMSCs failed to form embryoid bodies and died afterwards (data not shown). OCT4, NANOG, and SOX2 expression was barely detectable in all of the colonies analyzed, and no expression of VASA was detected. Intriguingly, VASA expression was present in the initial mixed population isolated from testis biopsies, ruling out the possibility that the lack of VASA expression might be due to the absence of a germline population in the starting sample. When we evaluated the mesenchymal features of the testis-derived colonies, we found that not only did the cells express all the classical markers of MSCs (CD90, CD73, and CD104) but also they differentiated into cells of mesodermal origin with ease. Interestingly, we found the tMSCs to be positive for AP, another MSC marker, which was never shown before. The heterogeneous expression of AP among the cells is in line with their mesenchymal origin [36]. With a small biopsy, tMSCs are easily derived and exhibit a relatively extended life span compared to other "classical" MSCs [36], making these testicular mesenchymal stem cells amenable to expansion for therapeutic purposes, an attractive proposition for regenerative medicine.

A growing body of evidence has demonstrated that MSCs act through a paracrine effect by secreting soluble factors and microvesicles [37, 38]. MVs derived from mesenchymal stem cells can reprogram target cells suggesting that they could be exploited in regenerative medicine to repair damaged tissues, and in particular, they have been demonstrated to be efficacious in preventing acute renal injury [22, 39, 40]. MVs isolated from MSCs were successfully incorporated by IMCD3, in which the GFP staining is already present 4 h postincubation. The GFP$^+$ signal increases over the time, demonstrating that the incorporation of MVs is time dependent. IMCD3 is an epithelial cell line derived from the inner medullary collecting ducts of the murine kidney; this observation may be important in light of a possible use for tMSC-MVs in the repair of renal injury. Finally, the statistically relevant expression of the two mesenchymal markers vimentin and CD90 confirms that the tMSC-MVs are definitively derived from a mesenchymal population.

5. Conclusions

In conclusion, we have demonstrated for the first time that mesenchymal stem cells isolated from small testis biopsies are positive for AP expression and are able to secrete MVs that can be successfully taken up by renal cells. Further analyses are required to evaluate the relevant biological activity of these new tMSC-derived MVs, with the possibility of exploiting their role and contribution in the repair of various chronic and acute diseases, as well as in nephrotoxicity testing *in vitro*.

Authors' Contributions

Letizia De Chiara designed and performed the experiments, analyzed the data, and wrote the paper. Elvira Smeralda Famulari performed the experiments. Sharmila Fagoonee helped in manuscript writing. Saskia VanDaleen gave a technical support. Stefano Buttiglieri helped in analyzing and interpreting the data. Alberto Revelli helped in the manuscript evaluation and contributed reagents and materials. Emanuela Tolosano and Lorenzo Silengo helped in the manuscript evaluation and gave conceptual advices. Ans M. M. van Pelt helped in the manuscript evaluation, gave expert critical opinion, and provided a technical support. Fiorella Altruda supervised the development of the work, helped in the data interpretation, and edited the paper.

Acknowledgments

This study was supported by Telethon Project GGP14028, Advanced Life Science in Italy (Alisei) (awarded to Fiorella Altruda).

References

[1] M. Owen and A. J. Friedenstein, "Stromal stem cells: marrow-derived osteogenic precursors," *Ciba Foundation Symposium*, vol. 136, pp. 42–60, 1988.

[2] C. T. Vangsness Jr., H. Sternberg, and L. Harris, "Umbilical cord tissue offers the greatest number of harvestable mesenchymal stem cells for research and clinical application: a literature review of different harvest sites," *Arthroscopy: The Journal of Arthroscopic & Related Surgery*, vol. 31, no. 9, pp. 1836–1843, 2015.

[3] F. De Francesco, G. Ricci, F. D'Andrea, G. F. Nicoletti, and G. A. Ferraro, "Human adipose stem cells: from bench to bedside," *Tissue Engineering Part B: Reviews*, vol. 21, no. 6, pp. 572–584, 2015.

[4] E. Cordeiro-Spinetti, W. de Mello, L. S. Trindade, D. D. Taub, R. S. Taichman, and A. Balduino, "Human bone marrow mesenchymal progenitors: perspectives on an optimized in vitro manipulation," *Frontiers in Cell and Developmental Biology*, vol. 2, 2014.

[5] B. T. Phillips, K. Gassei, and K. E. Orwig, "Spermatogonial stem cell regulation and spermatogenesis," *Philosophical Transactions of the Royal Society B: Biological Sciences*, vol. 365, no. 1546, pp. 1663–1678, 2010.

[6] D. G. de Rooij, M. Okabe, and Y. Nishimune, "Arrest of spermatogonial differentiation in jsd/jsd, Sl17H/Sl17H, and cryptorchid mice," *Biology of Reproduction*, vol. 61, no. 3, pp. 842–847, 1999.

[7] M. C. Nagano, "Homing efficiency and proliferation kinetics of male germ line stem cells following transplantation in

mice," *Biology of Reproduction*, vol. 69, no. 2, pp. 701–707, 2003.

[8] M. Yamada, L. De Chiara, and M. Seandel, "Spermatogonial stem cells: implications for genetic disorders and prevention," *Stem Cells and Development*, vol. 25, no. 20, pp. 1483–1494, 2016.

[9] K. Guan, K. Nayernia, L. S. Maier et al., "Pluripotency of spermatogonial stem cells from adult mouse testis," *Nature*, vol. 440, no. 7088, pp. 1199–1203, 2006.

[10] M. Kanatsu-Shinohara, K. Inoue, J. Lee et al., "Generation of pluripotent stem cells from neonatal mouse testis," *Cell*, vol. 119, no. 7, pp. 1001–1012, 2004.

[11] M. Seandel, D. James, S. V. Shmelkov et al., "Generation of functional multipotent adult stem cells from GPR125+ germ-line progenitors," *Nature*, vol. 449, no. 7160, pp. 346–350, 2007.

[12] K. Ko, N. Tapia, G. Wu et al., "Induction of pluripotency in adult unipotent germline stem cells," *Cell Stem Cell*, vol. 5, no. 1, pp. 87–96, 2009.

[13] S. Conrad, M. Renninger, J. Hennenlotter et al., "Generation of pluripotent stem cells from adult human testis," *Nature*, vol. 456, no. 7220, pp. 344–349, 2008.

[14] N. Golestaneh, M. Kokkinaki, D. Pant et al., "Pluripotent stem cells derived from adult human testes," *Stem Cells and Development*, vol. 18, no. 8, pp. 1115–1125, 2009.

[15] N. Tapia, M. J. Arauzo-Bravo, K. Ko, and H. R. Scholer, "Concise review: challenging the pluripotency of human testis-derived ESC-like cells," *Stem Cells*, vol. 29, no. 8, pp. 1165–1169, 2011.

[16] K. Ko, M. J. Araúzo-Bravo, N. Tapia et al., "Human adult germline stem cells in question," *Nature*, vol. 465, no. 7301, article E1, 2010.

[17] J. V. Chikhovskaya, S. K. M. van Daalen, C. M. Korver, S. Repping, and A. M. M. van Pelt, "Mesenchymal origin of multipotent human testis-derived stem cells in human testicular cell cultures," *Molecular Human Reproduction*, vol. 20, no. 2, pp. 155–167, 2014.

[18] J. V. Chikhovskaya, M. J. Jonker, A. Meissner, T. M. Breit, S. Repping, and A. M. M. van Pelt, "Human testis-derived embryonic stem cell-like cells are not pluripotent, but possess potential of mesenchymal progenitors," *Human Reproduction*, vol. 27, no. 1, pp. 210–221, 2012.

[19] N. Barkalina, C. Jones, M. J. A. Wood, and K. Coward, "Extracellular vesicle-mediated delivery of molecular compounds into gametes and embryos: learning from nature," *Human Reproduction Update*, vol. 21, no. 5, pp. 627–639, 2015.

[20] K. Mahmoudi, A. Ezrin, and C. Hadjipanayis, "Small extracellular vesicles as tumor biomarkers for glioblastoma," *Molecular Aspects of Medicine*, vol. 45, pp. 97–102, 2015.

[21] S. Bruno, C. Grange, F. Collino et al., "Microvesicles derived from mesenchymal stem cells enhance survival in a lethal model of acute kidney injury," *PloS One*, vol. 7, no. 3, article e33115, 2012.

[22] S. Gatti, S. Bruno, M. C. Deregibus et al., "Microvesicles derived from human adult mesenchymal stem cells protect against ischaemia-reperfusion-induced acute and chronic kidney injury," *Nephrology Dialysis Transplantation*, vol. 26, no. 5, pp. 1474–1483, 2011.

[23] F. T. Borges, L. A. Reis, and N. Schor, "Extracellular vesicles: structure, function, and potential clinical uses in renal diseases," *Brazilian Journal of Medical and Biological Research*, vol. 46, no. 10, pp. 824–830, 2013.

[24] S. C. Mizrak, J. V. Chikhovskaya, H. Sadri-Ardekani et al., "Embryonic stem cell-like cells derived from adult human testis," *Human Reproduction*, vol. 25, no. 1, pp. 158–167, 2010.

[25] H. Sadri-Ardekani, S. C. Mizrak, S. K. van Daalen et al., "Propagation of human spermatogonial stem cells in vitro," *JAMA*, vol. 302, no. 19, pp. 2127–2134, 2009.

[26] M. Kanatsu-Shinohara, N. Ogonuki, K. Inoue et al., "Long-term proliferation in culture and germline transmission of mouse male germline stem cells," *Biology of Reproduction*, vol. 69, no. 2, pp. 612–616, 2003.

[27] C. Xu, M. S. Inokuma, J. Denham et al., "Feeder-free growth of undifferentiated human embryonic stem cells," *Nature Biotechnology*, vol. 19, no. 10, pp. 971–974, 2001.

[28] L. De Chiara, S. Fagoonee, A. Ranghino et al., "Renal cells from spermatogonial germline stem cells protect against kidney injury," *Journal of the American Society of Nephrology: JASN*, vol. 25, no. 2, pp. 316–328, 2014.

[29] H. Shiura, R. Ikeda, J. Lee et al., "Generation of a novel germline stem cell line expressing a germline-specific reporter in the mouse," *Genesis*, vol. 51, no. 7, pp. 498–505, 2013.

[30] E. Raz, "The function and regulation of vasa-like genes in germ-cell development," *Genome Biology*, vol. 1, no. 3, 2000.

[31] M. Dominici, K. Le Blanc, I. Mueller et al., "Minimal criteria for defining multipotent mesenchymal stromal cells. The International Society for Cellular Therapy position statement," *Cytotherapy*, vol. 8, no. 4, pp. 315–317, 2006.

[32] S. Kern, H. Eichler, J. Stoeve, H. Kluter, and K. Bieback, "Comparative analysis of mesenchymal stem cells from bone marrow, umbilical cord blood, or adipose tissue," *Stem Cells*, vol. 24, no. 5, pp. 1294–1301, 2006.

[33] M. Sobiesiak, K. Sivasubramaniyan, C. Hermann et al., "The mesenchymal stem cell antigen MSCA-1 is identical to tissue non-specific alkaline phosphatase," *Stem Cells and Development*, vol. 19, no. 5, pp. 669–677, 2010.

[34] E. R. Balmayor, M. Flicker, T. Kaser, A. Saalmuller, and R. G. Erben, "Human placental alkaline phosphatase as a tracking marker for bone marrow mesenchymal stem cells," *BioResearch Open Access*, vol. 2, no. 5, pp. 346–355, 2013.

[35] R. Gonzalez, L. Griparic, V. Vargas et al., "A putative mesenchymal stem cells population isolated from adult human testes," *Biochemical and Biophysical Research Communications*, vol. 385, no. 4, pp. 570–575, 2009.

[36] A. D. Ho, W. Wagner, and W. Franke, "Heterogeneity of mesenchymal stromal cell preparations," *Cytotherapy*, vol. 10, no. 4, pp. 320–330, 2008.

[37] J. R. Lavoie and M. Rosu-Myles, "Uncovering the secretes of mesenchymal stem cells," *Biochimie*, vol. 95, no. 12, pp. 2212–2221, 2013.

[38] M. Gnecchi, Z. Zhang, A. Ni, and V. J. Dzau, "Paracrine mechanisms in adult stem cell signaling and therapy," *Circulation Research*, vol. 103, no. 11, pp. 1204–1219, 2008.

5

Molecular Mechanisms of Transdifferentiation of Adipose-Derived Stem Cells into Neural Cells

Liang Luo,[1,2,3] Da-Hai Hu,[1] James Q. Yin ⓘ,[2,3] and Ru-Xiang Xu ⓘ[2,3]

[1]*Department of Burns and Cutaneous Surgery, Xijing Hospital, Fourth Military Medical University, Xi'an, Shanxi 710032, China*
[2]*Stem Cell Research Center, Neurosurgery Institute of PLA Army, Beijing 100700, China*
[3]*Bayi Brain Hospital, General Hospital of PLA Army, Beijing 100700, China*

Correspondence should be addressed to James Q. Yin; jamesyingqw@sohu.com and Ru-Xiang Xu; drxuruxiang@126.com

Academic Editor: James Adjaye

Neurological diseases can severely compromise both physical and psychological health. Recently, adult mesenchymal stem cell- (MSC-) based cell transplantation has become a potential therapeutic strategy. However, most studies related to the transdifferentiation of MSCs into neural cells have had disappointing outcomes. Better understanding of the mechanisms underlying MSC transdifferentiation is necessary to make adult stem cells more applicable to treating neurological diseases. Several studies have focused on adipose-derived stromal/stem cell (ADSC) transdifferentiation. The purpose of this review is to outline the molecular characterization of ADSCs, to describe the methods for inducing ADSC transdifferentiation, and to examine factors influencing transdifferentiation, including transcription factors, epigenetics, and signaling pathways. Exploring and understanding the mechanisms are a precondition for developing and applying novel cell therapies.

1. Introduction

After the groundbreaking studies that succeeded in reprogramming mouse and human somatic cells into induced pluripotent stem cells (iPSCs) [1], researchers have made a great progress in refining reprogramming methods and applying this technology in the clinic to treat human diseases. However, for successful clinical applications, iPSCs must be more efficiently transdifferentiated into different cell types. Furthermore, both embryonic stem cells (ESCs) and iPSCs have potential tumorigenic risks *in vivo* [2, 3], which significantly limits their utility. Lineage-restricted stem cells, such as neural stem cells (NSCs) and adipose-derived mesenchymal stromal/stem cells (ADSCs), do not have this limitation [4, 5]. Recently, a direct reprogramming of one of the cell types into another (transdifferentiation) has become another area of intense study [6]. Transdifferentiation may supplement iPSC technology and avoid the problems of differentiating iPSCs and ESCs into mature cell types. More importantly, this approach would reduce the risk of

teratogenesis after incomplete reprogramming and the likelihood of immune rejection and other complications associated with allogeneic transplantations.

Traditionally, nervous system tissue has been considered difficult to regenerate because mature neural cells do not proliferate or differentiate. Consequently, identification of a specific cell capable of neuronal differentiation has generated immense interest. Zuk et al. [7] first found that ADSCs isolated from the adipose stromo-vascular fraction have the capacity for multilineage differentiation. Safford et al. reported that mouse and human ADSCs (hADSCs) could be made to transdifferentiate into neural-like cells [8]. During the past decade, human adipose tissue has been identified as a source of adult multipotent ADSCs, which can transdifferentiate into a range of mesodermal, endodermal, and ectodermal cells [7, 9] in the presence of specific induction factors. These ADSCs have been shown to transdifferentiate into neurons [10, 11], oligodendrocytes [12], and Schwann cells [13]. Therefore, adipose tissue is a likely candidate source of stem cells capable of neural cell

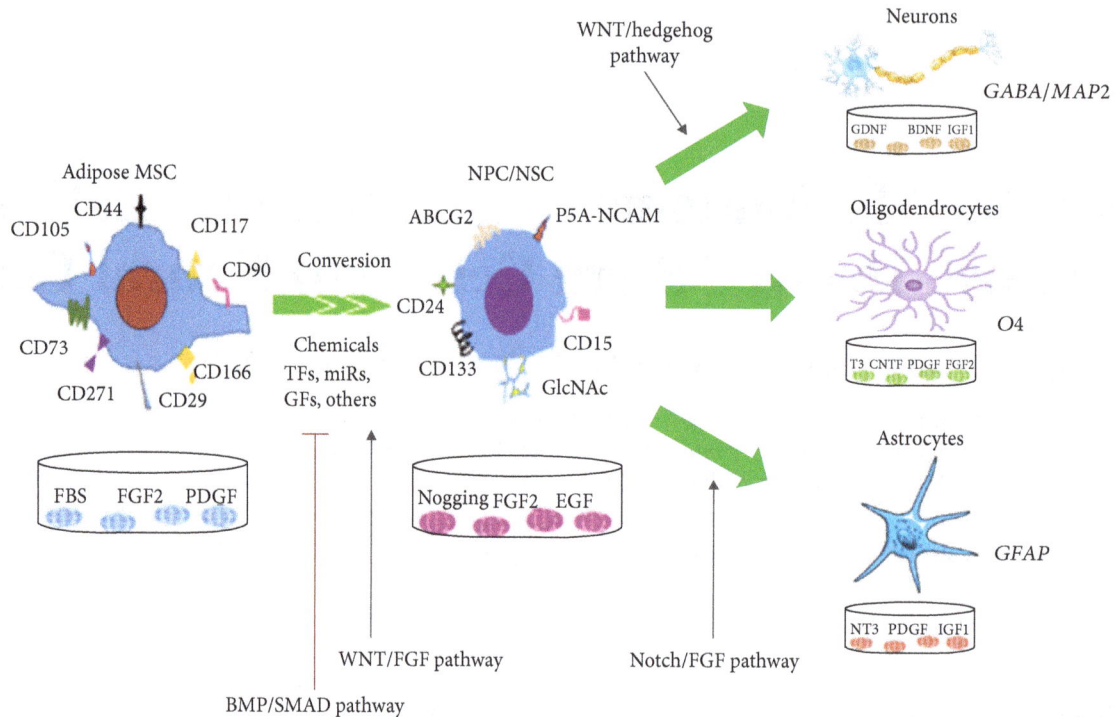

FIGURE 1: A schematic for the transdifferentiation of ADSCs into NSCs and neural cells, indicating relevant influences such as cell surface markers, transcriptional factors, culture media, and signaling pathways. The details can be seen in the text. TFs: transcription factors; miRs: microRNAs; GFs: growth factors; MSCs: mesenchymal stem cells; PSA-NCAM: polysialic acid neural cell adhesion molecule; GlcNAc: N-acetylglucosamine; PDGF: platelet-derived growth factor; IGF: insulin-like growth factor; CNTF: ciliary neurotrophic factor; GABA: γ-aminobutyric acid; GDNF: glial-derived neurotrophic factor; BDNF: brain-derived neurotrophic factor; T3: 3,5,3′-triiodothyronine; NT3: neurotrophin-3.

transdifferentiation in a short period of time and may potentially strengthen their clinical application. No other tissues appear more practical than adipose tissue, and adequate numbers of ADSCs can easily be isolated and expanded for clinical therapies [14].

Although ADSCs are ideal donor cells for treating neuronal diseases, the outcomes of most *in vivo* ADSC studies have been relatively disappointing. Better understanding of the molecular mechanisms of ADSC transdifferentiation is a key step in optimizing ADSC-neural system therapy. The aim of this review is to discuss the recent literature regarding the molecular mechanisms of ADSC transdifferentiation. We review the epigenetic factors, transcription factors (TFs), and signaling pathways that modulate ADSC transdifferentiation, as well as the development and transdifferentiation of ADSC-derived neural cells.

2. Characteristics of ADSCs and NSCs and Methods for Inducing Transdifferentiation

In 2006, the committee of the International Society for Cellular Therapy established the following minimum criteria for characterizing human mesenchymal stem cells (MSCs), and ADSCs comply with these criteria [15]: (1) the cells should adhere to plastic in culture; (2) more than 95% of them must express CD105, CD73, and CD90 but not express (<2%) CD34, CD45, CD14 or CD11b, CD79α or CD19, or

HLA-DR molecules; and (3) they should be able to differentiate into osteoblasts, adipocytes, and chondrocytes [16]. Recently, several new markers, such as CD146, CD271, SSEA1/4, and CD44, have been identified, and CD271 has been proposed as one of the most specific MSC markers (Figure 1) [17, 18].

Traditionally, MSCs can be obtained from bone marrow stem cells (BMSCs), but their expansion is limited and the population is small, comprising only 0.01~0.0001% of bone marrow cells in adult individuals [19]. However, ADSCs represent more than 1% of the adipose cell population, producing at least 100 times more MSCs than those from bone marrow [20]. Unlike BMSCs, which are difficult to obtain, adipose tissue biopsies can be obtained by relatively safe, popular liposuction procedures, one of the usual plastic surgeries performed in the United States (http://www.surgery.org) [21]. ADSCs are therefore an attractive source of cells for genetic, cellular, and molecular analyses and for clinical applications. Most neurological diseases, such as nerve injury and neurodegenerative disorders, are due to the loss or dysfunction of neural cells [22]. However, if we can obtain a sufficient supply of NSC/NPCs (neural progenitor cells) from transdifferentiated ADSCs, the problem can be solved to a great extent.

To achieve this purpose, one should first identify NSC/NPCs with relatively definitive markers. Recently, many cell surface and intracellular molecules have been identified: the

TABLE 1: List of transdifferentiation efficiency of ADSCs into NSCs.

Classification	Induction method	Duration	Efficiencies	CFE	Evaluation methods	Authors (year)
Growth factors and cytokines	B27, EGF, FGF	10–20 days	47.6~71.2%	<54% colony	ICC (Nestin, Fibr), qRT, EPA	Hermann et al. (2004) [33]
	B27, EGF, FGF	8–11 days	0.79%	Not mentioned	ICC/FCM (MAP2ab, GFAP, CD133), RT	Kang et al. (2004) [34]
	N2, B27, BME, NEAA, bFGF, EGF	22 days	>95%	Not mentioned	ICC, qRT, EPA	Feng et al. (2014) [35]
	B27, EGF, FGF	6 days	~15.4%	Not mentioned	ICC (Ki67, Nestin)	Yang et al. (2015) [36]
	B27, EGF, FGF	7 days	>80%	Not mentioned	ICC (Nestin, Sox2, Map2, NF-68)	Darvishi et al. (2017) [11]
	B27, N2, bFGF, EGF	7–10 days	$1/1 \times 10^{-7}$	$1/1 \times 10^{-7}$	ICC (Sox2, Nestin, Tuj1), qRT, EPA	Petersen et al. (2018) [37]
Small molecular & growth factors	SB431542 (SB), LDN193189 (L), noggin (N)	20 days	>85%	Not mentioned	FCM (NCAM, Nestin, Ki67)	Park et al. (2017) [10]
Transcription factors	OCT4, KLF4, SOX2, c-MYC	30 days	0.01%	0.01%	ICC (Sox1, Sox2, Nestin, Pax6, CD133, Ki67), EPA, TEA	Cairns et al. (2016) [30]
	Sox2	14 days	—	Not mentioned	ICC (Sox2, Pax6, Nestin)	Qin et al. (2015) [38]
Others	Lentivirus-GFP	10 days	—	Not mentioned	ICC (Nestin, NeuN, GFAP)	Zhang et al. (2014) [39]

ICC: immunocytochemistry; qRT: quantitative real-time polymerase chain reaction; EPA: electrophysiology assay; RT: reverse transcription; TEA: tissue engineering assay; CFE: colony formation efficiency.

stage-specific embryonic antigen-1 (SSEA-1/Lewis X/CD15) [23], CD24 [24], p75 receptor [25], ABCG2 [26], brain-specific chondroitin sulfate proteoglycans [27], O-glycans, and PSA-NCAM [28] have been utilized to purify a population of cells from neural tissues (Figure 1). On the other hand, several markers, such as CD133, NESTIN, SOX1/2, PAX6, MUSASHI-1, and VIMENTIN [29], have been often taken as markers to identify *in vitro* NSC-like cells derived from other types of cells.

The evaluation methods for transdifferentiation of ADSCs into NSCs measure the colony formation efficiency (CFE), induced conversion efficiency, and total conversion time. The estimates of neural stem cell derivation efficiencies obtained by different induction methods are summarized in Tables 1 and 2. One may conclude that most studies claim that the conversion efficiency of ADSC transdifferentiation into NSCs is very high (>10%) and that the conversion time is short (<14 d). However, these so-called high-efficiency methods have not been rigorously scrutinized, and most of these methods have not provided the colony formation efficiencies. Therefore, we think that the majority of "NSCs" reported in these articles were probably not NSCs or NPCs but rather were mostly NSC-like cells, which are like an intermediate-state cell that is a type cell of the intermediate process of transdifferentiating from ADSCs into NSCs. In contrast, some inefficient methods, such as those reported by Cairns and his colleague, may represent the true efficiency achieved so far [30] (Table 1); they reported that the CFE was

0.01% during the 30-day induced conversion from ADSCs to NSCs, for which they used a classic induction method using OSKM transcription factors.

Some reports have shown that somatic cells, such as mouse or human fibroblasts, can directly transdifferentiate into functional neurons [31, 32]. However, in the studies of ADSC transdifferentiation into neural cells, the data provided only weak evidence and indirect observations, such as cell polarity and relevant protein marker expression at appropriate locations. Few studies have strictly demonstrated that ADSCs can generate functional neurons; in most cases, the reported results rely too much on the morphological changes and/or neuronal marker expression as part of the cell identification criteria. Overall, researchers must provide more convincing proof of neuronal transdifferentiation, including depolarization, synapse formation and function, and a delayed-rectifier type of K^+ and Na^+ current. If transplanted, the transdifferentiated neurons must also contact and communicate with other neural cells. Furthermore, behavioral experiments should be conducted after transplantation.

The ultimate goal of ADSC use is to generate the cell population of interest for clinical transplantation. For ADSCs to become ideal for neurological disease therapy, they must generate a sufficient number of functional and high-quality neural cells. To this end, there are three approaches: (1) directed induction of ADSCs to neural cells; (2) first, induction of ADSCs to NSCs and then induction of those into other neural cells; and (3) conversion of ADSCs to iPS

TABLE 2: List of protocols inducing the transdifferentiation of ADSCs into neural cells.

Class	Factors	Species of ADSCs	Targeted cell type	References
Transcription factors	OSKM	Human	NPCs, NCs	[40]
	Sox2	Mouse	NSC-like cells	[38]
	Nurr-1	Rat	NCs	[41]
Growth factors and cytokines	bFGF and EGF	Human/mouse/rat	NSCs, NCs	Almost all references
	PDGF	Human/mouse/rat	NSCs, NCs	[9, 35, 42]
	BDNF	Human/mouse/rat	NSCs, NCs	[11, 43–48]
	LIF	Human	Schwann-like cells	[46]
	Heregulin-beta	Human	Schwann-like cells	[42]
	GGF-2	Rat	NCs	[9]
	GDNF	Rat	NCs	[11, 45]
	CNTF	Rat	NSCs, neurons	[11]
	NT-3	Rat	NSCs, neurons	[11, 44, 48]
Small molecules (epigenetic)	VPA	Mouse/human	NCs	[8, 49]
	SB431542/dorsomorphin	Human	Neurons	[50]
Signaling factors	Retinoic acid	Human/mouse/rat	NSCs, NCs	[11, 35, 40, 45, 47, 51–53]
	Forskolin	Human/mouse/rat	NSCs, NCs	[8, 9, 45, 46, 54]
	cAMP	Human	NCs	[49]
	IBMX	Human/mouse/rat	NSCs, NCs	[43, 49, 55, 56]
Hormones	Hydrocortisone	Mouse	NCs	[8]
	Dexamethasone	Rat	Schwann-like cells	[55]
	Insulin	Human/mouse/rat	NSCs, NCs	[8, 43, 45, 55, 56]
	Indomethacin	Human/mouse/rat	NSCs, NCs	[43, 55, 56]
Other factors	Conditioned medium	Human	NCs	[57]
	Rat sciatic nerve leachate	Rat	Schwann-like cells	[55]
	Alginate hydrogel	Human	Neurons	[58]
	Electrical stimulation	Rat	NCs	[59]
*Controversial chemical	BHA (butylated hydroxyanisole)	Human/mouse/rat	NSCs, NCs	[8, 45, 51, 60]
	BME (2-mercaptoethanol)	Human	NCs	[51]
	BHA/BME/DMSO/	Human/mouse/rat	NCs	[7, 61–63]

*The protocol to induce neural transdifferentiation of ADSCs using some chemical (such as DMSO, BHA (butylated hydroxyanisole), and BME (2-mercaptoethanol)) has been questioned by many researchers [64], so we list these items separately.

cells and induction of those into neural cells. At a first glance, method (1) appears to be the best, but it has not yet produced fully functional neural cells. Another drawback of method (1) is that the induced nerve cells do not proliferate. Method (3) has been developed with forced expression of defined factors using multiple viral vectors. However, such iPS cells contain a large number of viral vector integrations, which may cause unpredictable genetic dysfunction. Thus, a comprehensive consideration of these factors suggests that method (2) may be the best of the three.

In summary, combinations of TFs, small molecules, nutrients, and cytokines can induce ADSCs to transdifferentiate into neural-like cells (Tables 1 and 2). Furthermore, there are still some problems in validating the method for inducing transdifferentiation of ADSCs: few related studies of ADSC transdifferentiation to neural cells were conducted *in vivo*, and most of these studies have not included functional assessments, such as electrophysiology;

therefore, the optimal combination of factors remains to be established.

3. Epigenetic Regulation of Transdifferentiation of ADSCs into Neural Cells

Epigenetic factors are known to play a pivotal role in determining stem cell fate and differentiation. These factors include chromatin remodeling, histone modification, DNA methylation, and noncoding RNA regulation. At present, there are challenging problems to solve in transdifferentiation of ADSCs, and the key to solving these problems is to achieve an in-depth understanding of epigenetic mechanisms of transdifferentiation.

Transdifferentiation of cells is accompanied by drastic changes in gene expression and epigenetic profiles. MSC transdifferentiation into neural cells should include 2 major events: (1) the disruption of the apparent steady state of the original cell's epigenetic modification and (2) the establishment of homeostasis of NSCs or neural cell-specific modifications. ADSCs are also strictly guarded by an epigenetic barrier, and they acquire more pluripotency by crossing that barrier with the help of relevant reprogramming factors of neural cells, which include several key transcription factors (TFs) [65]. Epigenetic researchers focus on covalent and noncovalent modifications of DNA and histones and the mechanisms by which such modifications affect chromatin structure and gene expression. Currently, a limited number of published studies of ADSC transdifferentiation mainly focus on histone modification, DNA methylation, and noncoding RNA regulation.

3.1. Histone Modification.
Histone posttranslational modifications include methylation, acetylation, phosphorylation, ubiquitylation, and other translational modifications of the tail end sites of the core histones [66]. The histone modification mechanisms underlying the transdifferentiation of ADSCs into neural cells are largely unknown. So far, a few papers have only focused on histone acetylation and methylation research.

Histone acetylation is one of the most abundant and dynamic histone modifications [67]. Generally, acetylation of histone tails represents a major regulatory mechanism during gene activation and repression. Actively transcribed regions of the genome tend to be hyperacetylated, whereas inactive regions are hypoacetylated.

Histone acetylation weakens the interaction between histone tails and DNA, which creates a space for factors that bind to the promoter regions and initiate gene transcription, and p300/CBP is also believed to be involved in the processes of MSC transdifferentiation [68, 69]. For example, during neurogenesis, Ngn1 binds to P300/CBP, which prevents differentiation into glial cells [70]. In contrast, the histone deacetylase (HADC) inhibitors TSA, VPA, MS-275, and NaB could induce neurogenic differentiation of hADSCs, as shown by RT-PCR and Western blot analysis, and most neuronal marker genes were expressed when neural-induced hADSCs were treated with the HDAC inhibitors individually. Furthermore, studies also discovered that expression of most Wnt-related genes was highly increased following treatment with the HDAC inhibitors. In short, the HDAC inhibitors could induce neurogenic differentiation of hADSCs by activating the canonical Wnt or noncanonical Wnt signaling pathways [71]. Another study also reports that histone deacetylase inhibitor valproic acid (VPA) enhances the neural differentiation of mesenchymal stem cells into neural cells. During MSC differentiation, histone deacetylase, HDAC2, is reduced in the VPA set, whereas HDAC1 remains unchanged [72]. Moreover, during human MSC differentiation, the Sox9 transcriptional apparatus activates its target gene expression through p300-mediated histone acetylation of chromatin. These findings suggest that lineage-specific transcription factors can interact with chromatin and activate associated transcription via regulation of chromatin modification [73]. Based on the above and previously published epigenetics studies, in general, a more global level of histone acetylation rather than any specific residue is critical [74].

In contrast to acetylation, there is a clear functional distinction between histone methylation marks, concerning both the exact histone residues and their degree of modification [75]. Thus, H3K9me3 and H4K20me3 are enriched near the boundaries of large heterochromatic domains, and H3K9me1 and H4K20me1 are found primarily in active genes [76]. It has been reported that lysine methylation is responsible for the transcriptionally silenced or active chromatin status, whether it occurs at H3K4, H3K9, H3K27, H3K20, H3K36, or H3K79 residues [66]. During neurogenic transdifferentiation of ADSCs, dynamic changes are observed in methylation of histones H3K4, H3K9, and H3K27 in the NES locus [49].

Taken together, these studies provide an insight into the epigenetic mechanisms of ADSC transdifferentiation into neural cells and suggest molecular models of how the key factors are linked to histone modifications in ADSCs. Histone acetylation/deacetylation and methylation/demethylation exist simultaneously in the process of transdifferentiation, and they closely link and regulate the entire transdifferentiation process, but most of the specific mechanisms of histone modification remain to be elucidated in ADSC transdifferentiation.

3.2. DNA Methylation.
DNA methylation is a crucial epigenetic mechanism and is essential for normal cellular functions and development, especially for the imprinting of specific genes, X chromosome inactivation, and cell type-specific gene expression [77]. DNA methylation typically occurs in a CpG dinucleotide context. A methyl group is added to cytosine within a CpG dinucleotide by DNA methyltransferases (DNMT) DNMT1, DNMT3a, and DNMT3b [78], and the status of CpG methylation in the genomes of ADSCs reflects their transdifferentiation potential [79].

Mesenchymal stem cells have the potential to transdifferentiate into NSCs or other neural cells. Changing the methylation status of lineage-specific genes may be a key step in the processes of neural cell generation. Using inhibitor and activator agents of DNA methylation and acetylation, scientists found that MSCs can be induced to express high levels of neural stem cell marker SOX2. Exposing these modified cells to a neural environment promoted efficient generation of neural stem-like cells as well as cells with neuronal and glial characteristics [80]. Studies found that the neural-specific enhancer regions of Nestin are demethylated during reprogramming and remethylated upon neurogenic differentiation [49].

On the other hand, attenuation of adipogenesis may be a key process during the transdifferentiation of ADSCs into neural cells. A nuclear hormone receptor, peroxisome proliferator-activated receptor-gamma (PPAR-γ), plays a crucial role in adipogenesis, in which TFs with chromatin remodeling activities sustain the role of epigenetic regulation [81]. Noer et al. analyzed the DNA methylation profiles of both adipogenic and nonadipogenic gene promoters in ADSCs. Studies in freshly isolated ADSCs found that

TABLE 3: miRNAs associated with differentiation and antiadipogenic effects.

miRNA	Target	References
miR-22	HDAC6	[85]
miR-27a/b, miR-130	PPAR	[86]
miR-138	EID1	[87]
miR-145	KLF4	[88]
miR-155	LEBPA and CEBPB	[89]
miR-215	FNDC3B and CTNNBIP1	[90]
miR-224	EGR2 and ACSL4	[91]
miR-369-5p	FABP4	[92]
miR-375	ADIPOR2	[93]

adipogenic gene (PPAR-γ2, leptin, FABP4, and LPL) promoters appear to be globally hypomethylated, whereas myogenic and endothelial cell regulatory regions tend to be more methylated [82]. However, in general, due to very few ADSC epigenetic studies, key methylation mechanisms in transdifferentiation of ADSCs into NSCs are still largely unknown.

3.3. Noncoding RNA Regulation. During cell differentiation, multiple genes must be expressed coordinately at precise levels, both spatially and temporally. Feedback and feedforward pathways are key regulatory strategies for maintaining this coordination. MicroRNAs are essential mediators in feedback and feedforward regulation.

Recently, miR-124 was found to be significantly upregulated during neurogenic transdifferentiation of ADSCs, and knockdown of miR-124 blocked ADSC neurogenic transdifferentiation. miR-124 modulates neurogenic transdifferentiation, in part, via the RhoA/ROCK1 signaling pathway [83]. Furthermore, ADSCs were transduced by lentiviral vectors containing miRNA-34a as the way to regenerate the sciatic nerve in a surgically induced sciatic nerve injury rat model. The results showed that transplantation of miRNA-34a-overexpressing adipose-derived stem cells significantly enhanced the restoration of nerve continuity and functional recovery [84].

Relatively few miRNAs were reported to be involved in ASDC transdifferentiation compared with those in studies of NSCs, so we summarized miRNAs associated with ASDC differentiation and antiadipogenic genes (Table 3); additionally, we list NSC-specific miRNAs in Table 4 for reference.

4. Key Transcription Factors Involved in ADSC Transdifferentiation

In 2006, the Yamanaka group showed that mouse fibroblast cells can be reprogrammed into iPSCs by overexpression of OCT4, SOX2, KLF4, and cMyc (OSKM) TFs [1]. Since then, many groups have studied the methods and mechanisms of the somatic cell reprogramming process by analyzing epigenetic and transcriptional changes at different time points after factor induction in different somatic cells. It has been reported that OSKM can reprogram ADSCs to iPSCs [104, 105].

To date, there have only been a few reports on ADSC transdifferentiation by TFs. After being transfected with TFs OCT3/4, SOX2, KLF4, and c-MYC and then further treated with neural-inducing medium, hADSCs switched to transdifferentiation toward neural cell lineages [40]. ADSCs can be converted into induced NSC-like cells with a single transcription factor, SOX2 [38]. Using a 3-step NSC-inducing protocol, highly purified NSCs can be derived from hADSCs by SOX1 activation [35]. Expression patterns of key transcription factors, such as PAX6, MASH1, NGN2, NeuroD1, TBR2, and TBR1, were changed during neurogenic transdifferentiation of hADSCs [60]. In general, relevant ADSC transdifferentiation research has been infrequently reported.

Although few transdifferentiation studies use ADSCs as a cell model, some elegant studies have detailed TF transfections and reprogramming methods, in which fibroblasts, which originate from the mesoderm, differentiate into neural cells or NSCs. These TFs include (but are not limited to) the following: SOX2, PAX6, BRN2 or BRN4, NG, ASCL1 and MYT1l, Nr2e1 (TLX), BMI1, FOXG1, and E47/TCF3 [106]. It is reasonable to suggest that these TFs may be essential for transforming ADSCs to neural cells by changing relevant epigenetic modifications or initiating specific programs. These findings also hint that overexpression of a few key factors can drive ADSCs to transdifferentiate directly into neural cells.

5. Signaling Pathways Implemented in ADSC Transdifferentiation

During transdifferentiation into neural cells, ADSCs are stimulated by xenobiotics or specific factors and the corresponding signaling pathways and TFs are activated, resulting in the partial methylation or acetylation of genomic regions and activation of further transdifferentiation processes. Below, we review the crucial signaling pathways in the transdifferentiation of ADSCs to neural cells (Figures 1 and 2).

5.1. WNT and β-Catenin Pathway. WNT proteins are a class of highly conserved glycoproteins with key roles in cell development and differentiation [107]. Activation of WNT/β-catenin signaling accelerates the transdifferentiation of MSCs while depressing commitment to the adipocytic lineage [108]. WNT signaling regulates adipocyte differentiation by repressing the expression of CEBPα and PPAR-γ, the central regulators of adipocyte differentiation. Recently, it was observed that WNT/β-catenin signaling was activated during the transdifferentiation of hADSCs into neural cells [35, 109]. Wnt5a promoted hADSC transdifferentiation into neural cells, binding to the Fz3/Fz5 receptor, and signaling by the Wnt5a-JNK pathway [109]. The expression of genes downstream of the WNT/β-catenin pathway, such as cyclin D1 and Stat3, increased [110], while BMP2 and BMP4 expression decreased during early differentiation [111]. Genetic studies have established that activated WNT/β-catenin signaling is crucial for neural cell development [112].

Moreover, the WNT/β-catenin pathway probably regulates NSC maintenance and differentiation throughout development [113]. In the WNT/β-catenin pathway,

TABLE 4: Neural stem cell- or neural cell-specific microRNAs.

miRNA	Effect on NSCs or neural cells	Target(s)	Ref.
miR-9	Neural stem cell self-renewal	TLX (NR2E1), REST, FoxG1, Her5, Her9	[94, 95]
miR-137	Promotion of proliferation and repression of differentiation	Ezh2, PcG, MeCP2	[96, 97]
let-7b	Inhibition of NSC proliferation and accelerated neural differentiation	Hmga2	[98–100]
miR-184	Promotion of neural stem cell proliferation and inhibition of differentiation by targeting Numb-like	MBD1	[101]
miR-124	Neuronal differentiation	REST (NRSF), PTBP	[102]
miR-132	Radial-glial stem cell self-renewal	CREB, Nurr1	[103]
miR-138	Synaptic plasticity	Lypla1	[103]

nonphosphorylated β-catenin is expressed in the NSC cytoplasm, then translocates to the nucleus and binds to the LEF/TCF TFs, and then activates the transcription of downstream genes, such as Neurod1 and Prox1, which are TFs specifically involved in neuronal differentiation [114]. Another study indicated that constitutive activation of the Wnt/β-catenin pathway in NSCs disrupted the proliferation and migration of neurons within the CNS [115]. Therefore, it is possible that the WNT/β-catenin pathway must be tightly controlled in a time- and cell type-specific manner. In short, activation of WNT/β-catenin signaling plays a crucial role in promoting the transdifferentiation of ADSCs towards a neural fate.

5.2. Notch Pathway. The Notch signaling pathway is highly conserved and exists in all vertebrates [116]. In hADSCs, Notch signaling maintains stem cell self-renewal and inhibits the differentiation into adipocytes [117]. If the Notch pathway is downregulated, hADSCs will transdifferentiate in many directions into cells including neural cells [118, 119], osteocytes [120], and other cell types. The type of transdifferentiated cells will be decided by the inducing environment. Notch is also a key regulator of cell transdifferentiation. Previous reports have indicated that Notch signaling occurs in proliferating hADSCs and is downregulated when cells are transdifferentiated to a neuronal phenotype [119]. On the other hand, Notch was found to be required for the expansion and self-renewal of NSCs in vitro and in vivo [121], and this signaling pathway is also a key regulator of stem cell lineage commitment and differentiation [121]. Notch receptor activation induces expression of the specific target genes hairy and enhancer of split 3 (HES3) and sonic hedgehog (Shh) through rapid activation of cytoplasmic signals, including Akt and STAT3, and promotes NSC survival [122]. These results indicate that Notch signaling affects NSC expansion *in vitro* and *in vivo*. Future studies will provide novel insights into how Notch accurately regulates ADSC transdifferentiation into neural cells and will elucidate common mechanisms of the Notch pathway regulation.

5.3. TGF-β and BMP Signaling. The transforming growth factor-β (TGF-β) superfamily comprises the TGF-β/activin/nodal and the bone morphogenetic protein (BMP) subfamilies. TGF-β family proteins are bifunctional regulators of proliferation or differentiation of stem cells [123]. Signaling gradients, activated by the BMPs, often generate alternative differentiation pathways.

The TGF-β family proteins are prototypes of multifunctional growth factors and control switches in regulating key events in hADSC and NSC proliferation, transdifferentiation, migration, and apoptosis [124]. The effects of BMP signaling on NSCs change with developmental stages and are varied. Some studies have identified a BMP signaling inhibitor, Noggin, that can lead to efficient generation of NPCs from human pluripotent cells [125]. Moreover, BMP2 is overexpressed in both type 1 and type 2 astrocytes, but it has no detectable expression in neurons and oligodendrocytes, which indicates that astrocytes may be a source of BMPs during NSC differentiation [126]. BMP5/7 is a regulator of neural stem cell development into mDA neurons in the brain [127] and is involved in neural induction through an interaction with calcineurin-regulated Smad1/5 proteins [128]. These studies indicate that the precise function of the BMP protein subfamily likely depends on the cell context-dependent signaling network.

In brief, BMP and TGF-β activate or inhibit cell proliferation, apoptosis, and differentiation. These seemingly contradictory TGF-β superfamily functions can be attributed to the level of gene expression, the cross-talk between TGF-β/Smad and other signaling pathways (Figure 2), and the stimulation of different TFs that influence the signaling pathways.

5.4. Sonic Hedgehog Pathway. Sonic hedgehog receptors consisting of patched (Ptch) and smoothened (SMO) are important in regulating vertebrate organogenesis. The Shh pathway controls cell division and maintains functions of stem cells. In ADSCs, the Shh pathway is involved in the maintenance of stem cell properties and decreases in proliferation during differentiation [51]. Moreover, Shh influences hADSC transdifferentiation during neurogenesis. Previous reports have shown that all hADSCs have the capacity for an active hedgehog pathway through expression of genes that are inhibited after neuronal induction [129]. Shh was often used with RA in induction medium during neural induction from hADSCs. One study showed that neuron-like cells were obtained from hADSCs by activating Shh, RA, and MAPK/ERK signaling and the neuron-like cells expressed the Nkx2.2, Pax6, Hb9, and Olig2 gene [130]. Using *in vivo* genetic fate mapping, both quiescent NSCs and transit-amplifying progenitor cells in the subventricular zone and subgranular zone were shown to respond to Shh signaling and contribute to the ongoing neurogenesis in the adult forebrain [131]. These results suggest that the Shh pathway directs lineage transdifferentiation of ADSCs

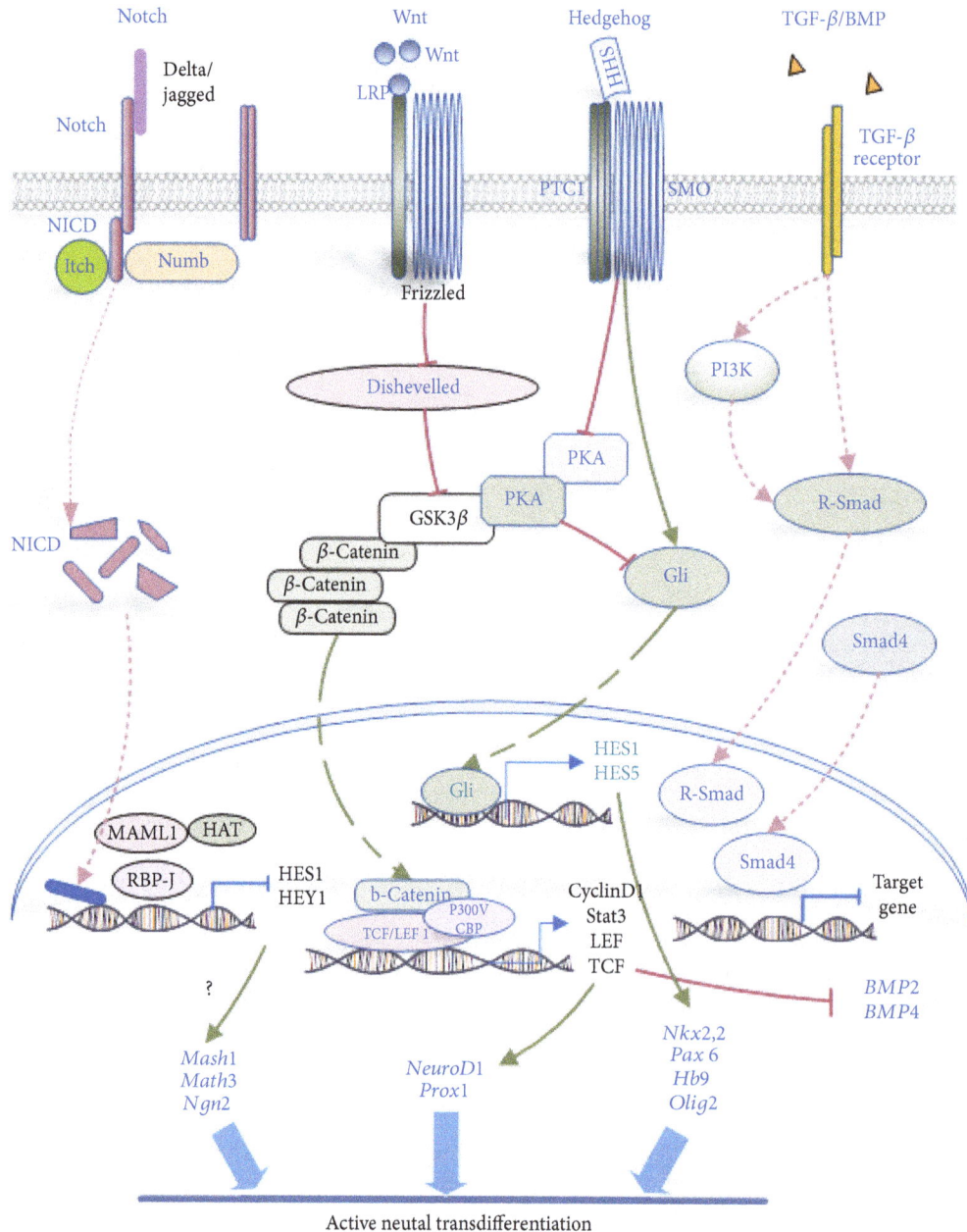

FIGURE 2: Overview of several important pathways involved in regulating the transdifferentiation of NSCs and neural cells. The Wnt, Notch, hedgehog, and TGF-β signaling pathways have been implicated in the transdifferentiation of neural cells. Activation or inhibition of these signaling pathways as well as their cross-talk may initiate cell conversion, maintain the self-renewal of stem cells, and drive their transdifferentiation. Akt: protein kinase B; Dvl: dishevelled; GFs: growth factors; GliR: Gli repressors; GSK3β: glycogen synthase 3 beta; LEF1: lymphoid-enhancing factor-1; NICD1: Notch intracellular domain-1; PI3K: phosphatidylinositol-3-kinase; PKA: protein kinase A; Ptch: patched; R-smad: receptor-regulated Smads; Shh: sonic hedgehog protein; SMO: smoothened; TCF: T cell factor transcription factor; Wnt: wingless.

and is likely involved in neuronal transdifferentiation of ADSCs (Figure 1).

6. Challenges and Issues for Transdifferentiation of ADSCs into Neural Cells

Ample evidence suggests that the ADSC is an ideal cell for regenerative medicine and immunosuppressive cellular therapies. However, to date, few groups have provided clear evidence that ADSCs can transdifferentiate into mature or functional neuronal cells *in vivo* or *in vitro*. Expression of a delayed-rectifier type of K$^+$ current would indicate a more functional neuronal phenotype. So far, there has been no demonstration of neuronal depolarization or synaptic functioning in transdifferentiated cells cultured *in vitro*. The main reasons for this lack of evidence are the following challenges in ADSC transdifferentiation:

(1) ADSCs constitute a heterogeneous population, which itself is a challenge for ADSC transdifferentiation. ADSCs from different donors have different characteristics, including age of the cell donor and use of fat from different parts of the body, which could affect the reproducibility of experiments. Another consequence of ADSC heterogeneity may be the presence of other stem cell types in the isolated adipose tissues. More importantly, there could be some problems with current induction methods, and ADSCs have never been completely converted into true neural cells because one or more programs specific for natural neural cells have not been activated.

(2) Until now, there has been no single, universal ADSC marker and no specific neural or NSC marker. The lack of a specific ADSC marker means that there is no way to obtain a highly purified ADSC population. The heterogeneity of ADSC populations combined with different protocols of cell isolation and expansion restricts the ability to precisely analyze and identify specific properties of stem cells. Similarly, because of a lack of specific neural markers, it is difficult to assess the results of ADSC transdifferentiation into NSC, which should be based on 2 or more types of markers, such as a combination of a surface marker and a TF marker (e.g., Nestin, Pax6, and Sox2).

(3) Under normal culture conditions, ADSCs can spontaneously express some neural markers [132] or change morphology and related neural marker expression levels [133, 134]. This phenomenon requires further studies to elucidate the relevance of markers or morphology to ADSC transdifferentiation.

(4) For the induction of ADSCs to NSCs, some studies only used immunocytochemistry or flow cytometry methods to identify whether ADSCs transdifferentiate into NSCs. We recommend that the assessment of ASC transdifferentiation into NSCs must use colony formation efficiency to avoid false-positive results due to the reasons mentioned above.

(5) In most publications, the majority of methods for measuring the induction efficiency use marker expression of NSCs and neural cells. Some studies do not even provide the statistical data of multiple sets of experiments. For the reasons mentioned in 2, we recommend using more than three well-recognized antibodies/markers to verify or assess the differentiation efficiency. In addition, due to the popularity of whole-genome sequencing and cost reduction, we recommend using RNA-seq to assess the quality of differentiation.

(6) Up to now, ADSCs have directly been used in many therapeutic studies and clinical trials, and the majority of these studies and trials used nontransdifferentiated cell types. Clearly, cell therapy of ADSCs transdifferentiated to functional neural cells should be more effective for neurological disorders; however, to improve the efficiency of clinical-grade ADSC transdifferentiation and to provide sufficient number of high-quality clinical transdifferentiated cells in a short time, we must face these challenges squarely when the relevant technologies are applied to clinical therapy.

Ultimately, we must do more experiments to establish a strict control of cell differentiation and more rigorous work to verify our hypothesis.

7. Conclusion

It would be a mistake to conclude that a functional neuron has been obtained solely based on observing a neural-like morphology or the expression of several neuronal markers during transdifferentiation. Instead, we must do more to validate neural cell function. Genuine neural cell differentiation should yield full cell functionality, which can be demonstrated through the expression of transcriptomes of neuronal genes and electrophysiology.

Neural cells can be generated from MSCs, but current approaches show low efficiency and are complex. No convincing method for the directed transdifferentiation of human ADSCs toward functional neural cells has been reported. The current situation severely limits the usage of these cells as a model for tissue engineering or cell therapy.

In conclusion, several tasks should be addressed in future studies:

(i) To clarify the molecular mechanisms underlying ADSC transdifferentiation into NSCs

(ii) To verify the function of neurons induced from ADSCs more strictly, using a variety of methods to verify the existence of K^+ and Na^+ ion channels and the establishment of synaptic networks after transplantation

(iii) To require better characterization, including a clear definition of a set of markers determining ADSCs and NSCs

(iv) To develop better methods for inducing the transdifferentiation of ADSCs into functional NSCs on a clinical scale

(v) To investigate the safety of ADSC-derived NSCs and their descendant neural cells in patients

We hope that in the near future, new methods for inducing transdifferentiation will improve the existing ADSC transdifferentiation techniques.

Acknowledgments

This work was supported by the National Key Scientific Program of China (Grant no. 201ICB964902), the Military Twelfth Five-Year Key Sci-Tech Research Projects (Grant no. BWS12J010), and the China Postdoctoral Science Foundation (no. 2014M562574).

References

[1] K. Takahashi and S. Yamanaka, "Induction of pluripotent stem cells from mouse embryonic and adult fibroblast cultures by defined factors," *Cell*, vol. 126, no. 4, pp. 663–676, 2006.

[2] A. S. Lee, C. Tang, M. S. Rao, I. L. Weissman, and J. C. Wu, "Tumorigenicity as a clinical hurdle for pluripotent stem cell therapies," *Nature Medicine*, vol. 19, no. 8, pp. 998–1004, 2013.

[3] H. Tao, X. Chen, A. Wei et al., "Comparison of teratoma formation between embryonic stem cells and parthenogenetic embryonic stem cells by molecular imaging," *Stem Cells International*, vol. 2018, Article ID 7906531, 9 pages, 2018.

[4] L. Barkholt, E. Flory, V. Jekerle et al., "Risk of tumorigenicity in mesenchymal stromal cell–based therapies—bridging scientific observations and regulatory viewpoints," *Cytotherapy*, vol. 15, no. 7, pp. 753–759, 2013.

[5] A. Mohr and R. Zwacka, "The future of mesenchymal stem cell-based therapeutic approaches for cancer - from cells to ghosts," *Cancer Letters*, vol. 414, pp. 239–249, 2018.

[6] A. Cieslar-Pobuda, V. Knoflach, M. V. Ringh et al., "Transdifferentiation and reprogramming: overview of the processes, their similarities and differences," *Biochimica et Biophysica Acta (BBA) - Molecular Cell Research*, vol. 1864, no. 7, pp. 1359–1369, 2017.

[7] P. A. Zuk, M. Zhu, P. Ashjian et al., "Human adipose tissue is a source of multipotent stem cells," *Molecular Biology of the Cell*, vol. 13, no. 12, pp. 4279–4295, 2002.

[8] K. M. Safford, K. C. Hicok, S. D. Safford et al., "Neurogenic differentiation of murine and human adipose-derived stromal cells," *Biochemical and Biophysical Research Communications*, vol. 294, no. 2, pp. 371–379, 2002.

[9] P. J. Kingham, D. F. Kalbermatten, D. Mahay, S. J. Armstrong, M. Wiberg, and G. Terenghi, "Adipose-derived stem cells differentiate into a Schwann cell phenotype and promote neurite outgrowth in vitro," *Experimental Neurology*, vol. 207, no. 2, pp. 267–274, 2007.

[10] J. Park, N. Lee, J. Lee et al., "Small molecule-based lineage switch of human adipose-derived stem cells into neural stem cells and functional GABAergic neurons," *Scientific Reports*, vol. 7, no. 1, article 10166, 2017.

[11] M. Darvishi, T. Tiraihi, S. A. Mesbah-Namin, A. Delshad, and T. Taheri, "Motor neuron transdifferentiation of neural stem cell from adipose-derived stem cell characterized by differential gene expression," *Cellular and Molecular Neurobiology*, vol. 37, no. 2, pp. 275–289, 2017.

[12] C. Paíno, M. Muñoz, L. Barrio, D. González Nieto, and L. Velosillo, "Myelinating oligodendrocytes generated by direct cell reprogramming from adult rat adipose tissue," in *XII European Meeting on Glial Cells in Health and Disease*, pp. 11-12, Medimond, Bilbao, Spain, 2015.

[13] X. Fu, Z. Tong, Q. Li et al., "Induction of adipose-derived stem cells into Schwann-like cells and observation of Schwann-like cell proliferation," *Molecular Medicine Reports*, vol. 14, no. 2, pp. 1187–1193, 2016.

[14] F. Simonacci, N. Bertozzi, and E. Raposio, "Off-label use of adipose-derived stem cells," *Annals of Medicine and Surgery*, vol. 24, pp. 44–51, 2017.

[15] G. A. Ferraro, H. Mizuno, and N. Pallua, "Adipose stem cells: from bench to bedside," *Stem Cells International*, vol. 2016, Article ID 6484038, 2 pages, 2016.

[16] M. Tobita, S. Tajima, and H. Mizuno, "Adipose tissue-derived mesenchymal stem cells and platelet-rich plasma: stem cell transplantation methods that enhance stemness," *Stem Cell Research & Therapy*, vol. 6, no. 1, p. 215, 2015.

[17] F. J. Lv, R. S. Tuan, K. M. C. Cheung, and V. Y. L. Leung, "Concise review: the surface markers and identity of human mesenchymal stem cells," *Stem Cells*, vol. 32, no. 6, pp. 1408–1419, 2014.

[18] G. Pachón-Peña, C. Donnelly, C. Ruiz-Cañada et al., "A glycovariant of human CD44 is characteristically expressed on human mesenchymal stem cells," *Stem Cells*, vol. 35, no. 4, pp. 1080–1092, 2017.

[19] J. Leibacher and R. Henschler, "Biodistribution, migration and homing of systemically applied mesenchymal stem/stromal cells," *Stem Cell Research & Therapy*, vol. 7, no. 1, p. 7, 2016.

[20] C. Siciliano, A. Bordin, M. Ibrahim et al., "The adipose tissue of origin influences the biological potential of human adipose stromal cells isolated from mediastinal and subcutaneous fat depots," *Stem Cell Research*, vol. 17, no. 2, pp. 342–351, 2016.

[21] J. M. Gimble, S. P. Ray, F. Zanata et al., "Adipose derived cells and tissues for regenerative medicine," *ACS Biomaterials Science & Engineering*, vol. 3, no. 8, pp. 1477–1482, 2016.

[22] J. Brettschneider, K. D. Tredici, V. M. Y. Lee, and J. Q. Trojanowski, "Spreading of pathology in neurodegenerative diseases: a focus on human studies," *Nature Reviews Neuroscience*, vol. 16, no. 2, pp. 109–120, 2015.

[23] P. H. Vincent, E. Benedikz, P. Uhlen, O. Hovatta, and E. Sundstrom, "Expression of pluripotency markers in nonpluripotent human neural stem and progenitor cells," *Stem Cells and Development*, vol. 26, no. 12, pp. 876–887, 2017.

[24] J. D. Tingling, S. Bake, R. Holgate et al., "CD24 expression identifies teratogen-sensitive fetal neural stem cell subpopulations: evidence from developmental ethanol exposure and orthotopic cell transfer models," *PloS one*, vol. 8, no. 7, article e69560, 2013.

[25] E. Tomellini, C. Lagadec, R. Polakowska, and X. Le Bourhis, "Role of p 75 neurotrophin receptor in stem cell biology: more than just a marker," *Cellular and Molecular Life Sciences*, vol. 71, no. 13, pp. 2467–2481, 2014.

[26] B. Wee, A. Pietras, T. Ozawa et al., "ABCG2 regulates self-renewal and stem cell marker expression but not tumorigenicity or radiation resistance of glioma cells," *Scientific Reports*, vol. 6, no. 1, article 25956, 2016.

[27] A. Purushothaman, K. Sugahara, and A. Faissner, "Chondroitin sulfate "wobble motifs" modulate maintenance and differentiation of neural stem cells and their progeny," *Journal of Biological Chemistry*, vol. 287, no. 5, pp. 2935–2942, 2012.

[28] H. Sabelström, M. Stenudd, and J. Frisén, "Neural stem cells in the adult spinal cord," *Experimental Neurology*, vol. 260, pp. 44–49, 2014.

[29] M. Ruggieri, G. Riboldi, S. Brajkovic et al., "Induced neural stem cells: methods of reprogramming and potential therapeutic applications," *Progress in Neurobiology*, vol. 114, pp. 15–24, 2014.

[30] D. M. Cairns, K. Chwalek, Y. E. Moore et al., "Expandable and rapidly differentiating human induced neural stem cell lines for multiple tissue engineering applications," *Stem Cell Reports*, vol. 7, no. 3, pp. 557–570, 2016.

[31] K. L. Ring, L. M. Tong, M. E. Balestra et al., "Direct reprogramming of mouse and human fibroblasts into multipotent neural stem cells with a single factor," *Cell Stem Cell*, vol. 11, no. 1, pp. 100–109, 2012.

[32] O. L. Wapinski, T. Vierbuchen, K. Qu et al., "Hierarchical mechanisms for direct reprogramming of fibroblasts to neurons," *Cell*, vol. 155, no. 3, pp. 621–635, 2013.

[33] A. Hermann, R. Gastl, S. Liebau et al., "Efficient generation of neural stem cell-like cells from adult human bone marrow stromal cells," *Journal of Cell Science*, vol. 117, no. 19, pp. 4411–4422, 2004.

[34] S. K. Kang, L. A. Putnam, J. Ylostalo et al., "Neurogenesis of Rhesus adipose stromal cells," *Journal of Cell Science*, vol. 117, no. 18, pp. 4289–4299, 2004.

[35] N. Feng, Q. Han, J. Li et al., "Generation of highly purified neural stem cells from human adipose-derived mesenchymal stem cells by Sox 1 activation," *Stem Cells and Development*, vol. 23, no. 5, pp. 515–529, 2014.

[36] E. Yang, N. Liu, Y. Tang et al., "Generation of neurospheres from human adipose-derived stem cells," *BioMed Research International*, vol. 2015, Article ID 743714, 10 pages, 2015.

[37] E. D. Petersen, J. R. Zenchak, O. V. Lossia, and U. Hochgeschwender, "Neural stem cells derived directly from adipose tissue," *Stem Cells and Development*, vol. 27, no. 9, pp. 637–647, 2018.

[38] Y. Qin, C. Zhou, N. Wang, H. Yang, and W. Q. Gao, "Conversion of adipose tissue-derived mesenchymal stem cells to neural stem cell-like cells by a single transcription factor, Sox 2," *Cellular Reprogramming*, vol. 17, no. 3, pp. 221–226, 2015.

[39] Y. Zhang, N. Liu, Y. Tang et al., "Efficient generation of neural stem cell-like cells from rat adipose derived stem cells after lentiviral transduction with green fluorescent protein," *Molecular Neurobiology*, vol. 50, no. 2, pp. 647–654, 2014.

[40] X. Qu, T. Liu, K. Song, X. Li, and D. Ge, "Differentiation of reprogrammed human adipose mesenchymal stem cells toward neural cells with defined transcription factors," *Biochemical and Biophysical Research Communications*, vol. 439, no. 4, pp. 552–558, 2013.

[41] Y. Yang, T. Ma, J. Ge et al., "Facilitated neural differentiation of adipose tissue-derived stem cells by electrical stimulation and Nurr-1 gene transduction," *Cell Transplantation*, vol. 25, no. 6, pp. 1177–1191, 2016.

[42] S. Razavi, N. Ahmadi, M. Kazemi, M. Mardani, and E. Esfandiari, "Efficient transdifferentiation of human adipose-derived stem cells into Schwann-like cells: a promise for treatment of demyelinating diseases," *Advanced Biomedical Research*, vol. 1, no. 1, p. 12, 2012.

[43] C. Ying, W. Hu, B. Cheng, X. Zheng, and S. Li, "Neural differentiation of rat adipose-derived stem cells in vitro," *Cellular and Molecular Neurobiology*, vol. 32, no. 8, pp. 1255–1263, 2012.

[44] Y. Tang, H. He, N. Cheng et al., "PDGF, NT-3 and IGF-2 in combination induced transdifferentiation of muscle-derived stem cells into Schwann cell-like cells," *PloS One*, vol. 9, no. 1, article e73402, 2014.

[45] J. Chen, Y. X. Tang, Y. M. Liu et al., "Transplantation of adipose-derived stem cells is associated with neural differentiation and functional improvement in a rat model of intracerebral hemorrhage," *CNS Neuroscience & Therapeutics*, vol. 18, no. 10, pp. 847–854, 2012.

[46] S. Razavi, M. Mardani, M. Kazemi et al., "Effect of leukemia inhibitory factor on the myelinogenic ability of Schwann-like cells induced from human adipose-derived stem cells," *Cellular and Molecular Neurobiology*, vol. 33, no. 2, pp. 283–289, 2013.

[47] E. Anghileri, S. Marconi, A. Pignatelli et al., "Neuronal differentiation potential of human adipose-derived mesenchymal stem cells," *Stem Cells and Development*, vol. 17, no. 5, pp. 909–916, 2008.

[48] W. Ji, X. Zhang, L. Ji, K. Wang, and Y. Qiu, "Effects of brain-derived neurotrophic factor and neurotrophin-3 on the neuronal differentiation of rat adipose-derived stem cells," *Molecular Medicine Reports*, vol. 12, no. 4, pp. 4981–4988, 2015.

[49] J. L. Boulland, M. Mastrangelopoulou, A. C. Boquest et al., "Epigenetic regulation of nestin expression during neurogenic differentiation of adipose tissue stem cells," *Stem Cells and Development*, vol. 22, no. 7, pp. 1042–1052, 2013.

[50] V. Madhu, A. S. Dighe, Q. Cui, and D. N. Deal, "Dual inhibition of activin/nodal/TGF-β and BMP signaling pathways by SB431542 and dorsomorphin induces neuronal differentiation of human adipose derived stem cells," *Stem Cells International*, vol. 2016, Article ID 1035374, 13 pages, 2016.

[51] A. Cardozo, M. Ielpi, D. Gómez, and A. P. Argibay, "Differential expression of Shh and BMP signaling in the potential conversion of human adipose tissue stem cells into neuron-like cells in vitro," *Gene Expression*, vol. 14, no. 6, pp. 307–319, 2010.

[52] F. Hu, X. Wang, G. Liang et al., "Effects of epidermal growth factor and basic fibroblast growth factor on the proliferation and osteogenic and neural differentiation of adipose-derived stem cells," *Cellular Reprogramming*, vol. 15, no. 3, pp. 224–232, 2013.

[53] L. Bahmani, M. F. Taha, and A. Javeri, "Coculture with embryonic stem cells improves neural differentiation of adipose tissue-derived stem cells," *Neuroscience*, vol. 272, pp. 229–239, 2014.

[54] S. Jang, H. H. Cho, Y. B. Cho, J. S. Park, and H. S. Jeong, "Functional neural differentiation of human adipose tissue-derived stem cells using bFGF and forskolin," *BMC Cell Biology*, vol. 11, no. 1, p. 25, 2010.

[55] Y. Liu, Z. Zhang, Y. Qin et al., "A new method for Schwann-like cell differentiation of adipose derived stem cells," *Neuroscience Letters*, vol. 551, pp. 79–83, 2013.

[56] P. H. Ashjian, A. S. Elbarbary, B. Edmonds et al., "In vitro differentiation of human processed lipoaspirate cells into early neural progenitors," *Plastic and Reconstructive Surgery*, vol. 111, no. 6, pp. 1922–1931, 2003.

[57] D. Lo Furno, R. Pellitteri, A. C. E. Graziano et al., "Differentiation of human adipose stem cells into neural

phenotype by neuroblastoma- or olfactory ensheathing cells-conditioned medium," *Journal of Cellular Physiology*, vol. 228, no. 11, pp. 2109–2118, 2013.

[58] Z. Khosravizadeh and R. Sh, "Neuronal markers expression of induced human adipose-derived stem cells in alginate hydrogel," *Iranian Journal of Reproductive Medicine*, vol. 13, pp. 61-62, 2015.

[59] L. Jaatinen, S. Salemi, S. Miettinen, J. Hyttinen, and D. Eberli, "The combination of electric current and copper promotes neuronal differentiation of adipose-derived stem cells," *Annual Review of Biomedical Engineering*, vol. 43, no. 4, pp. 1014–1023, 2015.

[60] A. J. Cardozo, D. E. Gomez, and P. F. Argibay, "Neurogenic differentiation of human adipose-derived stem cells: relevance of different signaling molecules, transcription factors, and key marker genes," *Gene*, vol. 511, no. 2, pp. 427–436, 2012.

[61] D. Woodbury, E. J. Schwarz, D. J. Prockop, and I. B. Black, "Adult rat and human bone marrow stromal cells differentiate into neurons," *Journal of Neuroscience Research*, vol. 61, no. 4, pp. 364–370, 2000.

[62] Y. Y. Hsueh, Y. J. Chang, C. W. Huang et al., "Synergy of endothelial and neural progenitor cells from adipose-derived stem cells to preserve neurovascular structures in rat hypoxic-ischemic brain injury," *Scientific Reports*, vol. 5, article 14985, 2015.

[63] Y. A. Romanov, A. N. Darevskaya, N. V. Merzlikina, and L. B. Buravkova, "Mesenchymal stem cells from human bone marrow and adipose tissue: isolation, characterization, and differentiation potentialities," *Bulletin of Experimental Biology and Medicine*, vol. 140, no. 1, pp. 138–143, 2005.

[64] A. P. Croft and S. A. Przyborski, "Formation of neurons by non-neural adult stem cells: potential mechanism implicates an artifact of growth in culture," *Stem Cells*, vol. 24, no. 8, pp. 1841–1851, 2006.

[65] J. M. Encinas and C. P. Fitzsimons, "Gene regulation in adult neural stem cells. Current challenges and possible applications," *Advanced Drug Delivery Reviews*, vol. 120, pp. 118–132, 2017.

[66] B. Huang, G. Li, and X. H. Jiang, "Fate determination in mesenchymal stem cells: a perspective from histone-modifying enzymes," *Stem Cell Research & Therapy*, vol. 6, no. 1, p. 35, 2015.

[67] C. Alabert, Z. Jasencakova, and A. Groth, "Chromatin replication and histone dynamics," in *DNA Replication*, vol. 1042 of Advances in Experimental Medicine and Biology, pp. 311–333, 2017.

[68] K. Baumann, "Post-translational modifications: crotonylation versus acetylation," *Nature Reviews Molecular Cell Biology*, vol. 16, no. 5, p. 265, 2015.

[69] L. Luo, W. J. Chen, J. Q. Yin, and R. X. Xu, "EID3 directly associates with DNMT3A during transdifferentiation of human umbilical cord mesenchymal stem cells to NPC-like cells," *Scientific Reports*, vol. 7, no. 1, article 40463, 2017.

[70] N. Tiwari and B. Berninger, "Transcriptional and epigenetic control of astrogliogenesis," in *Essentials of Noncoding RNA in Neuroscience*, pp. 177–195, Elsevier, 2017.

[71] S. Jang and H.-S. Jeong, "Histone deacetylase inhibition-mediated neuronal differentiation via the Wnt signaling pathway in human adipose tissue-derived mesenchymal stem cells," *Neuroscience Letters*, vol. 668, pp. 24–30, 2018.

[72] M. Talwadekar, S. Fernandes, V. Kale, and L. Limaye, "Valproic acid enhances the neural differentiation of human placenta derived-mesenchymal stem cells in vitro," *Journal of Tissue Engineering and Regenerative Medicine*, vol. 11, no. 11, pp. 3111–3123, 2017.

[73] T. Furumatsu, M. Tsuda, K. Yoshida et al., "Sox 9 and p 300 cooperatively regulate chromatin-mediated transcription," *The Journal of Biological Chemistry*, vol. 280, no. 42, pp. 35203–35208, 2005.

[74] C. Feller, I. Forne, A. Imhof, and P. B. Becker, "Global and specific responses of the histone acetylome to systematic perturbation," *Molecular Cell*, vol. 57, no. 3, pp. 559–571, 2015.

[75] C. Carlberg and F. Molnár, "The histone code," in *Human Epigenomics*, pp. 75–88, Springer, 2018.

[76] A. Barski, S. Cuddapah, K. Cui et al., "High-resolution profiling of histone methylations in the human genome," *Cell*, vol. 129, no. 4, pp. 823–837, 2007.

[77] Y. Ozkul and U. Galderisi, "The impact of epigenetics on mesenchymal stem cell biology," *Journal of Cellular Physiology*, vol. 231, no. 11, pp. 2393–2401, 2016.

[78] J. Hsieh and X. Zhao, "Genetics and epigenetics in adult neurogenesis," *Cold Spring Harbor Perspectives in Biology*, vol. 8, no. 6, article a018911, 2016.

[79] M. Berdasco, C. Melguizo, J. Prados et al., "DNA methylation plasticity of human adipose-derived stem cells in lineage commitment," *The American Journal of Pathology*, vol. 181, no. 6, pp. 2079–2093, 2012.

[80] A. R. Alexanian, "Epigenetic modulators promote mesenchymal stem cell phenotype switches," *The International Journal of Biochemistry & Cell Biology*, vol. 64, pp. 190–194, 2015.

[81] N. Saidi, M. Ghalavand, M. S. Hashemzadeh, R. Dorostkar, H. Mohammadi, and A. Mahdian-shakib, "Dynamic changes of epigenetic signatures during chondrogenic and adipogenic differentiation of mesenchymal stem cells," *Biomedicine & Pharmacotherapy*, vol. 89, pp. 719–731, 2017.

[82] A. Noer, A. L. Sorensen, A. C. Boquest, and P. Collas, "Stable CpG hypomethylation of adipogenic promoters in freshly isolated, cultured, and differentiated mesenchymal stem cells from adipose tissue," *Molecular Biology of the Cell*, vol. 17, no. 8, pp. 3543–3556, 2006.

[83] Y. Wang, D. Wang, and D. Guo, "MiR-124 promote neurogenic transdifferentiation of adipose derived mesenchymal stromal cells partly through RhoA/ROCK1, but not ROCK2 signaling pathway," *PloS One*, vol. 11, no. 1, article e0146646, 2016.

[84] X. He, Q. Ao, Y. Wei, and J. Song, "Transplantation of miRNA-34a overexpressing adipose-derived stem cell enhances rat nerve regeneration," *Wound Repair and Regeneration*, vol. 24, no. 3, pp. 542–550, 2016.

[85] S. Huang, S. Wang, C. Bian et al., "Upregulation of miR-22 promotes osteogenic differentiation and inhibits adipogenic differentiation of human adipose tissue-derived mesenchymal stem cells by repressing *HDAC6* protein expression," *Stem Cells and Development*, vol. 21, no. 13, pp. 2531–2540, 2012.

[86] E. K. Lee, M. J. Lee, K. Abdelmohsen et al., "miR-130 suppresses adipogenesis by inhibiting peroxisome proliferator-activated receptor γ expression," *Molecular Biology of the Cell*, vol. 31, no. 4, pp. 626–638, 2011.

[87] Z. Yang, C. Bian, H. Zhou et al., "MicroRNA hsa-miR-138 inhibits adipogenic differentiation of human adipose

tissue-derived mesenchymal stem cells through adenovirus EID-1," *Stem Cells and Development*, vol. 20, no. 2, pp. 259–267, 2011.

[88] K. Aji, Y. Zhang, A. Aimaiti et al., "MicroRNA-145 regulates the differentiation of human adipose-derived stem cells to smooth muscle cells via targeting Krüppel-like factor 4," *Molecular Medicine Reports*, vol. 15, no. 6, pp. 3787–3795, 2017.

[89] S. Liu, Y. Yang, and J. Wu, "TNFα-induced up-regulation of miR-155 inhibits adipogenesis by down-regulating early adipogenic transcription factors," *Biochemical and Biophysical Research Communications*, vol. 414, no. 3, pp. 618–624, 2011.

[90] Y. Peng, H. Li, X. Li et al., "MicroRNA-215 impairs adipocyte differentiation and co-represses FNDC3B and CTNNBIP1," *The International Journal of Biochemistry & Cell Biology*, vol. 79, pp. 104–112, 2016.

[91] Y. Peng, H. Xiang, C. Chen et al., "MiR-224 impairs adipocyte early differentiation and regulates fatty acid metabolism," *The International Journal of Biochemistry & Cell Biology*, vol. 45, no. 8, pp. 1585–1593, 2013.

[92] S. Bork, P. Horn, M. Castoldi, I. Hellwig, A. D. Ho, and W. Wagner, "Adipogenic differentiation of human mesenchymal stromal cells is down-regulated by microRNA-369-5p and up-regulated by microRNA-371," *Journal of Cellular Physiology*, vol. 226, no. 9, pp. 2226–2234, 2011.

[93] M. Kraus, T. Greither, C. Wenzel, D. Bräuer-Hartmann, M. Wabitsch, and H. M. Behre, "Inhibition of adipogenic differentiation of human SGBS preadipocytes by androgen-regulated microRNA miR-375," *Molecular and Cellular Endocrinology*, vol. 414, pp. 177–185, 2015.

[94] A. S. Yoo, A. X. Sun, L. Li et al., "MicroRNA-mediated conversion of human fibroblasts to neurons," *Nature*, vol. 476, no. 7359, pp. 228–231, 2011.

[95] C. Delaloy, L. Liu, J. A. Lee et al., "MicroRNA-9 coordinates proliferation and migration of human embryonic stem cell-derived neural progenitors," *Cell Stem Cell*, vol. 6, no. 4, pp. 323–335, 2010.

[96] G. Sun, P. Ye, K. Murai et al., "miR-137 forms a regulatory loop with nuclear receptor TLX and LSD1 in neural stem cells," *Nature Communications*, vol. 2, no. 1, p. 529, 2011.

[97] M. J. Hill, J. G. Donocik, R. A. Nuamah, C. A. Mein, R. Sainz-Fuertes, and N. J. Bray, "Transcriptional consequences of schizophrenia candidate miR-137 manipulation in human neural progenitor cells," *Schizophrenia Research*, vol. 153, no. 1–3, pp. 225–230, 2014.

[98] C. Zhao, G. Sun, S. Li et al., "MicroRNA *let-7b* regulates neural stem cell proliferation and differentiation by targeting nuclear receptor TLX signaling," *Proceedings of the National Academy of Sciences of the United States of America*, vol. 107, no. 5, pp. 1876–1881, 2010.

[99] C. Zhao, G. Q. Sun, P. Ye, S. Li, and Y. Shi, "MicroRNA let-7d regulates the TLX/microRNA-9 cascade to control neural cell fate and neurogenesis," *Scientific Reports*, vol. 3, no. 1, article 1329, 2013.

[100] K.-R. Yu, J. H. Shin, J. J. Kim et al., "Rapid and efficient direct conversion of human adult somatic cells into neural stem cells by HMGA2/let-7b," *Cell Reports*, vol. 10, no. 3, pp. 441–452, 2015.

[101] C. Liu, Z. Q. Teng, N. J. Santistevan et al., "Epigenetic regulation of miR-184 by MBD1 governs neural stem cell proliferation and differentiation," *Cell Stem Cell*, vol. 6, no. 5, pp. 433–444, 2010.

[102] L. P. Lim, N. C. Lau, P. Garrett-Engele et al., "Microarray analysis shows that some microRNAs downregulate large numbers of target mRNAs," *Nature*, vol. 433, no. 7027, pp. 769–773, 2005.

[103] Y. Shi, X. Zhao, J. Hsieh et al., "MicroRNA regulation of neural stem cells and neurogenesis," *Journal of Neuroscience*, vol. 30, no. 45, pp. 14931–14936, 2010.

[104] P. A. Tat, H. Sumer, K. L. Jones, K. Upton, and P. J. Verma, "The efficient generation of induced pluripotent stem (iPS) cells from adult mouse adipose tissue-derived and neural stem cells," *Cell Transplantation*, vol. 19, no. 5, pp. 525–536, 2010.

[105] N. Sun, N. J. Panetta, D. M. Gupta et al., "Feeder-free derivation of induced pluripotent stem cells from adult human adipose stem cells," *Proceedings of the National Academy of Sciences*, vol. 106, no. 37, pp. 15720–15725, 2009.

[106] P. Bielefeld, M. Schouten, P. J. Lucassen, and C. P. Fitzsimons, "Transcription factor oscillations in neural stem cells: implications for accurate control of gene expression," *Neurogenesis*, vol. 4, no. 1, article e1262934, 2017.

[107] M. Visweswaran, S. Pohl, F. Arfuso et al., "Multi-lineage differentiation of mesenchymal stem cells - to Wnt, or not Wnt," *The International Journal of Biochemistry & Cell Biology*, vol. 68, pp. 139–147, 2015.

[108] J. K. Van Camp, S. Beckers, D. Zegers, and W. Van Hul, "Wnt signaling and the control of human stem cell fate," *Stem Cell Reviews*, vol. 10, no. 2, pp. 207–229, 2014.

[109] S. Jang, J. S. Park, and H. S. Jeong, "Neural differentiation of human adipose tissue-derived stem cells involves activation of the Wnt5a/JNK signalling," *Stem Cells International*, vol. 2015, Article ID 178618, 7 pages, 2015.

[110] N. Bizen, T. Inoue, T. Shimizu, K. Tabu, T. Kagawa, and T. Taga, "A growth-promoting signaling component cyclin D1 in neural stem cells has antiastrogliogenic function to execute self-renewal," *Stem Cells*, vol. 32, no. 6, pp. 1602–1615, 2014.

[111] M. Kléber, H.-Y. Lee, H. Wurdak et al., "Neural crest stem cell maintenance by combinatorial Wnt and BMP signaling," *The Journal of Cell Biology*, vol. 169, no. 2, pp. 309–320, 2005.

[112] A. N. Bowman, R. van Amerongen, T. D. Palmer, and R. Nusse, "Lineage tracing with Axin2 reveals distinct developmental and adult populations of Wnt/β-catenin-responsive neural stem cells," *Proceedings of the National Academy of Sciences of the United States of America*, vol. 110, no. 18, pp. 7324–7329, 2013.

[113] R. Nusse and H. Clevers, "Wnt/β-catenin signaling, disease, and emerging therapeutic modalities," *Cell*, vol. 169, no. 6, pp. 985–999, 2017.

[114] M. B. Wisniewska, "Physiological role of β-catenin/TCF signaling in neurons of the adult brain," *Neurochemical Research*, vol. 38, no. 6, pp. 1144–1155, 2013.

[115] N. C. Inestrosa and L. Varela-Nallar, "Wnt signalling in neuronal differentiation and development," *Cell and Tissue Research*, vol. 359, no. 1, pp. 215–223, 2015.

[116] S. J. Bray, "Notch signalling in context," *Nature Reviews Molecular Cell Biology*, vol. 17, no. 11, pp. 722–735, 2016.

[117] T. Osathanon, K. Subbalekha, P. Sastravaha, and P. Pavasant, "Notch signalling inhibits the adipogenic differentiation of single-cell-derived mesenchymal stem cell clones isolated

from human adipose tissue," *Cell Biology International*, vol. 36, no. 12, pp. 1161–1170, 2012.

[118] P. J. Kingham, C. Mantovani, and G. Terenghi, "Notch independent signalling mediates Schwann cell-like differentiation of adipose derived stem cells," *Neuroscience Letters*, vol. 467, no. 2, pp. 164–168, 2009.

[119] A. J. Cardozo, D. E. Gómez, and P. F. Argibay, "Transcriptional characterization of Wnt and Notch signaling pathways in neuronal differentiation of human adipose tissue-derived stem cells," *Journal of Molecular Neuroscience*, vol. 44, no. 3, pp. 186–194, 2011.

[120] W. Jing, Z. Xiong, X. Cai et al., "Effects of γ-secretase inhibition on the proliferation and vitamin D 3 induced osteogenesis in adipose derived stem cells," *Biochemical and Biophysical Research Communications*, vol. 392, no. 3, pp. 442–447, 2010.

[121] K. Venkatesh, L. V. K. Reddy, S. Abbas et al., "NOTCH signaling is essential for maturation, self-renewal, and tri-differentiation of *in vitro* derived human neural stem cells," *Cellular Reprogramming*, vol. 19, no. 6, pp. 372–383, 2017.

[122] P. E. Ludwig, F. G. Thankam, A. A. Patil, A. J. Chamczuk, and D. K. Agrawal, "Brain injury and neural stem cells," *Neural Regeneration Research*, vol. 13, no. 1, pp. 7–18, 2018.

[123] E. A. Meyers and J. A. Kessler, "TGF-β family signaling in neural and neuronal differentiation, development, and function," *Cold Spring Harbor Perspectives in Biology*, vol. 9, no. 8, article a022244, 2017.

[124] N. Kakudo, S. Kushida, K. Suzuki et al., "Effects of transforming growth factor-beta 1 on cell motility, collagen gel contraction, myofibroblastic differentiation, and extracellular matrix expression of human adipose-derived stem cell," *Human Cell*, vol. 25, no. 4, pp. 87–95, 2012.

[125] S. M. Chambers, Y. Mica, G. Lee, L. Studer, and M. J. Tomishima, "Dual-SMAD inhibition/WNT activation-based methods to induce neural crest and derivatives from human pluripotent stem cells," in *Human Embryonic Stem Cell Protocols*, Methods in molecular biology, Humana Press, New York, NY, USA, 2013.

[126] J. G. Hu, Y. X. Zhang, Q. Qi et al., "Expression of BMP-2 and BMP-4 proteins by type-1 and type-2 astrocytes induced from neural stem cells under different differentiation conditions," *Acta Neurobiologiae Experimentalis*, vol. 72, no. 1, pp. 95–101, 2012.

[127] V. M. Jovanovic, A. Salti, H. Tilleman et al., "BMP/SMAD pathway promotes neurogenesis of midbrain dopaminergic neurons *in vivo* and in human induced pluripotent and neural stem cells," *The Journal of Neuroscience*, vol. 38, no. 7, pp. 1662–1676, 2018.

[128] I. De Almeida, N. M. M. Oliveira, R. A. Randall, C. S. Hill, J. M. McCoy, and C. D. Stern, "Calreticulin is a secreted BMP antagonist, expressed in Hensen's node during neural induction," *Developmental Biology*, vol. 421, no. 2, pp. 161–170, 2017.

[129] F. T. Xu, H. M. Li, Q. S. Yin et al., "Effect of ginsenoside Rg1 on proliferation and neural phenotype differentiation of human adipose-derived stem cells in vitro," *Canadian Journal of Physiology and Pharmacology*, vol. 92, no. 6, pp. 467–475, 2014.

[130] Y. Liqing, G. Jia, C. Jiqing et al., "Directed differentiation of motor neuron cell-like cells from human adipose-derived stem cells in vitro," *Neuroreport*, vol. 22, no. 8, pp. 370–373, 2011.

[131] E. Llorens-Bobadilla and A. Martin-Villalba, "Adult NSC diversity and plasticity: the role of the niche," *Current Opinion in Neurobiology*, vol. 42, pp. 68–74, 2017.

[132] D. Blecker, M. I. Elashry, M. Heimann, S. Wenisch, and S. Arnhold, "New insights into the neural differentiation potential of canine adipose tissue-derived mesenchymal stem cells," *Anatomia, Histologia, Embryologia*, vol. 46, no. 3, pp. 304–315, 2017.

[133] M. I. Arribas, A. B. Ropero, J. A. Reig et al., "Negative neuronal differentiation of human adipose-derived stem cell clones," *Regenerative Medicine*, vol. 9, no. 3, pp. 279–293, 2014.

[134] B. C. Heng, P. Saxena, and M. Fussenegger, "Heterogeneity of baseline neural marker expression by undifferentiated mesenchymal stem cells may be correlated to donor age," *Journal of Biotechnology*, vol. 174, pp. 29–33, 2014.

6

Icariin Promotes the Migration of BMSCs In Vitro and In Vivo via the MAPK Signaling Pathway

Feng Jiao ⓘ,[1] **Wang Tang,**[2] **He Huang,**[1] **Zhaofei Zhang,**[1] **Donghua Liu,**[1] **Hongyi Zhang,**[1] **and Hui Ren**[3]

[1]*Guangzhou Hospital of Integrated Traditional and Western Medicine, China*
[2]*Guangzhou University of Chinese Medicine, China*
[3]*The First Affiliated Hospital of Guangzhou University of Traditional Chinese Medicine, China*

Correspondence should be addressed to Feng Jiao; twjiaofeng123@163.com

Academic Editor: Zengwu Shao

Bone marrow-derived mesenchymal stem cells (BMSCs) are widely used in tissue engineering for regenerative medicine due to their multipotent differentiation potential. However, their poor migration ability limits repair effects. Icariin (ICA), a major component of the Chinese medical herb Herba Epimedii, has been reported to accelerate the proliferation, osteogenic, and chondrogenic differentiation of BMSCs. However, it remains unknown whether ICA can enhance BMSC migration, and the possible underlying mechanisms need to be elucidated. In this study, we found that ICA significantly increased the migration capacity of BMSCs, with an optimal concentration of 1 μmol/L. Moreover, we found that ICA stimulated actin stress fiber formation in BMSCs. Our work revealed that activation of the MAPK signaling pathway was required for ICA-induced migration and actin stress fiber formation. In vivo, ICA promoted the recruitment of BMSCs to the cartilage defect region. Taken together, these results show that ICA promotes BMSC migration in vivo and in vitro by inducing actin stress fiber formation via the MAPK signaling pathway. Thus, combined administration of ICA with BMSCs has great potential in cartilage defect therapy.

1. Introduction

Osteoarthritis (OA), known as degenerative arthritis or joint disease, may lead to the loss of cartilage [1, 2]. Lack of vessels, nerves, and local progenitor cells leads to difficulty in repairing cartilage. With the development of cell therapies, cell-based repair, which includes treatments with chondrocytes and bone marrow-derived mesenchymal stem cells (BMSCs), has recently attracted considerable attention from researchers. Although autologous chondrocyte implantation for the cartilage treatment is a practical solution, the limited sources and dedifferentiation of chondrocytes cultured in vitro restrict its application [3, 4]. In contrast, BMSCs are easy to obtain, have abundant sources, and exhibit strong reproductive activity. BMSCs can be directed to differentiate into many types of cells damaged by disease under certain conditions. Moreover, BMSCs can secrete active components that promote wound healing [5, 6]. However, BMSCs must

successfully migrate to the wound to participate in repair processes. The low recruitment of BMSCs to target tissue deters their repair effect [7, 8]. Based on all these characteristics, enhancing the migration ability of BMSCs may be a promising research direction for treating cartilage defects.

Cell-based repair involves migration of stem cells from the sites where they colonize to the wound. The process of migration is regulated by several distinct but interacting signaling pathways. Among these, the mitogen-activated protein kinase (MAPK) signaling pathway has been widely researched [9, 10] and has been confirmed to regulate microtubules and actin filaments; the latter of which can produce pushing (protrusive) forces or pulling (contractile) forces that are particularly important for whole-cell migration [11–13]. These findings provide new directions for the medicine screening.

Herba Epimedii (HEP) is a widely used traditional Chinese herb in the treatment of OA [14]. Icariin (ICA), the major pharmacologically active component of HEP, was proven to be an efficient accelerator of cartilage tissue engineering. ICA can accelerate the formation of cartilage matrix and chondroid tissue [15, 16]. Moreover, it has been found that ICA exerts multiple effects on BMSCs by activating MAPK signal pathway, including its ability to promote the proliferation and osteogenic, chondrogenic, and adipogenic differentiation [17–19]. Nonetheless, whether ICA has the potential to promote the migration of BMSCs and whether the possible underlying mechanism occurs via the MAPK signaling pathway remain unclear.

In this study, we assessed the effect of ICA on BMSC migration and its underlying mechanisms. In addition, BMSCs were injected via the ear vein of rabbits with knee articular cartilage defects to investigate the effect of ICA on BMSC migration in vivo.

2. Materials and Methods

2.1. Materials. Three-month-old female New Zealand rabbits (2 ± 0.5 kg) were purchased from the Center of Experimental Animals at Guangzhou University of Chinese Medicine. All animals were treated according to the animal guidelines of Guangzhou University of Chinese Medicine. Experimental measurements were carried out in the Laboratory of Orthopaedics and Traumatology of Chinese Medicine of the Lingnan Medical Research Center at Guangzhou University of Chinese Medicine.

2.2. Cell Culture. BMSCs were isolated and cultured from the bone marrow of 3-month-old female New Zealand rabbits. The cells were cultured in alpha minimum essential medium (MEM) containing 10% fetal bovine serum and 1% penicillin-streptomycin in an incubator at 5% CO_2 at 37°C. The culture flask was washed with phosphate-buffered saline (PBS) to remove nonadherent cells after 72 h. When grown to 80–90% confluence, the BMSCs were trypsinized and passaged, and the medium was replaced every 2 days.

To determine whether the isolated BMSCs possess multipotent differentiation ability in vitro, BMSCs at passage 3 were grown in osteogenic medium consisting of alpha MEM containing 10% fetal bovine serum, 1% penicillin-streptomycin, 0.2% ascorbate, 1% β-glycerophosphate, and 0.01% dexamethasone or chondrogenic medium containing 0.01% dexamethasone, 0.3% ascorbate, 1% insulin-transferrin-selenium (ITS) + supplement, 0.1% sodium pyruvate, 0.1% proline, and 1% TGF-β3 for 14 days. The medium was replaced every three days. The cells were then washed with PBS and then fixed with 4% paraformaldehyde for 10 min. Osteogenic cells were stained with alkaline phosphatase and alizarin red. Chondrogenic cells were stained with alcian blue. Photographs were taken using an inverted microscope with a camera.

2.3. Cell Counting Kit-8 (CCK-8) Assay. Cell proliferation was measured using the CCK-8 assay. BMSCs at passage 4 were seeded in 96-well plates at a density of 5×10^3 cells with four replicates for each group. The groups were as follows: 0 μM ICA, 0.01 μM ICA, 0.1 μM ICA, 1 μM ICA, 10 μM ICA, and 100 μM ICA. Cell proliferation was measured at 12, 24, 36, 48, 72, and 76 h after incubation. The CCK-8 solution was changed after the different intervals of incubation. Then, the plates were then incubated at 37°C for an additional 40 min. The optical density was determined at 520 nm using a microplate reader.

2.4. Scratch Wound-Healing Assay. BMSCs at passage 4 were seeded in 6-well plates at a density of 2×10^5 cells per well. When the cells grew to 95% confluence, the medium was aspirated out of the well, and cells were serum-starved for 12 h. A scratch wound was created with a micropipette tip, and the cells were washed twice with PBS to remove cellular debris and floating cells, followed by incubation with vehicle. The control group was treated with culture medium, and the experimental groups were treated with different doses of ICA. The remaining wound area was observed and photographed using an inverted microscope with a camera at 0, 12, and 24 h.

2.5. Transwell Migration Assay. BMSCs were subjected to serum deprivation for 12 h before being cultured on a polycarbonate porous membrane insert with 8 μm pores (Corning Costar, Shanghai, China). The cell density was adjusted to 1×10^6 cells/mL with alpha MEM containing fetal bovine serum. The cells were divided into the following groups: (1) control group (0 μM ICA in both the upper and lower chambers); (2) 0.1 μM ICA group (upper chamber: 0 μM ICA, lower chamber: 0.1 μM ICA); (3) 1 μM ICA group (upper chamber: 0 μM ICA, lower chamber: 1 μM ICA); and (4) 10 μM group (upper chamber: 0 μM ICA, lower chamber: 10 μM ICA). One hundred microliters of cell suspension were added to the upper chamber, and alpha MEM was added to the lower chamber. The cells were allowed to migrate for 24 h; after which, the polycarbonate membrane was removed, fixed with 70% ethanol for 30 min, and stained with 0.1% crystal violet for 30 min. BMSCs were counted under a fluorescence microscope.

2.6. Rhodamine-Phalloidin Staining. BMSCs were grown in 24-well plates with glass coverslips at a density of 100 cells per well. BMSCs in the control group were treated with alpha MEM, while those in the experimental group were incubated with ICA. After treatment, the cells were washed with PBS, fixed with 4% paraformaldehyde for 10 min, washed with PBS, permeabilized with 0.5% Triton X-100 for 5 min, and incubated with 100 nM rhodamine-phalloidin prepared in 1% bovine serum albumin (BSA). Cells were counterstained with Prolong Gold AntiFade Reagent with DAPI for 30 seconds after washing with PBS. Photographs were taken with a confocal laser scanning microscope.

2.7. Western Blotting. After incubation in growth medium or growth medium containing 1 μM ICA for 30, 60, and 120 min, cells were washed three times with cold PBS and suspended in 60 μL of cell lysis buffer containing protease inhibitors (Beyotime, China). The suspension was centrifuged at 15,000 rpm for 20 min at 4°C, and the supernatant was reserved. The concentration of protein in the sample was measured by a BCA protein quantitation kit, and 10%

sodium dodecyl sulfate–polyacrylamide gel electrophoresis (SDS-PAGE) was used to separate aliquots of lysates containing an equal amount of protein ($20\,\mu g$) followed by transfer onto polyvinylidene fluoride (PVDF) membranes. The membranes were washed with Tris-buffered saline (TBST), blocked for 1 h at room temperature in TBST containing 5% dry milk, and incubated overnight with specific primary antibodies (phospho-p38, phospho-ERK1/2, and phospho-JNK) at 4°C. Next, the membranes were incubated with secondary antibodies for 1 h at room temperature. Blots were visualized using a standard enhanced chemiluminescence system.

2.8. Immunofluorescence Assay. BMSCs at passage 3 were seeded in 12-well culture plates. When the cells grew to 60% confluence, the medium was aspirated from the plates and replaced with $10\,\mu M$ $5'$-bromo-2-deoxyuridine (BrdU) for 48 h. After the media were aspirated, the cells were covered completely with cold 70% ethanol and fixed for 5 min at room temperature. The cells were then blocked with 5% normal goat serum and incubated with BrdU antibody overnight at 4°C. After rinsing three times with PBS for 5 min each, the cells were incubated in fluorochrome-conjugated secondary antibody diluted in Antibody Dilution Buffer for 1 h at room temperature in the dark. In addition, sufficient Prolong Gold AntiFade Reagent with DAPI was applied to cover cells in the 12-well culture plates. Fluorescence microscopy was employed to observe the rate of BrdU labeling.

2.9. Cartilage Defect Model. Fifteen three-month-old healthy female New Zealand white rabbits ($2.5 \pm 0.3\,kg$) were randomly divided into the normal control group, BMSC group, and ICA + BMSC group. After anesthesia, the knee joint was exposed, and a full-thickness cylindrical cartilage defect of 4 mm in diameter and 3 mm in depth (reaching the bone marrow exude) was created in the patellar groove using a standard-size stainless steel biopsy punch. In addition, 4×10^5 U penicillin was intramuscularly injected after the operation. Two hours after surgery, rabbits in the experimental group were injected with BMSCs that had been incubated with ICA for 72 h, and rabbits in the BMSC group were injected with BMSCs without ICA pretreatment via the ear vein; the normal control group was injected with PBS. The BMSCs were all labeled with BrdU before injection. The rabbits were housed in separate hutches and allowed to move freely.

2.10. Immunohistochemical Staining of BrdU. The regenerated tissues of all groups were collected 4 weeks after surgery. The sample was fixed in 4% paraformaldehyde for 48 h, decalcified in 10% EDTA for 4 weeks until a needle could impale the tissues, paraffin embedded, and sectioned. After the sections were dewaxed and rehydrated, the slides were submersed in 1× citrate unmasking solution and heated in a microwave until boiling, after which they were maintained for 10 min at a subboiling temperature (95–98°C). After cooling on a bench top for 30 min and three PBS washes for 5 min each, the sections were incubated in 3% hydrogen peroxide for 10 min. The solution was then replaced with BrdU primary antibody for overnight incubation at 4°C. The sections

were washed again and incubated with secondary antibody. Then, the sections were washed with PBS and coverslipped. Photographs were taken using an inverted phase contrast microscope. Positively stained BMSCs were quantified in three random areas of each section.

2.11. Statistical Analysis. Statistical analyses were performed using the SPSS 24.0 software. The results were presented as the mean ± standard deviation. Differences among groups were tested by one-way analysis of variance (ANOVA). $P < 0.05$ was considered to indicate a statistically significant difference.

3. Results

3.1. Identification of BMSCs. BMSCs were obtained from rabbits, and their multipotent differentiation ability was detected by osteoplastic and chondrogenic differentiation. BMSCs developed into osteoblasts and chondrocytes after incubation with differentiation solution for 14 days. Osteoplastic cells were detected by alizarin red and alkaline phosphatase, and chondrogenic cells were detected by alcian blue staining. These results showed that many cells remained BMSCs after three generations of subculture (Figure 1).

3.2. Effect of ICA on the Proliferation of BMSCs. To investigate the effect of ICA on BMSC proliferation, we added different doses of ICA and then measured cell proliferation by the CCK-8 assay after 12, 24, 36, 48, 72, and 96 h. As shown in Figure 2, ICA did not noticeably promote BMSC proliferation. There were no statistically significant differences among the groups (Figure 2).

3.3. ICA Accelerates the Migration of BMSCs. The ability of ICA to promote BMSC migration was examined through the wound-healing assay and Transwell migration assay. In the wound-healing assay, many BMSCs in the groups treated with 0.1, 1, and $10\,\mu M$ ICA but few cells in the control group migrated to the scratch wound at 12 and 24 h after creating the scratch. Among all these groups, the remaining wound area in the group treated with $1\,\mu M$ ICA was the smallest, and the difference was statistically significant ($P < 0.05$). However, BMSC migration in the $100\,\mu M$ ICA group was not noticeably promoted compared with that in the control group (Figures 3(a) and 3(b)). As shown in Figure 3(c), the number of cells that migrated to the lower chamber in the 0.1 and $1\,\mu M$ ICA groups was much higher than that in the control group ($P < 0.05$). Although there was no significant difference in BMSC migration between the $1\,\mu M$ and $0.1\,\mu M$ ICA groups, more migrating cells were observed after culture with $1\,\mu M$ ICA than with $0.1\,\mu M$ ICA. These results show that $1\,\mu M$ ICA stimulates BMSC migration.

3.4. ICA Promotes the Migration of BMSCs Probably by Stimulating Actin Stress Fiber Formation. The cytoskeleton is a network of fibers composed of proteins contained within the cytoplasm in all cells of all domains of life, most notably in eukaryotic cells. The cytoskeleton of eukaryotes has three major components: microfilaments, microtubules, and intermediate filaments. By contrast, intermediate

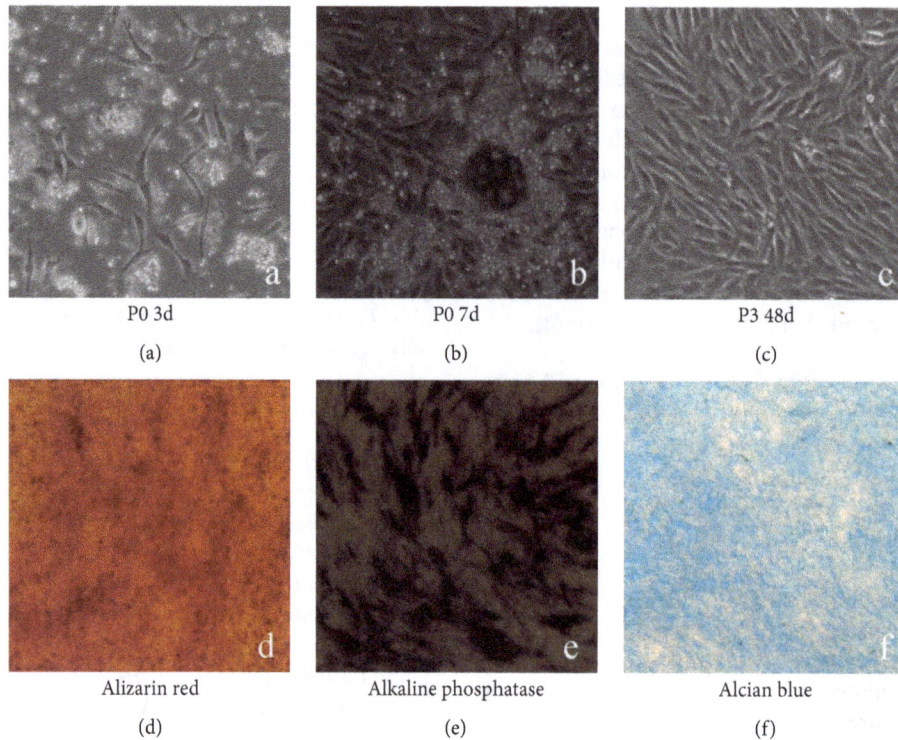

FIGURE 1: Characteristics of rabbit BMSCs. (a) Few BMSCs grew via static adherence cultured in growth medium in the primary phase. (b) The growth of BMSCs from embryoid body (EB) formation, reaching 80% confluence at day 7. (c) BMSCs at passage 3, reaching confluence 90% after incubation for 48 h. (d) Osteoplastic differentiation revealed by alizarin red staining after 2 weeks. (e) Osteoplastic differentiation revealed by alkaline phosphatase staining after 2 weeks. (f) Chondrogenic differentiation revealed by alcian blue staining after 2 weeks.

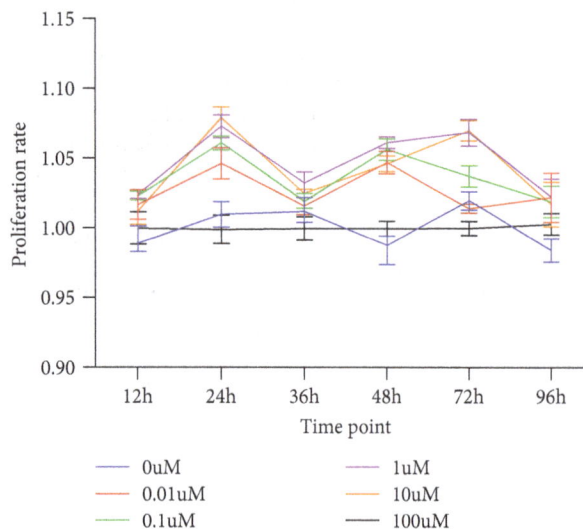

FIGURE 2: Effect of ICA on the proliferation of BMSCs. BMSCs were treated with various concentrations of ICA (0, 0.01, 0.1, 1, 10, and 100 μM) for 12, 24, 36, 48, 72, and 96 h. The proliferation rate of BMSCs was assessed by the CCK-8 assay.

filaments consist of actin protein, which is the primary force-generating machinery in the cell and can produce pushing forces that can power diverse motility processes. To study the effect of ICA on actin proteins in BMSCs,

rhodamine-phalloidin was used to stain actin protein. After ICA treatment (1 μM), the formation of intermediate filaments was apparently increased compared with that in the control group (Figure 3(e)).

3.5. ICA Upregulates Protein Expression of the MAPK Signaling Pathway. There are many signaling pathways involved in BMSC migration, but the MAPK signaling pathway is the most crucial. To examine whether ICA can upregulate the MAPK signaling pathway, cells were treated with ICA (1 μM) for 30, 60, or 120 min, and the expressions of p-P38, extracellular regulated kinase (ERK or p42/p44 MAPK), and jun amino-terminal kinases/stress-activated protein kinase (JNK) were detected by Western blot. We found that p-P38, ERK, and JNK were increased after ICA treatment (Figure 4).

3.6. MAPK Signaling Pathway Participates in the Migration of BMSCs Induced by ICA. To further determine the role of the MAPK signaling pathway in the migration of BMSCs induced by ICA, migration was analysed by a scratch wound-healing assay and rhodamine-phalloidin staining in the presence of the P38-specific inhibitor SB202190, the ERK-specific inhibitor PD98059, or the JNK-specific inhibitor SP600125. As shown in Figure 5(a), in the scratch wound-healing assay, the inhibitor groups exhibited significantly reduced ICA-induced migration of BMSCs. Similar results were also obtained for rhodamine-phalloidin staining. After treatment with ICA in the presence of the three

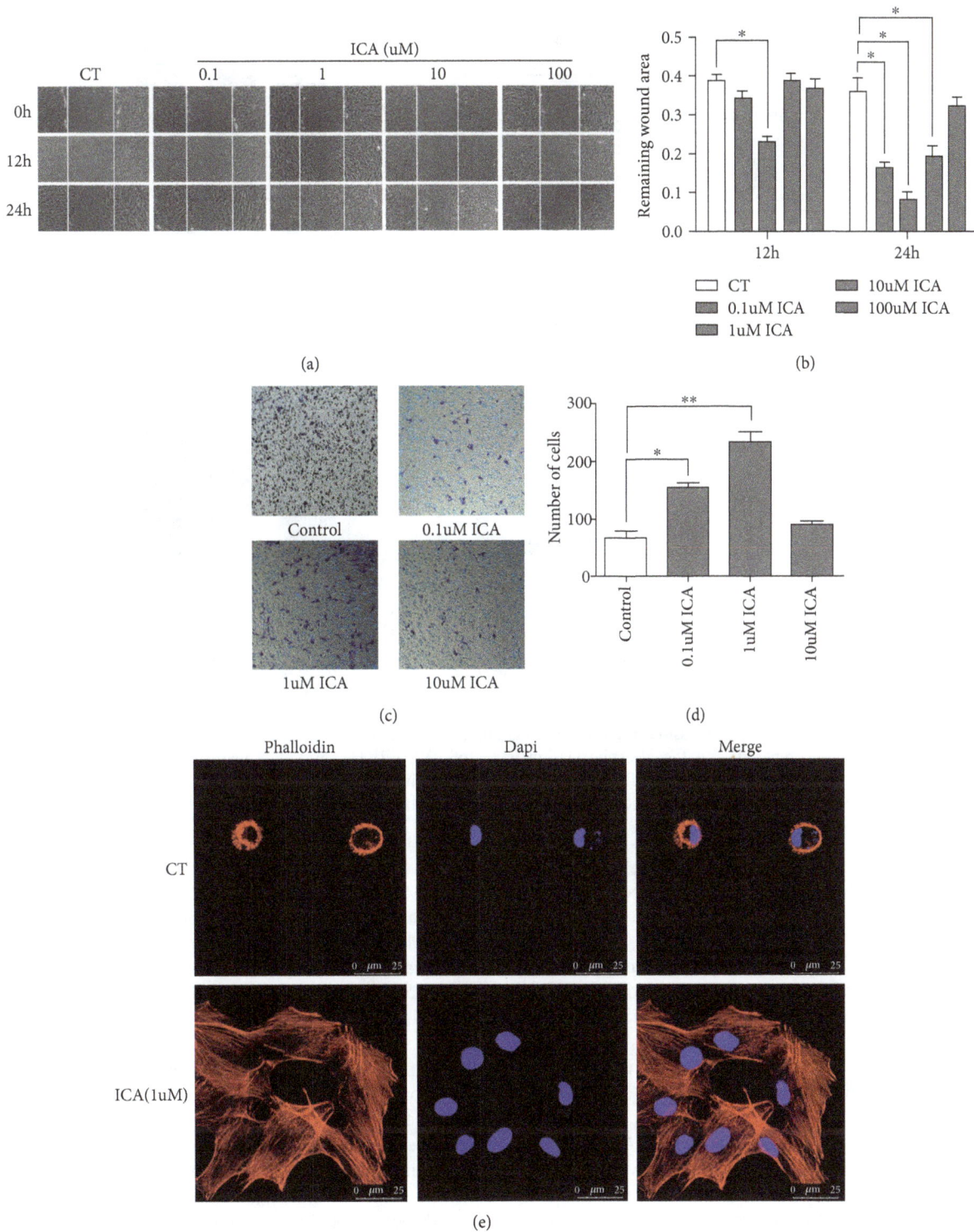

(a)

(b)

(c)

(d)

(e)

FIGURE 3: ICA promotes the migration of BMSCs in vitro. (a) Scratch wound-healing assay of BMSCs treated with ICA (0, 0.1, 1, 10, and 100 μM). Phase contrast images were captured after 12 and 24 h. (b) Quantitative analysis of the remaining wound area in Figure 3(a). Three random fields of each group were selected, and the remaining area of wound was measured using Image J. (c) Transwell migration assay of BMSCs treated with ICA (0.1, 1, and 10 μM). The number of BMSCs in the outside bottom chamber was calculated. (d) Quantitative analysis of the migrated cells. The results are shown as the mean value of 5 random fields. (e) ICA stimulated actin stress fiber formation of BMSCs. Data are shown as the mean $\pm$ SD of three independent experiments. $^{*}P < 0.05$, $^{**}P < 0.01$ compared with the group control.

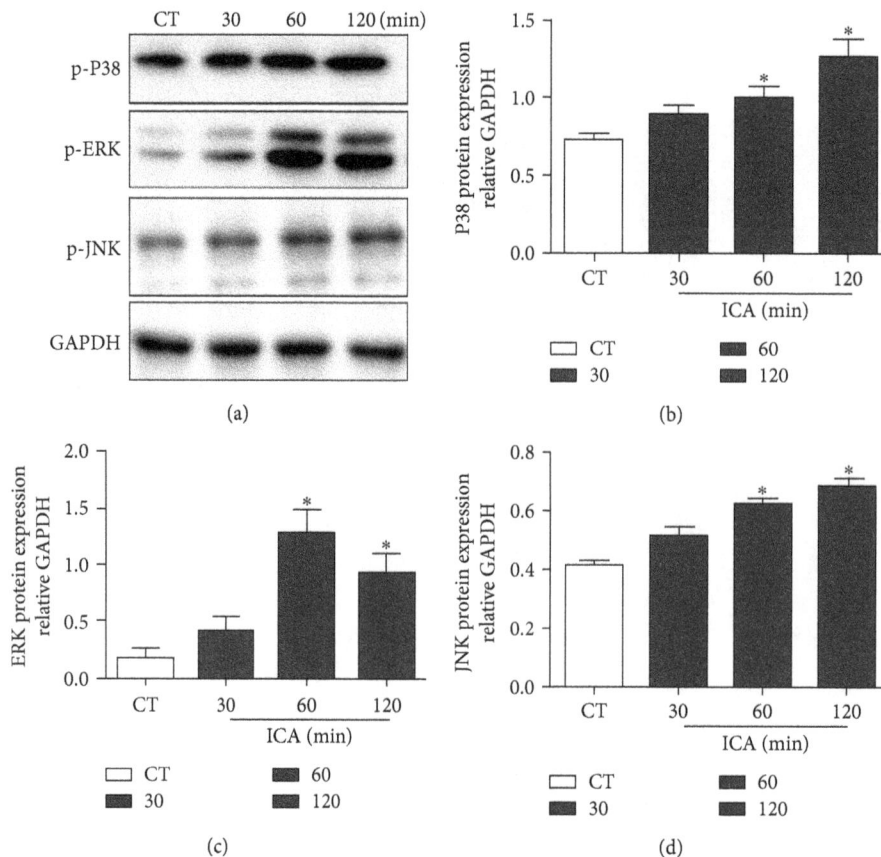

(a)

(b)

(c)

(d)

FIGURE 4: ICA upregulates the protein expression of the MAPK signaling pathway. BMSCs were treated with ICA for 30, 60, and 120 min. Total protein extracts were prepared, and the phosphorylation levels of P38, ERK1/2, and JNK were detected by Western blot. The experiment was repeated at least three times to verify the result. (a) Representative bands of P38, ERK 1/2, and P38. The internal reference was GAPDH. (b, c, d) Densitometric analysis of immunoblotting of phosphorylated-P38, ERK1/2, and JNK compared by one-way ANOVA. Data are shown as the mean ± SD of three independent experiments. $^*P < 0.05$ compared with the group control.

inhibitors, BMSCs had less actin stress fiber formation (Figure 5(b)).

3.7. ICA Improves the Homing Rates of BrdU-Labeled BMSCs. To ensure that most of the BMSCs were labeled by BrdU, an immunofluorescence assay was performed. BMSCs were cultured with $10 \mu M$ BrdU for 72 h. Positive cells were labeled with red fluorescence in the nucleus, and the percentage of BrdU-positive cells was $95 \pm 2.1\%$ (Figures 6(a) and 6(b)). The BrdU$^+$ cells in the tissues undergoing repair were detected by an immunofluorescence assay at 4 weeks after surgery. As shown in Figure 6(c), there were more BrdU-positive cells in the group that received ICA-treated BMSCs than in the group that received control BMSCs, suggesting that the combination of ICA and BMSCs led to improved migration. Moreover, the distribution of BrdU$^+$ cells in the group that received ICA-treated BMSCs was more extensive and uniform than that in the group that received control BMSCs.

4. Discussion

With the development of cell-based therapies, BMSCs have attracted the attention of researchers for the treatment of

OA. As the ideal seed cells for tissue engineering, BMSCs play important roles in the rehabilitation and regeneration of tissue. BMSCs not only have extensive proliferative ability but also retain multilineage mesenchymal differentiation potential [3, 20]. However, the restorative effect of BMSCs is determined by their homing rate, and these cells generally showed limited engraftment upon in vivo implantation due to the hostile microenvironment within the injured tissue [21, 22]. Therefore, increasing the homing rate of BMSCs should improve their therapeutic effects. In the present study, we hypothesized that ICA might promote cell migration. To determine the optimal concentration of ICA for the induction of BMSC migration, concentrations from $0.01 \mu M$ to $100 \mu M$ were tested in the CCK-8 assay. We found that ICA had no positive effect on BMSC proliferation, which conflicts with other reports [23], most likely due to differences in the species from which the tested cells were obtained. The wound-healing assay and Transwell migration assay showed that $1 \mu M$ ICA induced more BMSC migration than other concentrations of ICA. We further showed that ICA promoted the migration of BMSCs probably by stimulating actin stress fiber formation.

Although the underlying mechanism of BMSC migration has not yet been clarified, multiple cell signaling pathways

(a)

(b)

(c)

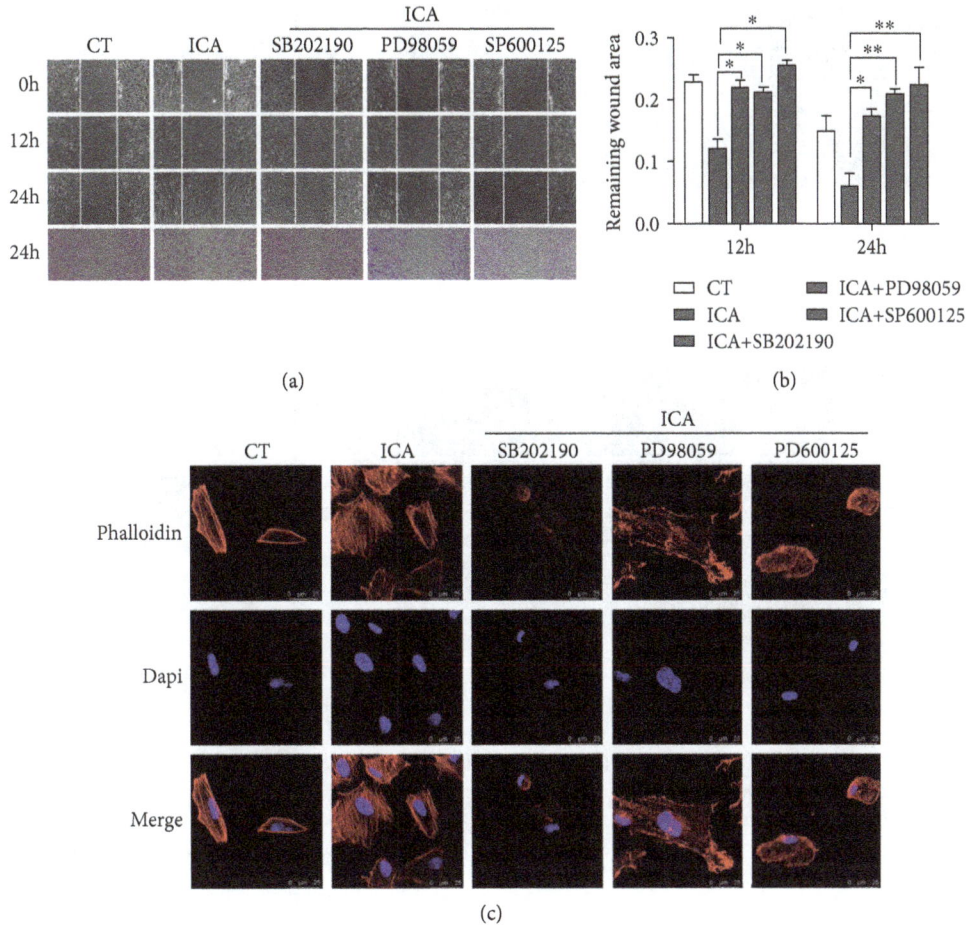

FIGURE 5: Effect of MAPK inhibitors on the wound-healing assay and rhodamine-phalloidin staining to determine the role of the MAPK signaling pathway in ICA-induced migration. (a) Activation of the MAPK signaling pathway was required for ICA-induced BMSC migration in the scratch wound-healing assay. BMSCs were treated with ICA ($1 \mu M$) in the presence of three inhibitors. The wounds were evaluated at 12 and 24 h after scratching. (b) Statistical data analysis of the remaining wound area. (c) ICA induces actin stress fiber formation by upregulating the MAPK signaling pathway. BMSCs were pretreated with the three inhibitors for 1 h. Then, rhodamine-phalloidin staining was performed after treatment with ICA.

have been implicated in the regulation of BMSC migration. The MAPK signaling pathway plays a key role in the process of BMSC migration [24]. The MAPK protein family includes ERK, p38 kinase, and JNK. Extensive evidence has shown that changes in osmotic stress, heat shock, and proinflammatory cytokines can activate the MAPK signaling pathway [10]. When activated, MAPK signaling can enhance myosin light-chain kinase (MLCK) activity, which leads to increased MLC phosphorylation. The phosphorylation of MLC is associated with actin stress fiber formation in the cell body [12]. Our in vitro results suggested that ICA enhanced ERK, p38 kinase, and JNK phosphorylations, and inhibition of them decreased BMSC migration and actin stress fiber formation. These data further verified the complex pleiotropic mechanisms by which BMSC migration is regulated.

To date, many strategies have been developed to improve the homing of BMSCs to the injured site [25–27]. First, BMSCs were genetically engineered to change the genotype of its progeny to improve their homing ability [28]. Second, cytokines were used to induce homing receptor expression in BMSCs to promote their migration [29]. Third, a magnetic system was designed to guide the superparamagnetic iron oxide nanoparticle- (SPION-) labeled cells precisely to the lesion location [30]. However, the safety of the first two methods remains doubtful due to the varying effects [31, 32], and the weakness of the third method is that SPION can cause oxidative damage in tissues. Compared with other strategies, ICA treatment, which by itself was reported to accelerate the formation of cartilage matrix and chondroid tissue, could exert positive effects on BMSCs [19, 23, 33]. In the present study, we successfully labeled the BMSCs with BrdU. The immunofluorescence assay of repairing tissues with the participation of the BrdU-labeled BMSCs showed that ICA could increase the recruitment of BMSCs into the cartilage defect region. Moreover, the distribution of BrdU$^+$ cells in the group that received ICA-treated BMSCs was more extensive and uniform than that in the group that received control BMSCs. This finding demonstrates that ICA-treated BMSCs may become a very promising strategy for the repair of cartilage defects and will increase the possibilities for treatment of other diseases requiring high homing rates.

(a)

(b)

(c)

(d)

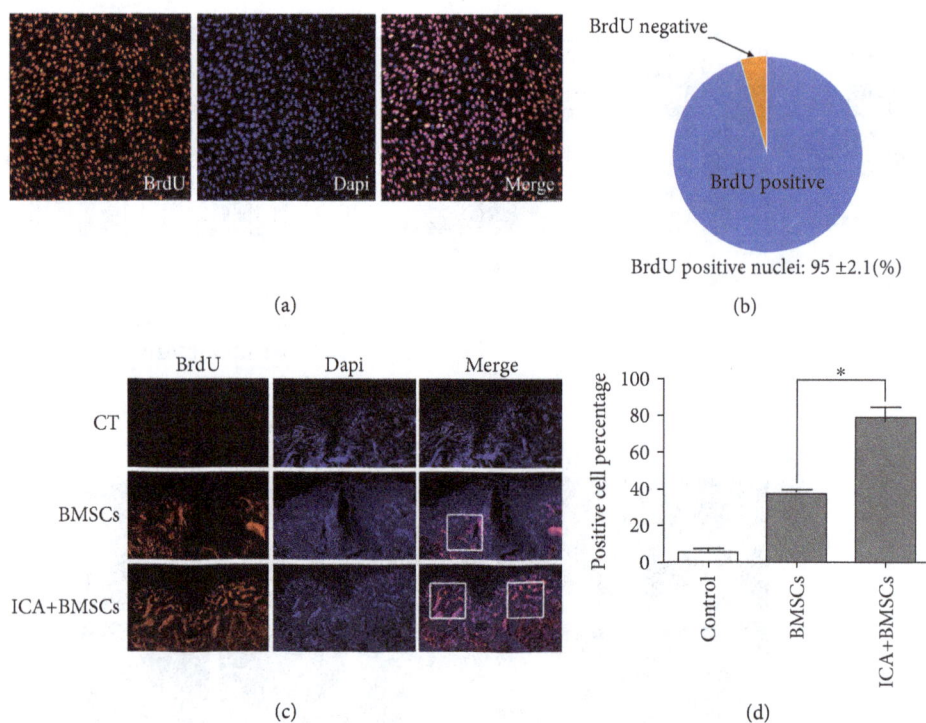

FIGURE 6: The migration of BrdU-labeled BMSCs in vivo. (a) To observe the migration of BMSCs in vivo, BMSCs were labeled with BrdU. All cells stained with DAPI were shown in blue, while BrdU-positive cells were labeled with red fluorescence. (b) The labeling efficiency of BrdU was $95 \pm 2.1\%$. (c) BrdU$^+$ cells were detected by an immunofluorescence assay at 4 weeks after surgery. The number of BMSCs treated with ICA in the repairing tissue is much greater than that in the group injected with control BMSCs. (d) Statistical data analysis of the positive cell percentage in Figure 6(c). $^*P < 0.05$ compared with the BMSC control.

Although the repairing effect of ICA combined with BMSCs was not detected, the gross appearance showed better results. In future studies, the long-term effects of transplanted ICA-treated BMSCs should be investigated in more detail.

5. Conclusion

In summary, the data reported herein show that ICA promotes BMSC migration in vivo and in vitro. In addition, the mechanism of ICA-induced BMSC migration involves the promotion of actin stress fiber formation via the MAPK signaling pathway. Hence, combined therapy of BMSCs with ICA may confer better results in the treatment of cartilage defects and may be a challenging direction for further study.

Acknowledgments

This study was supported by the Traditional Chinese Medicine Bureau of Guangdong Province (no. 20171220).

References

[1] A. M. Lubis and V. K. Lubis, "Adult bone marrow stem cells in cartilage therapy," *Acta Medica Indonesiana*, vol. 44, no. 1, pp. 62–68, 2012.

[2] K. E. Wescoe, R. C. Schugar, C. R. Chu, and B. M. Deasy, "The role of the biochemical and biophysical environment in chondrogenic stem cell differentiation assays and cartilage tissue engineering," *Cell Biochemistry and Biophysics*, vol. 52, no. 2, pp. 85–102, 2008.

[3] J. Gao, J. Q. Yao, and A. I. Caplan, "Stem cells for tissue engineering of articular cartilage," *Proceedings of the Institution of Mechanical Engineers, Part H: Journal of Engineering in Medicine*, vol. 221, no. 5, pp. 441–450, 2007.

[4] M. Mata, L. Milian, M. Oliver et al., "In vivo articular cartilage regeneration using human dental pulp stem cells cultured in an alginate scaffold: a preliminary study," *Stem Cells International*, vol. 2017, Article ID 8309256, 9 pages, 2017.

[5] M. F. Pittenger, A. M. Mackay, S. C. Beck et al., "Multilineage potential of adult human mesenchymal stem cells," *Science*, vol. 284, no. 5411, pp. 143–147, 1999.

[6] H. Nakagawa, S. Akita, M. Fukui, T. Fujii, and K. Akino, "Human mesenchymal stem cells successfully improve skin-substitute wound healing," *British Journal of Dermatology*, vol. 153, no. 1, pp. 29–36, 2005.

[7] E. Chavakis, C. Urbich, and S. Dimmeler, "Homing and engraftment of progenitor cells: a prerequisite for cell therapy," *Journal of Molecular and Cellular Cardiology*, vol. 45, no. 4, pp. 514–522, 2008.

[8] J. M. Karp and G. S. Leng Teo, "Mesenchymal stem cell homing: the devil is in the details," *Cell Stem Cell*, vol. 4, no. 3, pp. 206–216, 2009.

[9] C. Huang, Z. Rajfur, C. Borchers, M. D. Schaller, and

K. Jacobson, "JNK phosphorylates paxillin and regulates cell migration," *Nature*, vol. 424, no. 6945, pp. 219–223, 2003.

[10] M. Krishna and H. Narang, "The complexity of mitogen-activated protein kinases (MAPKs) made simple," *Cellular and Molecular Life Sciences*, vol. 65, no. 22, pp. 3525–3544, 2008.

[11] T. Svitkina, "The actin cytoskeleton and actin-based motility," *Cold Spring Harbor Perspectives in Biology*, vol. 10, no. 1, 2018.

[12] K. B. Reddy, S. M. Nabha, and N. Atanaskova, "Role of MAP kinase in tumor progression and invasion," *Cancer Metastasis Reviews*, vol. 22, no. 4, pp. 395–403, 2003.

[13] Y. Shi, Y. Y. Xia, L. Wang, R. Liu, K. S. Khoo, and Z. W. Feng, "Neural cell adhesion molecule modulates mesenchymal stromal cell migration via activation of MAPK/ERK signaling," *Experimental Cell Research*, vol. 318, no. 17, pp. 2257–2267, 2012.

[14] D. Zheng, S. Peng, S. H. Yang et al., "The beneficial effect of icariin on bone is diminished in osteoprotegerin-deficient mice," *Bone*, vol. 51, no. 1, pp. 85–92, 2012.

[15] D. Li, T. Yuan, X. Zhang et al., "Icariin: a potential promoting compound for cartilage tissue engineering," *Osteoarthritis and Cartilage*, vol. 20, no. 12, pp. 1647–1656, 2012.

[16] L. Zhang, X. Zhang, K. F. Li et al., "Icariin promotes extracellular matrix synthesis and gene expression of chondrocytes in vitro," *Phytotherapy Research*, vol. 26, no. 9, pp. 1385–1392, 2012.

[17] S. Zhang, P. Feng, G. Mo et al., "Icariin influences adipogenic differentiation of stem cells affected by osteoblast-osteoclast co-culture and clinical research adipogenic," *Biomedicine & Pharmacotherapy*, vol. 88, pp. 436–442, 2017.

[18] Y. Wu, L. Xia, Y. Zhou, Y. Xu, and X. Jiang, "Icariin induces osteogenic differentiation of bone mesenchymal stem cells in a MAPK-dependent manner," *Cell Proliferation*, vol. 48, no. 3, pp. 375–384, 2015.

[19] Z. C. Wang, H. J. Sun, K. H. Li, C. Fu, and M. Z. Liu, "Icariin promotes directed chondrogenic differentiation of bone marrow mesenchymal stem cells but not hypertrophy in vitro," *Experimental and Therapeutic Medicine*, vol. 8, no. 5, pp. 1528–1534, 2014.

[20] E. L. S. Fong, C. K. Chan, and S. B. Goodman, "Stem cell homing in musculoskeletal injury," *Biomaterials*, vol. 32, no. 2, pp. 395–409, 2011.

[21] C. Toma, W. R. Wagner, S. Bowry, A. Schwartz, and F. Villanueva, "Fate of culture-expanded mesenchymal stem cells in the microvasculature: in vivo observations of cell kinetics," *Circulation Research*, vol. 104, no. 3, pp. 398–402, 2009.

[22] B. M. Gleeson, K. Martin, M. T. Ali et al., "Bone marrow-derived mesenchymal stem cells have innate procoagulant activity and cause microvascular obstruction following intracoronary delivery: amelioration by antithrombin therapy," *Stem Cells*, vol. 33, no. 9, pp. 2726–2737, 2015.

[23] S. Qin, W. Zhou, S. Liu, P. Chen, and H. Wu, "Icariin stimulates the proliferation of rat bone mesenchymal stem cells via ERK and p38 MAPK signaling," *International Journal of Clinical and Experimental Medicine*, vol. 8, no. 5, pp. 7125–7133, 2015.

[24] M. M. Kavurma and L. M. Khachigian, "ERK, JNK, and p38 MAP kinases differentially regulate proliferation and migration of phenotypically distinct smooth muscle cell subtypes," *Journal of Cellular Biochemistry*, vol. 89, no. 2, pp. 289–300, 2003.

[25] B. R. Son, L. A. Marquez-Curtis, M. Kucia et al., "Migration of bone marrow and cord blood mesenchymal stem cells in vitro is regulated by stromal-derived factor-1-CXCR4 and hepatocyte growth factor-c-met axes and involves matrix metalloproteinases," *Stem Cells*, vol. 24, no. 5, pp. 1254–1264, 2006.

[26] A. P. Lykov, Y. V. Nikonorova, N. A. Bondarenko et al., "Proliferation, migration, and production of nitric oxide by bone marrow multipotent mesenchymal stromal cells from Wistar rats in hypoxia and hyperglycemia," *Bulletin of Experimental Biology and Medicine*, vol. 159, no. 4, pp. 443–445, 2015.

[27] S. Bobis-Wozowicz, K. Miekus, E. Wybieralska et al., "Genetically modified adipose tissue–derived mesenchymal stem cells overexpressing CXCR4 display increased motility, invasiveness, and homing to bone marrow of NOD/SCID mice," *Experimental Hematology*, vol. 39, no. 6, pp. 686–696.e4, 2011.

[28] H. Lin, X. Luo, B. Jin, H. Shi, and H. Gong, "The effect of EPO gene overexpression on proliferation and migration of mouse bone marrow-derived mesenchymal stem cells," *Cell Biochemistry and Biophysics*, vol. 71, no. 3, pp. 1365–1372, 2015.

[29] Y. Li, X. Y. Yu, S. G. Lin, X. H. Li, S. Zhang, and Y. H. Song, "Insulin-like growth factor 1 enhances the migratory capacity of mesenchymal stem cells," *Biochemical and Biophysical Research Communications*, vol. 356, no. 3, pp. 780–784, 2007.

[30] D. Tukmachev, O. Lunov, V. Zablotskii et al., "An effective strategy of magnetic stem cell delivery for spinal cord injury therapy," *Nanoscale*, vol. 7, no. 9, pp. 3954–3958, 2015.

[31] A. Saraf and A. Mikos, "Gene delivery strategies for cartilage tissue engineering," *Advanced Drug Delivery Reviews*, vol. 58, no. 4, pp. 592–603, 2006.

[32] F. Buket Basmanav, G. T. Kose, and V. Hasirci, "Sequential growth factor delivery from complexed microspheres for bone tissue engineering," *Biomaterials*, vol. 29, no. 31, pp. 4195–4204, 2008.

[33] Q. Wei, M. C. He, M. H. Chen et al., "Icariin stimulates osteogenic differentiation of rat bone marrow stromal stem cells by increasing TAZ expression," *Biomedicine & Pharmacotherapy*, vol. 91, pp. 581–589, 2017.

7

D-Mannose Enhanced Immunomodulation of Periodontal Ligament Stem Cells via Inhibiting IL-6 Secretion

Lijia Guo ⓘ,[1] Yanan Hou ⓘ,[2] Liang Song ⓘ,[3] Siying Zhu ⓘ,[4] Feiran Lin ⓘ,[4] and Yuxing Bai ⓘ[1]

[1]*Department of Orthodontics School of Stomatology, Capital Medical University, Beijing, China*
[2]*Department of Orthodontics, Peking University School of Stomatology, The Third Dental Center, Beijing, China*
[3]*Department of Stomatology, The Fifth People's Hospital of Shanghai, Fudan University, Shanghai, China*
[4]*Laboratory of Tissue Regeneration and Immunology and Department of Periodontics, Beijing Key Laboratory of Tooth Regeneration and Function Reconstruction, School of Stomatology, Capital Medical University, Beijing, China*

Correspondence should be addressed to Yuxing Bai; byuxing@ccmu.edu.cn

Academic Editor: Dandan Wang

Periodontal ligament stem cell- (PDLSC-) mediated periodontal tissue regeneration has recently been proposed for the new therapeutic method to regenerate lost alveolar bone and periodontal ligament. It was reported that both autogenic and allogeneic PDLSCs could reconstruct damaged periodontal tissues but the regeneration effects were not consistent. The effective methods to improve the properties of PDLSCs should be further considered. In this study, we investigated if D-mannose could affect the immunomodulatory properties of hPDLSCs. After being pretreated with D-mannose, hPDLSCs could inhibit T cell proliferation and affect T cell differentiation into Treg cells. We found that less IL-6 could be detected in D-mannose-pretreated hPDLSCs. In the D-mannose pretreatment group, induced Treg cell number would decrease if increased IL-6 levels could be detected. Our data uncovered a previously unrecognized function of D-mannose to regulate the immunomodulatory function of PDLSCs and that IL-6 might play a key role in this process. The results provided a property method to improve PDLSC-based periodontal regeneration.

1. Introduction

Periodontitis, as one of the major oral infectious diseases, has high incidence in human. Periodontitis could cause damage to periodontal tissues, such as gingiva recession, attachment loss, alveolar bone loss, and teeth loss [1]. There is still no efficient therapy to recover the lost tissue. Stem cell-mediated periodontal tissue reconstruction is a promising strategy. Recently, periodontal ligament stem cells (PDLSCs) have received more and more attention in periodontal tissue reconstruction because of its multiple differentiation capacity and immunomodulation [2].

Recently, mesenchymal stem cells (MSCs) have been confirmed to have immunosuppressive and immunomodulatory properties and are extensively used to treat autoimmune diseases. Under the stimulation of inflammatory cytokines in microenvironment, MSCs inhibit the activation and proliferation of a variety of immune cells. Nevertheless, the role of

MSCs on immune cells in different microenvironments remains partly unknown. More importantly, the diverse results suggested that the immunomodulatory functions of MSCs are involved in multiple factors. PDLSCs belong to one of various tooth-derived MSCs, which owned immunosuppressive abilities and mediate suppression by secreting inhibitory factors such as IFNγ, IDO, TGFβ1, and HGF [3–6]. PDLSCs could inhibit T cell proliferation though PGE2 and promote T cell differentiation into Treg cells [7, 8]. When minipigs are transplanted with periodontal defects, PDLSCs could remodel the local immune microenvironment and obtain new tissue regeneration [9]. However, the detailed mechanisms were unknown, which caused unstable therapeutic outcomes in periodontal tissue regeneration.

Glucose plays critical roles in cell metabolism during energy generation and storage. At same time, glucose participates in some pathogenic processes, such as diabetes and obesity. D-Mannose is one of the important proteins in the glycosylation. The blood concentration of D-mannose is less than one-fiftieth of that of glucose. However, D-mannose has not received much attention. D-Mannose is a kind of C-2 epimer of glucose, which has been reported to as an effective therapy for urinary tract infections [10–15]. Currently, the function of T cell regulation of D-mannose has been found. D-Mannose could stimulate Treg differentiation by promoting TGFβ signaling [16]. But whether D-mannose could affect immunomodulation of stem cell is still unknown. In this study, we cocultured T cells with D-mannose-pretreated human PDLSCs (hPDLSCs) to investigate the effect of D-mannose on hPDLSC immunomodulation function.

2. Materials and Method

2.1. Antibodies and Reagents. Purified anti-human CD3 (OKT3) and purified anti-human CD28 (CD28.2) were purchased from eBioscience. All fluorochrome-conjugated antibodies (anti-human CD4 (RPA-T4), anti-human CD45RA (HI100), anti-human CD25 (BC96), anti-human FoxP3 (PCH101), anti-human IFNγ, anti-human IL-4, anti-human IL-17, and anti-mouse IL-6 were from eBioscience. Recombinant human IL-2 (202-IL), human TGFβ1 (240-B), and human latent TGFβ1 (299-LT) were purchased from R&D Systems. Anti-TGFβ (1D11.16.8), anti-CD25 (PC-61.5.3), and their isotype control antibodies (MOPC-21, HRPN) were from Bio X Cell. PGE2, TGFβ, and IL-6 ELISA Ready-SET-Go! kits were purchased from eBioscience.

2.2. PDLSC Culture. PDLSCs were isolated and cultured from periodontal ligament tissues of periodontal healthy donors. The protocols for handling human tissues had been approved by the Research Ethical Committee of Capital Medical University. Healthy periodontal tissues from nine patients (age 18–36 years) were obtained. The periodontal ligament from the extracted teeth was separated from the surface of the roots and cut to small pieces. Then the small tissues were digested in 3 mg/ml collagenase type I (Worthington Biochemical, Freehold, NJ) and 4 mg/ml dispase (Roche Diagnostics, Basel, Switzerland) for 1 hour at 37°C. To get the single cells, all the cells were passed through a 70 μm strainer (BD Labware, Franklin Lakes, NJ). Then about 1×10^5 single cells were seeded into 10 cm culture dishes (Corning Costar, Cambridge, MA) with culture medium. The culture medium included α-modification of Eagle's medium (Gibco, Carlsbad, CA) and 10% fetal bovine serum (Equitech-Bio Inc., Kerrville, TX) supplemented with 100 mol/l ascorbic acid 2-phosphate (Wako Chemical, Tokyo), 2 mmol/l glutamine, 100 U/ml penicillin, and 100 μg/ml streptomycin (Invitrogen, Carlsbad, CA). Then the cells were incubated at 37°C in 5% carbon dioxide. The colony cells were passed on day 14. PDLSCs in the study were three to four passages. All cells used in this study were at 3-4 passages. For each experiment, the same passages of hPDLSCs were used.

2.3. Surface Marker of PDLSCs after Glucose or D-Mannose Treatment. PDLSCs were cultured in "complete" glucose-free α-MEM culture medium supplemented with 25 mM D-mannose (M-hPDLSCs) or in the normal culture medium supplemented with 25 mM glucose (G-hPDLSCs). Three days later, surface marker expressions were analyzed by FACS staining. The treated PDLSCs were harvested with 0.25% trypsin, and cell suspensions (1.0×10^6 cells) were incubated for 1 h at room temperature with monoclonal antibodies specific for CD90, CD45, CD44, CD73, and CD105 (BD Biosciences, Franklin Lakes, NJ, USA). Expression profiles of PDLSCs were analyzed by flow cytometry (BD Biosciences).

2.4. Osteogenic Differentiation Assay. PDLSCs were cultured in osteogenic medium. The inducing medium contained 2 mM β-glycerophosphate (Sigma-Aldrich, St. Louis, MO), 10 nM dexamethasone (Sigma-Aldrich, St Louis, MO), and 100 μM L-ascorbic acid 2-phosphate (Wako Chemicals USA, Richmond, VA). The total protein was collected from induced PDLSCs after ten days. The gene expression levels of BGLAP and ALPL were assayed by RT-PCR analysis. The primer set for PCR included BGLAP (sense, 5-CGCT ACCTGTATCAATGGCTGG-3, antisense, 5-CTCCTGAA AGCCGATGTGGTCA-3); ALPL (sense, 5-ATGGGATGG GTGTCTCCACA-3, antisense, 5-CCACGAAGGGGAACT TGTC-3); and GAPDH (sense, 5-AGCCGCATCTTCTTTT GCGTC-3, antisense, 5-TCATATTTGGCAGGTTTTT CT-3). To detect mineralized nodule formation, the cultured PDLSCs were stained with alizarin red after 4 weeks of induction.

2.5. Adipogenic Differentiation Assay. PDLSCs were cultured in adipogenic culture medium. The medium contained 500 μM isobutylmethylxanthine (Sigma-Aldrich, St. Louis, MO), 500 nM hydrocortisone (Sigma-Aldrich, St. Louis, MO), 60 μM indomethacin (Sigma-Aldrich, St. Louis, MO), 100 μM L-ascorbic acid 2-phosphate, and 10 μg/ml insulin (Sigma-Aldrich, St. Louis, MO). The gene expressions of peroxisome proliferator-activated receptor g (*PPAγG*) and FABP4 were analyzed via RT-PCR after adipogenic induction. The primer set for PCR included PPAγG (sense, 5-CTCCTATTGACCCAGAAAGC-3, antisense, 5-GTAGAG CTGAGTCTTCTCAG-3); FABP4 (sense, 5-GTCCAGGCT GGAATGCAGTG-3, antisense, 5-CACACAGACGTACA GAGTGG-3); and GAPDH (sense, 5-AGCCGCATCTT CTTTTGCGTC-3, antisense, 5-TCATATTTGGCAGGTT TTCT-3).

2.6. Alizarin Red Staining. After being induced for four weeks, the PDLSCs were fixed with 70% ethanol and stained with 2% alizarin red (Sigma-Aldrich). After being stained with alizarin red, the cells were destained for 30 min at room temperature with 10% cetylpyridinium chloride in 10 mM sodium phosphate and the calcium content was determined.

2.7. Oil Red O Staining. The cells were induced for 14 days in adipogenic medium and stained with Oil Red O (Sigma-Aldrich, St. Louis, MO). After being fixed with 4% paraformaldehyde, the cells were incubated with Oil Red O solution for 1 h. Then lipid droplets could be observed by microscopy.

2.8. Real-Time RT-PCR. Total RNA was derived from PDLSCs with an RNeasy mini kit (Qiagen). For real-time

RT-PCR, cDNA was synthesized with a high-capacity cDNA reverse transcription kit (Applied Biosystems). Quantitative real-time PCR was performed using TaqMan gene expression assay kits (Applied Biosystems). The gene expression levels were normalized to the expression of *Hprt*.

2.9. Peripheral Blood Mononuclear Cells and CD4+ T Cells.

Human peripheral blood mononuclear cells (PBMCs) from healthy volunteers were approved by the Research Ethical Committee of Capital Medical University. Blood samples were provided by the Capital Medical University School of Stomatology. All donors signed informed consent. Naive CD4+ T cells were purified by using Naive T Cell Isolation Kit II (Miltenyi Biotec). Then all the isolated cells were resuspended in T cell culture medium (Roswell Park Memorial Institute (RPMI)—1640 medium (GIBCO, Carlsbad, CA) with 10% FBS, 2 mmol/l glutamine, 20 mol/l HEPES, 100 U/ml penicillin, and 100 μg/ml streptomycin (Invitrogen). To stimulate the naive CD4+ T cells, the cells were cultured in the anti-human CD3 (5 μg/ml) precoated plate and soluble anti-human CD28 (2.5 μg/ml) plus IL-2 (10 ng/ml). Three days after stimulation, the cells were analyzed by FACS staining.

2.10. T Cells Cocultured with PDLSCs.

2×10^4 human PDLSCs were seeded in 24-well plates in triplicate, and cells adhered to the plates and stayed overnight. Then the glucose- or D-mannose-pretreated PDLSCs were cocultured with CD4+ T cells (T + G-hPDLSCS/T + M-hPDLSCs) for 3 days in T cell culture medium stimulated with soluble anti-human CD3 (5 μg/ml), anti-human CD28 (2.5 μg/ml), and IL-2 (10 ng/ml).

2.11. T Cell Proliferation Assay.

Activated T lymphocytes (1×10^6/well) were cocultured with or without 0.2×10^6 PDLSCs (pretreated with glucose or D-mannose) on 24-well multiplates with T cell-stimulated medium for 3 days. 1×10^4 cells were incubated with 5 mM carboxyfluorescein succinimidyl ester (CFSE, Invitrogen) for 10 min. Five volumes of ice-cold medium were added to stop the staining process. After being washed three times, T cells were cultured for 72 h and analyzed by CFSE flow cytometry. A percentage of divided cells were analyzed by FSC Express 3.0 software.

2.12. In Vitro Th1 and Th2 Induction by PDLSCs.

CD4+ T cells (1×10^6/well) were cocultured with 0.2×10^6 glucose- or D-mannose-pretreated PDLSCs on 24-well multiplates for 3 days in T cell culture medium stimulated with soluble anti-human CD3 (5 μg/ml), soluble anti-human CD28 (2.5 μg/ml), and IL-2 (10 ng/ml). After 3 days, cells in suspension were collected and detected Th1, Th2, Th17, and Treg via flow cytometry analysis. The concentrations of PGE2 and TGFβ1 in supernatant were analyzed by ELISA Ready-SET-Go! kits (eBioscience) following the manufacturer's instructions. Gene expression of Nos2 and IDO1 in cocultured PDLSCs were analyzed by RT-PCR.

2.13. Flow Cytometry Analysis.

Cells were incubated with PMA (10 ng/ml), ionomycin (250 ng/ml), and Golgi plug (1 : 1000 dilution; BD PharMingen) at 37°C for 4 h. For intracellular cytokine staining, cells were fixed with the fixation/permeabilization buffer solution (BD Biosciences). The collected T cells (1×10^6) were stained with anti-CD4-FITC, anti-IFNγ-PE, anti-IL-6-PerCP, anti-IL-4-APC, and anti-CD25-PerCP. For intranuclear staining, the cells were continuously treated with fixation/permeabilization buffer solution (eBioscience) and stained with anti-FoxP3-PacBlue antibodies (each 1 mg/ml; eBioscience). Cells were carried out on a FACSCalibur, and data were analyzed with FlowJo software.

2.14. Statistical Analysis.

All data were repeated in three to five independent experiments. Unless otherwise noted, statistical significance comparison was analyzed by two-tailed Student's *t*-test between two groups and by one-way ANOVA between more than two groups. Statistical analysis was performed with GraphPad Prism 6. *P* values less than 0.05 were determined statistically significant.

3. Results

3.1. D-Mannose-Pretreated PDLSCs Modulated T Cell Proliferation Better.

In order to examine the effects of D-mannose on hPDLSCs, we used D-mannose or glucose medium to culture hPDLSCs. Surface makers of hPDLSCs, CD44, CD73, CD90, and CD105 were detected by flow cytometry Figure 1(a) and there was no difference between the two groups. There were no significant differences in apoptosis and proliferation of hPDLSCs between D-mannose and glucose treatment. We have added the data in (Figures 1(b) and 1(c)). We also found that D-mannose-pretreated hPDLSCs had no difference compared with the glucose-pretreated group on osteogenic differentiation and adipogenic differentiation potentials (Figures 1(d)–1(i)). Then we cocultured mannose- or glucose-pretreated hPDLSCs with T cells, and the results showed that mannose-pretreated PDLSCs (M-hPDLSCs) had more inhibitory ability to proliferate T cells than G-hPDLSCs (Figures 1(j) and 1(k)).

3.2. More Regulatory T Cells Were Generated When Cocultured with D-Mannose-Pretreated PDLSCs.

To investigate how D-mannose affects hPDLSC immunomodulation function, T cells were cocultured with M-hPDLSCs or G-hPDLSCs. No difference was found in PGE2, TGFβ1, Nos2, and IDO1 between both groups (Figures 2(a)–2(d)). However, more FoxP3+ T cells could be found in the T + M-hPDLSCs coculture system, suggesting that M-hPDLSCs induced more T cells differentiated to Tregs (Figures 2(e) and 2(f)). Furthermore, less Th1 could be found in the M-hPDLSC coculture system (Figures 2(g) and 2(h)) compared with G-hPDLSCs and there was no significant difference in Th17 (Figures 2(g) and 2(i)) or Th2 (Figures 2(j) and 2(k)) between these two groups.

3.3. D-Mannose-Pretreated hPDLSCs Secret Less IL-6 and Induced More Tregs.

In order to know why the T cell M-hPDLSCs coculture system had more Tregs, we screened different cytokines (data not shown) and found that IL-6 was significantly lower in the T + M-hPDLSC coculture system. (Figure 3(a)). Interestingly, the number of Tregs increased

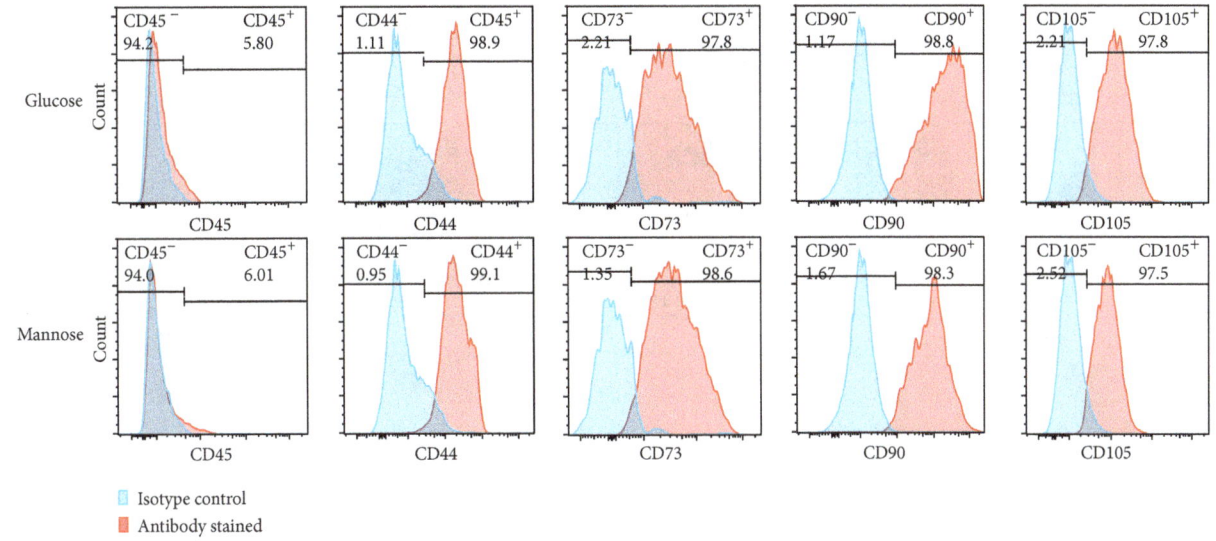

(a)

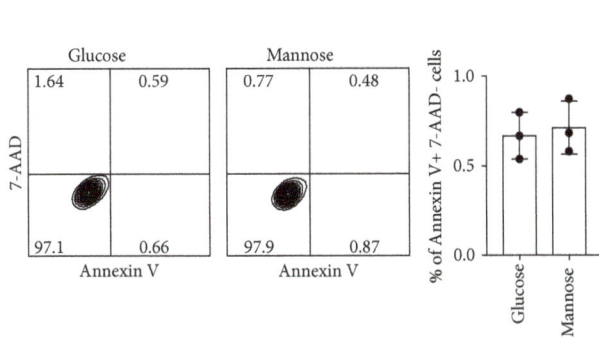

(b)

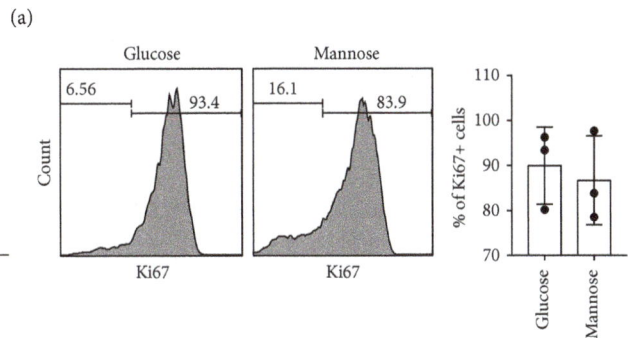

(c)

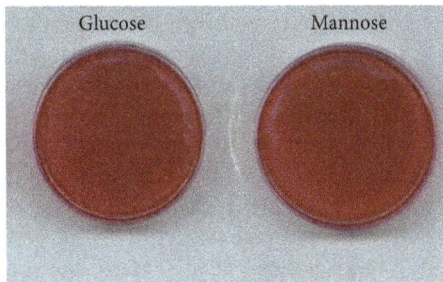

(d)

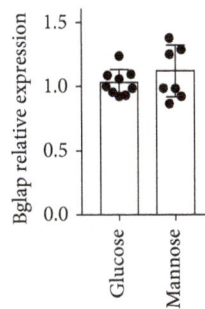

(e)

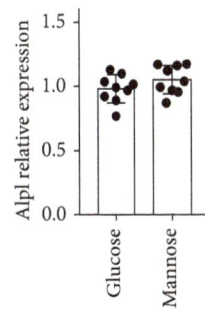

(f)

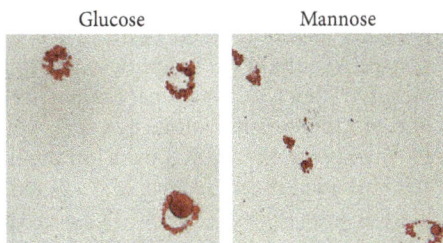

(g)

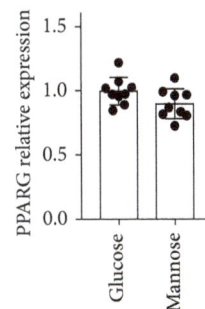

(h)

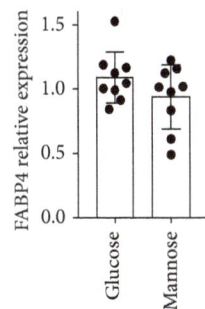

(i)

Figure 1: Continued.

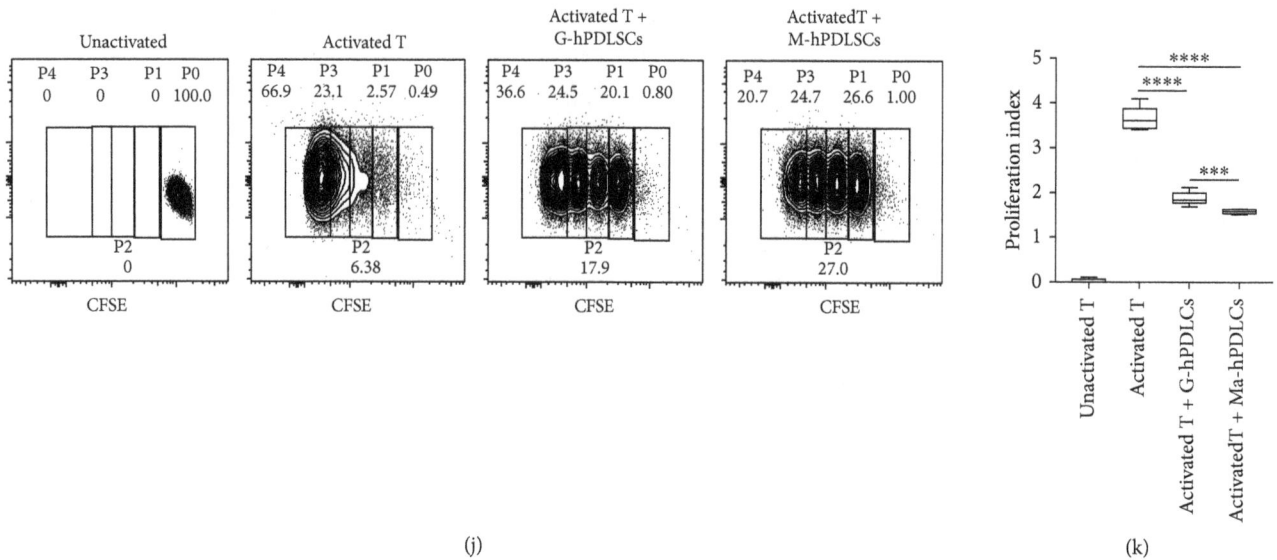

(j)

(k)

FIGURE 1: M-hPDLSCs have more inhibitory ability to proliferate T cells. (a) CD45, CD44, CD73, CD90, and CD105 have been detected by flow cytometry. There is no difference between M-hPDLSCs and G-hPDLSCs. (b, c) The apoptosis and proliferation of hPDLSCs between D-mannose and glucose treatment had no significant differences. (d–f) Osteogenic differentiation ability of M-hPDLSCs and G-PDLSCs has been detected. M-hPDLSCs and G-hPDLSCs were induced osteogenic differentiation. Alizarin red staining, BGLAP, and ALPL levels showed that M-PDLSCs have the same osteogenic differentiation ability as G-PDLSCs. (g–i) M-hPDLSCs and G-hPDLSCs were induced to adipogenic differentiation. Oil Red O staining, PPARG, and FABP4 levels showed that M-PDLSCs have the same adipogenic differentiation ability as G-hPDLSCs. (j, k) M-hPDLSCs and G-PDLSCs were cocultured with T cell to detect the effect of both on T cell proliferation. Both M-PDLSCs and G-PDLSCs could impair T cell proliferation. Compared with G-PDLSCs, M-hPDLSCs has more T cell proliferation inhibitory ability. Student's t test was used to analyze statistical significance. All error bars represent s.d. ($n = 9$). ***$P \leq 0.001$ and ****$P \leq 0.0001$.

after we neutralized IL-6 in T + G-hPDLSCs Figures 3(b) and 3(c) and decreased after we supply more IL-6 in the T + M-hPDLSC culture system (Figures 3(d) and 3(e)).

3.4. D-Mannose-Pretreated hPDLSCs Induced More Tregs In Vivo by Decreasing IL-6 Secretion. To verify previous results, we transplanted human T + G-hPDLSCs or human T + M-hPDLSC mixed cells with or without anti hIL-6 into nude mice. 2 days later, we extracted the spleen to examine T cells by flow cytometry. Without anti IL-6, the number of Tregs in the T + G-hPDLSCs group was much less than it in the T + M-hPDLSCs group. With anti hIL-6, the frequency of Tregs increased significantly in the T + G-hPDLSCs group (Figures 4(a) and 4(b)). These findings suggested that D-mannose could inhibit IL-6 in hPDLSCs to induce more Treg in vivo. On the other hand, more Th1 could be detected in the T + G-hPDLSCs group (Figures 4(c) and 4(d)) and IL-6 neutralizing could also reduce the number of Th17 (Figures 4(c) and 4(e)).

4. Discussion

Periodontitis is one of chronic infectious diseases destructing the alveolar bone and the supportive tissue of the teeth; it is also associated with a variety of systemic diseases such as diabetes, cardiovascular disease, and premature low birth weight [17–19]. The periodontal ligament comes from dental follicle, derived from neural crest cells, and PDLSCs play critical roles in periodontal ligament. PDLSCs could express the

stem cell markers such as CD105, CD166, STRO-1, and CD146/MUC18 and own the properties of self-renewal and multipotency differentiation to osteo-like cells, adipocytes [20, 21]. PDLSCs participated into the whole process of periodontal tissue regeneration.

PDLSC-mediated periodontal tissue regeneration has been proposed for the development of new periodontal tissue. It is reported that both autogeneic and allogeneic PDLSCs could reconstruct damaged periodontal tissues but the regeneration effects were not consistent [22, 23]. Although lots of studies confirm that MSCs, such as PDLSCs, are generally thought to be poorly immunogenic, PDLSC transplantation in periodontal tissue engineering would not eliminate host immune rejection against the donor cells. Recently, many studies reported that MSC-mediated bone regeneration could be regulated by the host immune system, especially T lymphocytes. Proliferation of allogeneic lymphocytes could be elicited in both differentiated and undifferentiated MSCs [24–27]. On the other hand, it is well known that MSCs own immunomodulatory properties both *in vitro* and *in vivo*. MSCs could suppress the proliferation and differentiation of Th1 and Th17 cells [28, 29], as well as their productions (IFNγ and interleukin 17), while MSCs could enhance Th2 cells and the production (IL-4) [30, 31]. So, the crosstalk between immune cells and PDLSCs decided the tissue regeneration effects.

Previous studies found that the immunomodulatory properties of PDLSCs partially depended on soluble factors, which could be produced by PDLSCs after being stimulated

(a)

(b)

(c)

(d)

(e)

(f)

(g)

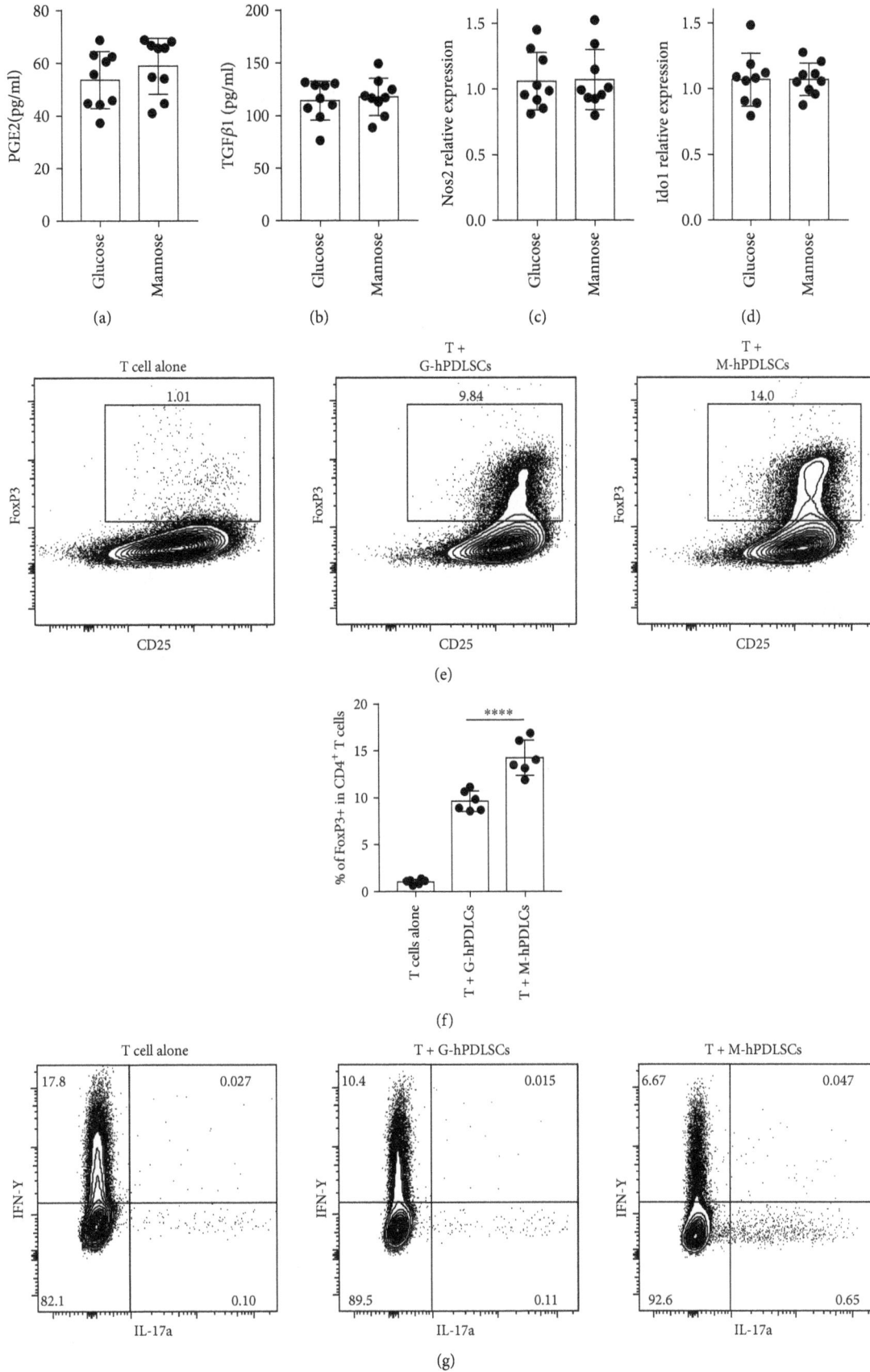

FIGURE 2: Continued.

(h)

(i)

(j)

(k)

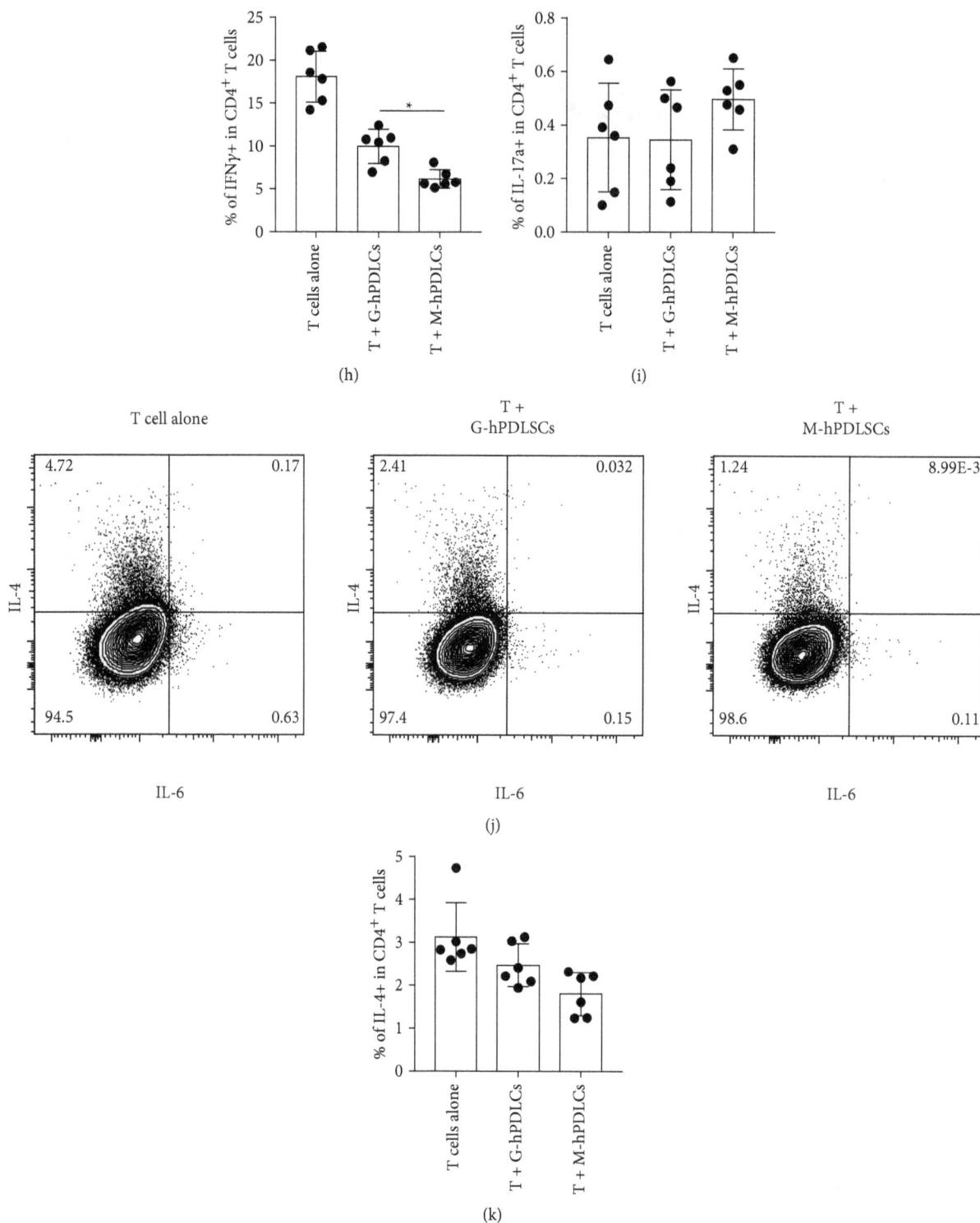

FIGURE 2: M-hPDLSCs induced more T cell differentiation into Tregs. (a, b) The results of ELISA showed that there was no difference in PGE2 and TGFβ1 between T + M-hPDLSCs and T + G-hPDLSCs. (c, d) RT-PCR results showed that there is no difference in Nos2 and Ido1 between T + M-hPDLSCs and T + G-hPDLSCs. (e, f) FoxP3 have been detected by flow cytometry. Compared with T + G-hPDLSCs, more FoxP3 was detected in T + M-hPDLSCs. (g, h) IFNγ and IL-17 have been detected by flow cytometry. More IFNγ could be detected in T + M-hPDLSCs. There was no difference in IL-17 between T + G-hPDLSCs and T + M-hPDLSCs. (j, k) There was no difference in IL-4 between T + G-hPDLSCs and T + M-hPDLSCs. Student's t-test was used to analyze statistical significance. All error bars represent s.d. ($n = 9$). *$P \leq 0.05$ and ****$P \leq 0.0001$.

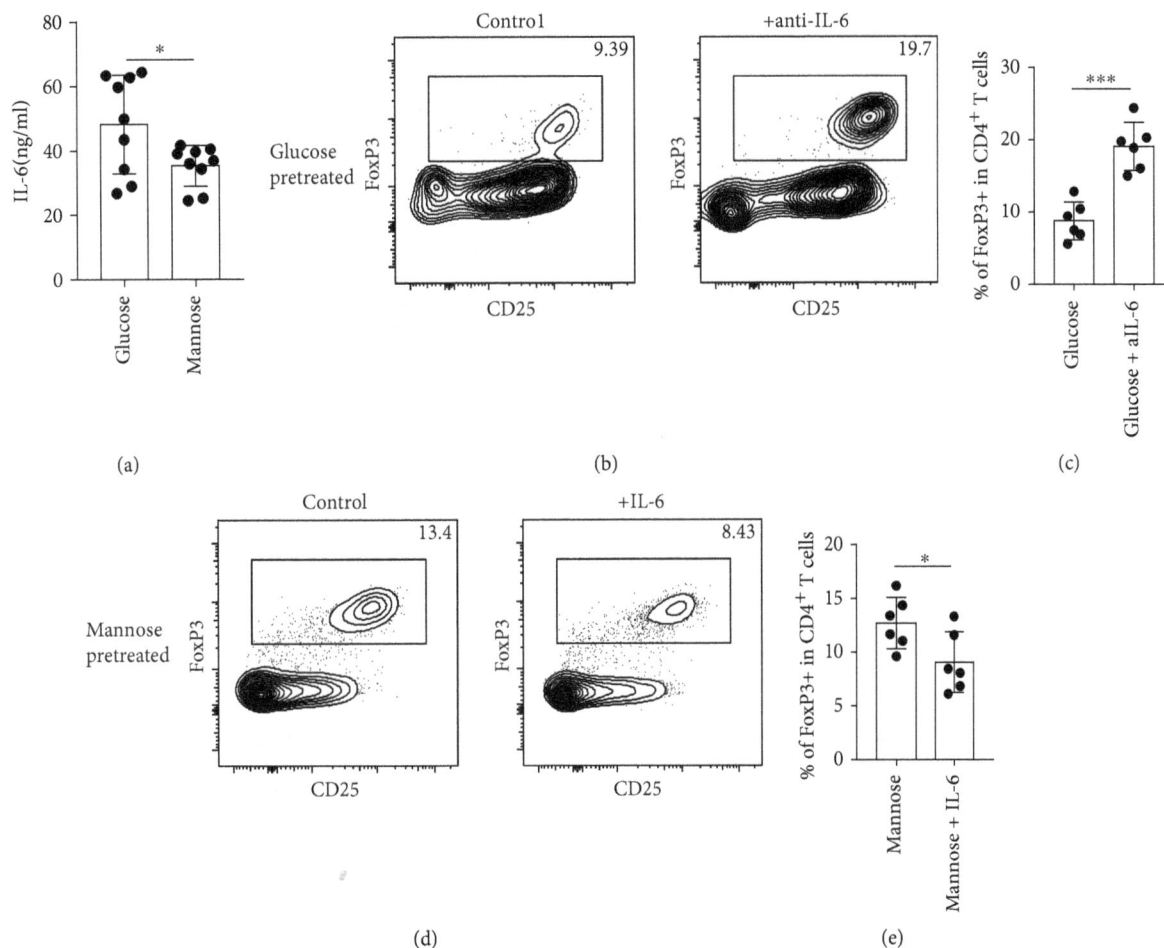

FIGURE 3: D-mannose inhibited IL-6 secretion of hPDLSCs to induce more T cell differentiation into Tregs. (a) Compared with T + G-hPDLSCs, less IL-6 could be detected in T + M-hPDLSCs. (b, c) Anti-IL-6 could increase the FoxP3 level in T + G-hPDLSCs. (d, e) Increased IL-6 could reduce the FoxP3 level in T + M-hPDLSCs. Student's t-test was used to analyze statistical significance. All error bars represent s.d. ($n = 9$). $^{*}P \leq 0.05$ and $^{***}P \leq 0.001$.

by activated PBMNCs. When PDLSCs were cocultured with activated PBMNCs, PDLSCs could produce more TGFβ1, indoleamine 2, 3-dioxygenase (IDO), and hepatocyte growth factor (HGF) [4]. hPDLSCs also could regulate the function of B cells. On the one hand, hPDLSCs could inhibit human B cell proliferation, differentiation, and chemotactic behavior. On the other hand, hPDLSCs could increase B cell viability by secreting interleukin-6. It was reported that the immunoregulatory capability of hPDLSCs to human B cells was through cell-to-cell contact manner, and programmed death-1 (PD-1) as well as its ligand (PD-L1) interaction was one of the critical ways in the process [32]. However, the interplay between host and transplanted PDLSCs during periodontal regeneration is unclear.

Recently, mannose was found as an important function in immune cell activity. D-Mannose could promote activation of the latent form of TGFβ and enhance naïve CD4^{+} T cell differentiation to Treg cells. However, the affection of D-mannose on the PDLSC characteristics was unclear. In this study, we found that D-mannose could affect hPDLSCs immunomodulation. hPDLSCs pretreated by D-mannose could inhibit T cell proliferation. As more results have shown,

hPDLSCs pretreated by D-mannose could induce more T cell differentiation into Tregs and IL-6 played a key role in this process. Less IL-6 has been detected in T + M-hPDLSCs. When we increased the IL-6 level, less Treg cells could be detected in T + M-hPDLSCs; and when IL-6 was reduced, the number of Treg cells was increased in T + G-hPDLSCs. As we know, TGFβ is an essential cytokine for inducing Foxp3+ Treg cells and enhanced TGFβ signaling is an underlying mechanism. In our current study, TGFβ levels between glucose- and D-mannose-pretreated groups had no significant difference.

IL-6 is a common cytokine and participates in almost every organ system's physiology. IL-6 could stimulate acute-phase responses, hematopoiesis, and immune reactions of the host to contribute to host defense. IL-6 plays an important role in the process of innate-acquired immune response. IL-6 could stimulate naïve CD4^{+} T cell differentiation [33]. It has been reported that IL-6 combined with TGFβ is necessary for the process of naïve CD4^{+} T cell differentiation into Th17 [34]. IL-6 also could inhibit Treg differentiation induced by TGFβ [35]. IL-6 plays a very important role in regulating Treg/Th17 balance. Breaking of the Treg/

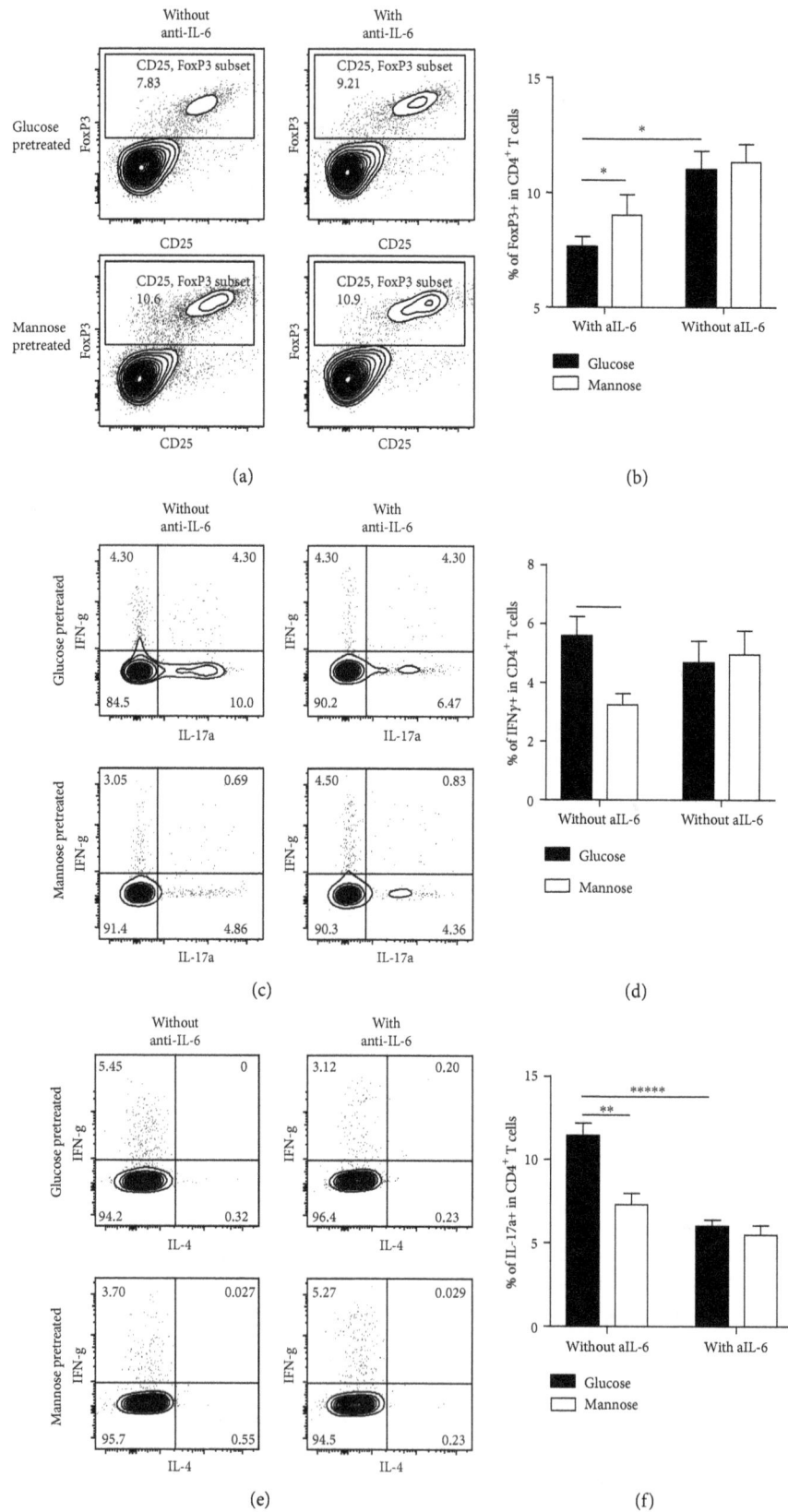

(a)

(b)

(c)

(d)

(e)

(f)

FIGURE 4: D-mannose inhibited IL-6 secretion of hPDLSCs to induce more T cell differentiation into Tregs in vivo. (a, b) IL-6 reduction could increase the number of FoxP3 and CD25 double positive cells in T + G-hPDLSC mixed cell-injected mice. (c, d) In vivo, compared with the T + G-hPDLSCs group, there was less Th1 cell in T + M-hPDLSC mixed cell-injected mice. (c, e) In vivo, IL-6 reduction could decrease the number of Th17 cell in T + G-hPDLSC mixed cell-injected mice. Student's t-test and one way ANOVA were used to analyze statistical significance. All error bars represent s.d. ($n = 9$). $^*P \leq 0.05$, $^{**}P \leq 0.01$, and $^{*****}P \leq 0.00001$.

Th17 balance could be responsible for the collapse of immunological tolerance [36]. Further in vivo results also verified the important function of IL-6 in the process of D-mannose-regulating hPDLSC-stimulating Treg differentiation from T cells. It was reported that integrin $\alpha v\beta 8$ and reactive oxygen species (ROS) were essential for D-mannose-treated activation of TGFβ T cells. However, how the detailed mechanism of D-mannose mediated IL-6 inhibition remains unknown.

In conclusion, our present results showed a new function of D-mannose on hPDLSC immunomodulation, exploring the important role of IL-6 in the process of D-mannose-regulating hPDLSC immunomodulation. Our findings provide more information for the basic immunological mechanisms of hexose sugars and provided the possible clinical applications of D-mannose.

Authors' Contributions

Lijia Guo and Yanan Hou contributed equally to this work.

Acknowledgments

This work was supported by grants from the National Nature Science Foundation of China (81600891 to Lijia Guo), Beijing Municipal Administration of Hospitals Clinical Medicine Development of Special Funding Support (ZYLX201703 to Yuxing Bai), Beijing Excellent Talent (2014000021469G251 to Lijia Guo), and Capital Characteristic Clinic Project (Z161100000516203 to Lijia Guo).

References

[1] B. L. Pihlstrom, B. S. Michalowicz, and N. W. Johnson, "Periodontal diseases," *Lancet*, vol. 366, no. 9499, pp. 1809–1820, 2005.

[2] H. Ikeda, Y. Sumita, M. Ikeda et al., "Engineering bone formation from human dental pulp- and periodontal ligament-derived cells," *Annals of Biomedical Engineering*, vol. 39, no. 1, pp. 26–34, 2011.

[3] N. Wada, D. Menicanin, S. Shi, P. M. Bartold, and S. Gronthos, "Immunomodulatory properties of human periodontal ligament stem cells," *Journal of Cellular Physiology*, vol. 219, no. 3, pp. 667–676, 2009.

[4] K. A. Cho, J. K. Lee, Y. H. Kim, M. Park, S. Y. Woo, and K. H. Ryu, "Mesenchymal stem cells ameliorate B-cell-mediated immune responses and increase IL-10-expressing regulatory B cells in an EBI3-dependent manner," *Cellular & Molecular Immunology*, 2017.

[5] D. Wang, S. P. Li, J. S. Fu, L. Bai, and L. Guo, "Resveratrol augments therapeutic efficiency of mouse bone marrow mesenchymal stem cell-based therapy in experimental autoimmune encephalomyelitis," *International Journal of Developmental Neuroscience*, vol. 49, pp. 60–66, 2016.

[6] R. A. Contreras, F. E. Figueroa, F. Djouad, and P. Luz-Crawford, "Mesenchymal stem cells regulate the innate and adaptive immune responses dampening arthritis progression," *Stem Cells International*, vol. 2016, 10 pages, 2016.

[7] R. Tang, F. Wei, L. Wei, S. Wang, and G. Ding, "Osteogenic differentiated periodontal ligament stem cells maintain their immunomodulatory capacity," *Journal of Tissue Engineering and Regenerative Medicine*, vol. 8, no. 3, pp. 226–232, 2014.

[8] D. Liu, J. Xu, O. Liu et al., "Mesenchymal stem cells derived from inflamed periodontal ligaments exhibit impaired immunomodulation," *Journal of Clinical Periodontology*, vol. 39, no. 12, pp. 1174–1182, 2012.

[9] A. D. Sawant, A. T. Abdelal, and D. G. Ahearn, "Purification and characterization of the anti-Candida toxin of Pichia anomala WC 65," *Antimicrobial Agents and Chemotherapy*, vol. 33, no. 1, pp. 48–52, 1989.

[10] B. Kranjčec, D. Papeš, and S. Altarac, "D-mannose powder for prophylaxis of recurrent urinary tract infections in women: a randomized clinical trial," *World Journal of Urology*, vol. 32, no. 1, pp. 79–84, 2014.

[11] S. Altarac and D. Papeš, "Use of D-mannose in prophylaxis of recurrent urinary tract infections (UTIs) in women," *BJU International*, vol. 113, no. 1, pp. 9-10, 2014.

[12] L. Domenici, M. Monti, C. Bracchi et al., "D-mannose: a promising support for acute urinary tract infections in women: a pilot study," *European Review for Medical and Pharmacological Sciences*, vol. 20, no. 13, pp. 2920–2925, 2016.

[13] J. R. Etchison and H. H. Freeze, "Enzymatic assay of D-mannose in serum," *Clinical Chemistry*, vol. 43, no. 3, pp. 533–538, 1997.

[14] A. Schneider, C. Thiel, J. Rindermann et al., "Successful prenatal mannose treatment for congenital disorder of glycosylation-Ia in mice," *Nature Medicine*, vol. 18, no. 1, pp. 71–73, 2011.

[15] G. Alton, M. Hasilik, R. Niehues et al., "Direct utilization of mannose for mammalian glycoprotein biosynthesis," *Glycobiology*, vol. 8, no. 3, pp. 285–295, 1998.

[16] D. Zhang, C. Chia, X. Jiao et al., "D-mannose induces regulatory T cells and suppresses immunopathology," *Nature Medicine*, vol. 23, no. 9, pp. 1036–1045, 2017.

[17] Z. Rutter-Locher, T. O. Smith, I. Giles, and N. Sofat, "Association between systemic lupus erythematosus and periodontitis: a systematic review and meta-analysis," *Frontiers in Immunology*, vol. 8, p. 1295, 2017.

[18] D. F. Kinane and G. J. Marshall, "Periodontal manifestations of systemic disease," *Australian Dental Journal*, vol. 46, no. 1, pp. 2–12, 2001.

[19] D. F. Kinane, P. G. Stathopoulou, and P. N. Papapanou, "Periodontal diseases," *Nature Reviews Disease Primers*, vol. 3, p. 17038, 2017.

[20] L. Huang, J. Liang, Y. Geng et al., "Directing adult human periodontal ligament-derived stem cells to retinal fate," *Investigative Ophthalmology & Visual Science*, vol. 54, no. 6, pp. 3965–3974, 2013.

[21] B. M. Seo, M. Miura, S. Gronthos et al., "Investigation of multipotent postnatal stem cells from human periodontal ligament," *Lancet*, vol. 364, no. 9429, pp. 149–155, 2004.

[22] Y. Liu, Y. Zheng, G. Ding et al., "Periodontal ligament stem cell-mediated treatment for periodontitis in miniature swine," *Stem Cells*, vol. 26, no. 4, pp. 1065–1073, 2008.

[23] G. Ding, Y. Liu, W. Wang et al., "Allogeneic periodontal ligament stem cell therapy for periodontitis in swine," *Stem Cells*, vol. 28, no. 10, pp. 1829–1838, 2010.

[24] C. D. Li, W. Y. Zhang, H. L. Li et al., "Mesenchymal stem cells derived from human placenta suppress allogeneic umbilical cord blood lymphocyte proliferation," *Cell Research*, vol. 15, no. 7, pp. 539–547, 2005.

[25] K. Le Blanc, C. Tammik, K. Rosendahl, E. Zetterberg, and O. Ringdén, "HLA expression and immunologic properties of differentiated and undifferentiated mesenchymal stem cells," *Experimental Hematology*, vol. 31, no. 10, pp. 890–896, 2003.

[26] F. Djouad, P. Plence, C. Bony et al., "Immunosuppressive effect of mesenchymal stem cells favors tumor growth in allogeneic animals," *Blood*, vol. 102, no. 10, pp. 3837–3844, 2003.

[27] Y. Liu, L. Wang, T. Kikuiri et al., "Mesenchymal stem cell-based tissue regeneration is governed by recipient T lymphocytes via IFN-γ and TNF-α," *Nature Medicine*, vol. 17, no. 12, pp. 1594–1601, 2011.

[28] M. Di Nicola, C. Carlo-Stella, M. Magni et al., "Human bone marrow stromal cells suppress T-lymphocyte proliferation induced by cellular or nonspecific mitogenic stimuli," *Blood*, vol. 99, no. 10, pp. 3838–3843, 2002.

[29] D. V. Krysko, G. Denecker, N. Festjens et al., "Macrophages use different internalization mechanisms to clear apoptotic and necrotic cells," *Cell Death and Differentiation*, vol. 13, no. 12, pp. 2011–2022, 2006.

[30] S. Aggarwal and M. F. Pittenger, "Human mesenchymal stem cells modulate allogeneic immune cell responses," *Blood*, vol. 105, no. 4, pp. 1815–1822, 2005.

[31] S. Zhao, R. Wehner, M. Bornhauser, R. Wassmuth, M. Bachmann, and M. Schmitz, "Immunomodulatory properties of mesenchymal stromal cells and their therapeutic consequences for immune-mediated disorders," *Stem Cells and Development*, vol. 19, no. 5, pp. 607–614, 2010.

[32] O. Liu, J. Xu, G. Ding et al., "Periodontal ligament stem cells regulate B lymphocyte function via programmed cell death protein 1," *Stem Cells*, vol. 31, no. 7, pp. 1371–1382, 2013.

[33] T. Tanaka, M. Narazaki, and T. Kishimoto, "IL-6 in inflammation, immunity, and disease," *Cold Spring Harbor Perspectives in Biology*, vol. 6, no. 10, article a016295, 2014.

[34] T. Korn, E. Bettelli, M. Oukka, and V. K. Kuchroo, "IL-17 and Th17 cells," *Annual Review of Immunology*, vol. 27, no. 1, pp. 485–517, 2009.

[35] E. Bettelli, Y. Carrier, W. Gao et al., "Reciprocal developmental pathways for the generation of pathogenic effector TH17 and regulatory T cells," *Nature*, vol. 441, no. 7090, pp. 235–238, 2006.

[36] A. Kimura and T. Kishimoto, "IL-6: regulator of Treg/Th17 balance," *European Journal of Immunology*, vol. 40, no. 7, pp. 1830–1835, 2010.

8

Synaptic Plasticity of Human Umbilical Cord Mesenchymal Stem Cell Differentiating into Neuron-like Cells In Vitro Induced by Edaravone

Yunpeng Shi,[1,2] **Chengrui Nan,**[1,2] **Zhongjie Yan,**[1,2] **Liqiang Liu,**[1,2] **Jingjing Zhou,**[3] **Zongmao Zhao**[1,2] **and Depei Li**[3]

[1]*Department of Neurosurgery, The Second Hospital of Hebei Medical University, Shijiazhuang, Hebei 050000, China*
[2]*Neuroscience Research Center, Hebei Medical University, Shijiazhuang, Hebei 050000, China*
[3]*Department of Anesthesiology and Critical Care, The University of Texas MD Anderson Cancer Center, Houston, TX 77030, USA*

Correspondence should be addressed to Zongmao Zhao; zzm692017@sina.com

Academic Editor: Weijun Su

Objective. The human umbilical cord mesenchymal stem cells (hUMSCs) are characterized with the potential ability to differentiate to several types of cells. Edaravone has been demonstrated to prevent the hUMSCs from the oxidative damage, especially its ability in antioxidative stress. We hypothesized that Edaravone induces the hUMSCs into the neuron-like cells. *Methods.* The hUMSCs were obtained from the human umbilical cord tissue. The differentiation of hUMSCs was induced by Edaravone with three different doses: 0.65 mg/ml, 1.31 mg/ml, and 2.62 mg/ml. Flow cytometry was used to detect the cell markers. Protein and mRNA levels of nestin, neuron-specific enolase (NSE), and glial fibrillary acidic protein (GFAP) were detected by Western blot and RT-PCR. The expression of synaptophysin (SYN), growth-associated protein 43 (GAP43), and postsynaptic density 95 (PSD95) was detected by Real-Time PCR. *Results.* As long as the prolongation of the culture, the hUMSCs displayed with the long strips or long fusiform to fat and then characterized with the radial helix growth. By using flow cytometry, the cultured hUMSCs at the 3rd, 5th, and 10th passages were expressed with CD73, CD90, and CD105 but not CD11b, CD19, CD34, CD45, and HLA-DR. Most of the hUMSCs cultured with Edaravone exhibited typical nerve-immediately characters including the cell body contraction, increased refraction, and protruding one or more elongated protrusions, which were not found in the control group without addition of Edaravone. NSE, nestin, and GFAP were positive in these neuron-like cells. Edaravone dose-dependently increased expression levels of NSE, nestin, and GFAP. After replacement of maintenance fluid, neuron-like cells continued to be cultured for five days. These neuron-like cells were positive for SYN, PSD95, and GAP43. *Conclusion.* Edaravone can dose-dependently induce hUMSCs to differentiate into neuron-like cells that expressed the neuronal markers including NSE, nestin, and GFAP and synaptic makers such as SYN, PSD95, and GAP43.

1. Introduction

Stem cells are characterized with self-renewal ability and multidirectional differentiation potential. For example, bone marrow, umbilical cord, and epidermis [1–3] were able to differentiate into various functional cells induced by different approaches [4]. In particular, mesenchymal stem cells (MSCs), as one of pluripotent stem cells, have been demonstrated to be capable to differentiate into pluripotent cells [5] including vascular endothelial cells [6], neuron-like cells [7, 8], corneal endothelial cell [9], and hepatocyte-like cells [10]. The differentiation ability probably explains why MSCs have been reported to play important roles in neuronal protection from the oxidative stress, inhibition of ischemia-induced necrosis, and apoptosis [11]. These evidences indicate the probability that the induction of MSC differentiation for neuronal protection would be an effective method for eliminating brain ischemia injury in a clinical setting. The human umbilical cord MSCs (hUMSCs) have the advantages of simple convenient preparation, feasible source, nontraumatic risk of infection, and its low immunogenicity and immunosuppression, so the hUMSCs turn to be an ideal source used as the engineering cells in studying stem cell differentiation.

Edaravone, a low-molecular weight agent, can scavenge oxygen free radicals and decrease the ability of the xanthine oxidase and hypoxanthine oxidase and reduce the formation of prostacyclin, thus enhance the tissue antioxidative capacity [12]. Edaravone can penetrate the blood-brain barrier, and it has been used in clinic to decrease the ischemia-induced injury in the brain such as acute cerebral infarction, cerebral hemorrhage, and even amyotrophic lateral sclerosis [13]. The early treatment of acute cerebral infarction with Edaravone can prevent the reduction of cerebral blood flow around the lesion area and increase the neuronal antioxidant ability. More importantly, Edaravone was reported to prevent the MSC damage from hypoxia and activate the potential for angiogenesis [14], but it is not known whether Edaravone can induce the differentiation of hUMSCs into the neuronal-like cells that would be explained as another mechanisms underlying its benefits to treat ischemia-induced neuronal injury. The aim of this study was to observe the effects of Edaravone on the differentiation of hUMSCs into neuron-like cells and to further explore the possible mechanisms.

As the main part of the neuron transmission of information, synapses are the structural basis of the interconnected transmission of information between neurons. It is the basic structure and functional unit of the neural loop. The establishment and maintenance of synapses depend on the corresponding expression of many genes. The number and density of synaptophysin (SYN) can indirectly reflect the number and density of synapses [15]. GAP43 (growth-associated protein 43) is closely related to axonal growth and is a key factor for axonal growth and elongation [16]. PSD95 (Postsynaptic density protein 95) is the most important scaffold protein on the postsynaptic membrane, which plays an important role in the process of synapse formation. We use Edaravone to induce hUMSCs to differentiate into nerve-like cells. We continue to culture the cells and detect the expression of specific synapse markers, SYN, GAP43, and PSD95, which lays the foundation for further cell electrophysiological study.

2. Materials and Methods

2.1. Materials and Chemicals. The umbilical cord was obtained from the Department of Obstetrics and Gynecology of the Second Affiliated Hospital of Hebei Medical University. All the participants signed the relevant consent letter to use the umbilical cord for the present research. The following reagents were obtained commercially: Edaravone (packing: 20 g, purity: 99.7%, batch no.: A06-131204) was provided by Jilin Province Boda Pharmaceutical Co. Ltd. FBS (BI, Israel); L-DMEM/F-12, H-DMEM/F-12 (GIBCO, Grand Island, USA); EDTA and DMSO (Sigma-Aldrich Co. LLC., St. Louis, MO 63178,USA); FITC-CD19, FITC-CD34, PE-CD11b, PE-CD73, PE-CD90, PE-CD45, and PE-CD105 (Becton, Dickinson and Company, Franklin Lakes, New Jersey 07417-1880); PS immunohistochemistry

kit (Beijing Zhongshan Golden Bridge Company, China); Taq PCR star mix (Genstar, China); EasyScript First-Strand cDNA synthesis supermix (TransGen Biotech, China); TB Green™ Premix Ex Taq™ II (Tli RNaseH Plus) (TaKaRa Japan); cell *RIPA* Lysis Buffer and phenylmethylsulfonyl fluoride (Solarbio, Beijing, China); polyclonal antibodies of neuron-specific enolase (NSE) and nestin (OriGene, USA); glial fibrillary acidic protein (GFAP) and glyceraldehyde-3-phosphate dehydrogenase (Affbiotech, USA); and polyclonal antibodies of synaptophysin, growth-associated protein 43, and postsynaptic density 95 (Abways, China).

2.2. Isolation and Culture of hUMSCs. The obtained umbilical cords were placed in H-DMEM/F12 culture medium under aseptic conditions, stored at 4°C, and then timely transported to a cell culture room to carry out the following steps. Each umbilical cord was rinsed thoroughly with D-Hank's medium. After removing the blood sample, umbilical artery, and umbilical vein, the umbilical cord mesenchymal tissue was cut into pieces of 1 mm^3 in size, digested with 0.2% collagenase II, and placed in a culture flask containing 2 ng/ml EGF, 20% FBS, 25 mM L-Glu, and 100 U/ml penicillin-streptomycin mixture at 37°C with 5% CO_2 and saturation humidity to obtain primary cells. Half of the culture medium was replaced every 24 h, and it was replenished every 3 days. When the cells achieved 80–90% confluency, the medium was removed, and cells were rinsed two times with PBS and then digested with trypsin (0.25%)–EDTA (0.2 g/l) into single cells for passaging at the ratio of 1 : 3. The culture medium was H-DMEM/F12 containing 100 U/ml of a penicillin-streptomycin mixture and 10% FBS.

2.3. Analysis of Cellular Phenotype of hUMSCs. In the logarithmic phase of growth, hUMSCs were digested with trypsin and rinsed with PBS, and then, the single cell suspension was aliquot into 10 tubes at 1×10^6 cells/tube. Separately, mouse anti-human monoclonal antibodies (5 μl/each) against CD11-PE, CD45-PE, CD73-PE, CD90-PE, CD105-PE, HLA-DR-PE, CD19-FITC, and CD34-FITC were added to the 8 tubes, while anti-mouse IgG1-PE and anti-mouse IgG1-FITC (each 7 μl) were added to the other two tubes as isotype controls. After mixing the contents thoroughly, the tubes were incubated at 4°C for 30 min. Thereafter, the cells were rinsed with PBS and then centrifuged. The supernatant was discarded, and the cells were resuspended with 400 μl of PBS for the followed analysis by flow cytometry.

2.4. Differentiation of hUMSCs into Neuron-like Cells. The hUMSCs were obtained at the 3rd passage of cells according to the logarithmic growth phase. The hUMSCs were separated into four groups including three groups treated with different dose of Edaravone (low-dose, LH; medium-dose, MD; and high-dose, HD) and one control group (Con). MSCs were placed in a cell culture chamber. When about 80% of the cells adhered to the wall, the whole culture solution was discarded. Neurobasal medium containing 50 ng/ml bFGF was first induced for 24 hours. After washing with PBS, LD, MD, and HD groups were, respectively, added with Edaravone concentrations of 0.65 mg/ml, 1.31 mg/ml, and

2.62 mg/ml for incubation with the Neurobasal medium. Then, the hUMSCs were induced in the incubator, and the morphological changes of the cells were observed by inverted phase contrast microscope.

2.5. Calculation of Positive Rate of Neuron-like Cells. Under the inverted microscope, 3 nonoverlapping fields were randomly selected; the total cell number and the number of neuron-like cells were counted, and the rate of neuron-like cells were calculated.

2.6. Immunochemistry Analysis. After incubation with Edaravone for 12 h, expression levels of neuronal-specific proteins NSE, nestin, and GFAP were detected by immunocytochemistry as follows. The cells were rinsed with PBS gently and fixed with 4% paraformaldehyde for 20 min at room temperature followed by the rinses with PBS three times for 5 min each time. The cell membranes were disrupted with 0.5% Triton-X-100 in PBS for 15 min at room temperature away from light and then incubated with 3% H_2O_2 at room temperature for 5 min. The cells were blocked by the normal goat serum at room temperature for 15 min. The blocked cells were induced by the primary antibodies against NSE, nestin, and GFAP at 4°C overnight. On the second day, the appropriate biotinylated secondary antibody was added for incubation at room temperature for 15 min, then followed by horseradish peroxidase-conjugated streptavidin at room temperature for 15 min. Finally, the cells were stained with freshly prepared DAB for 1 min and counterstained with hematoxylin before finally rinsed repeatedly with water. Under the inverted microscope, 3 nonoverlapping fields were randomly selected; the total cell number and the number of neuron-like cells were counted and the rate of neuron-like cells calculated.

2.7. RT-PCR Analysis. Total RNA was extracted by TRIpure Reagent (Aidlab Biotechnologies Co. Ltd., China) following the manufacturer's instructions and quantified with an Ultramicro ultraviolet visible light meter (Gene Company Limited, China). cDNA was synthesized from total RNA with Easy-Script First-Strand cDNA synthesis supermix (TransGen Biotech, China) following the manufacturer's instructions. Semiquantitative PCR was performed using Taq PCR star mix (Genstar, China) with the following reaction conditions: 1 cycle of 94°C for 3 min; 30 cycles of 94°C for 30 s, T_m (°C) for 30 s, and 72°C for 30 s; and a final extension at 72°C for 10 min. A 10 μl of each PCR product was analyzed by electrophoresis, and the gene expression levels were calculated using GAPDH as the internal control. The primers were designed using Primer 5.0 software and are shown: nestin: F-TCCA GAAACTCAAGCACCACT and R-TCCACCGTATCTTC CCACCT 342 bp, NSE: F-GGCACTCTACCAGGACTTTG and R-GCGATGACTCACCATAACCC 286 bp, GFAP: F-GTCCATGTGGAGCTTGAC and R-CATTGAGCAGGTC CTGGTAC 406 bp, and GAPDH: F-AGAAGGCTGGGGCT CATTTG and R-AGGGGCCATCCACAGTCTTC 258 bp.

2.8. Western Blot Analysis. Cell lysates were prepared with cell *RIPA* Lysis Buffer and phenylmethylsulfonyl fluoride, and protein concentrations were determined with an

Ultramicro ultraviolet visible light meter (Gene Company limited, China).Total protein (16 μg) of each lysate was electrophoresed in 10% SDS-PAGE gel and transferred to a polyvinylidene fluoride (PVDF) membrane (Solarbio, Beijing, China). The membranes were blocked by 10% nonfat milk for 2 h at room temperature and incubated with GFAP, nestin, and NSE primary antibodies at 4°C overnight. After rinsing with PBS for 10 min, the membranes were incubated with anti-rabbit IgG (1 : 2000, Affbiotech, USA) for 2 h at room temperature and visualized by Supersignal West Pico Chemiluminescent Substrate (Thermo Scientific, USA) using the Image alphaEaseFC system (Alpha Innotech, USA).

2.9. Continuous Culture of Neuron-like Cells. We chose a group of cells with the highest positive rate of nerve cell markers and stable expression. After 24 hours of induction, we clean it with PBS, replace the maintenance fluid, and continue training for five days. The maintenance fluid is formulated with Neurobasal medium containing 2% B27 and 50 ng/ml bFGF. The inverted phase contrast microscope dynamically observed the morphological changes of each group.

2.10. Real-Time PCR Analysis. Total RNA was extracted by TRIpure Reagent (Aidlab Biotechnologies Co. Ltd, China) following the manufacturer's instructions and quantified with Ultramicro ultraviolet visible light meter (Gene Company Limited, China). cDNA was synthesized from total RNA with EasyScript First-Strand cDNA synthesis supermix (TransGen Biotech, China) following the manufacturer's instructions. Real-Time PCR was performed using TB Green™ Premix Ex Taq™ II (Tli RNaseH Plus) by TaKaRa. The gene expression levels were calculated using GAPDH as the internal control. The primers were designed using Primer 5.0 software and are shown: SYN: F–CACTACTAC AGAGGGAAAATGAATG and R-CACGGTGCCCAGAC AGGT 108 bp, GAP43: F-GAAGGGGGAGGGTGATGC and R-CTTGGAGGACGGCGAGTTAT 130 bp, PSD95: F-GCGGAGCAACCCCAAAAG and R-GATGAACCCAA TGTCGTCGG 196 bp, and GAPDH: F-ACGGATTTGGT CGTATTGGG and R-GATGAACCCAATGTCGTCGG 210 bp.

2.11. Statistical Analysis. All the data were expressed as mean ± s.e. SPSS19.0 was used for statistical analysis. One-way ANOVA was used in three or more group comparison followed by SNK method within two separate groups. $P < 0.05$ was considered to be significantly different.

3. Results

3.1. Growth and Morphological Changes of hUMSCs. Primary cultured cells were passaged at the ratio of 1 : 1. After 12 hours of passage, most of the cells adhered to growth, and the cells were elongated or long fusiform (Figure 1(a)). With the increase of incubation time, the cells gradually became longer and adhered completely, and the morphology became flat. Cell growth was rapid, in about 5 days after passage can be completely adhere to the wall and grow. The cells had radial or spiral growth according to the ratio of 1 : 2 or 1 : 3 subculture. Continue to culture, the cells were overlapped

(a)

(b)

(c)

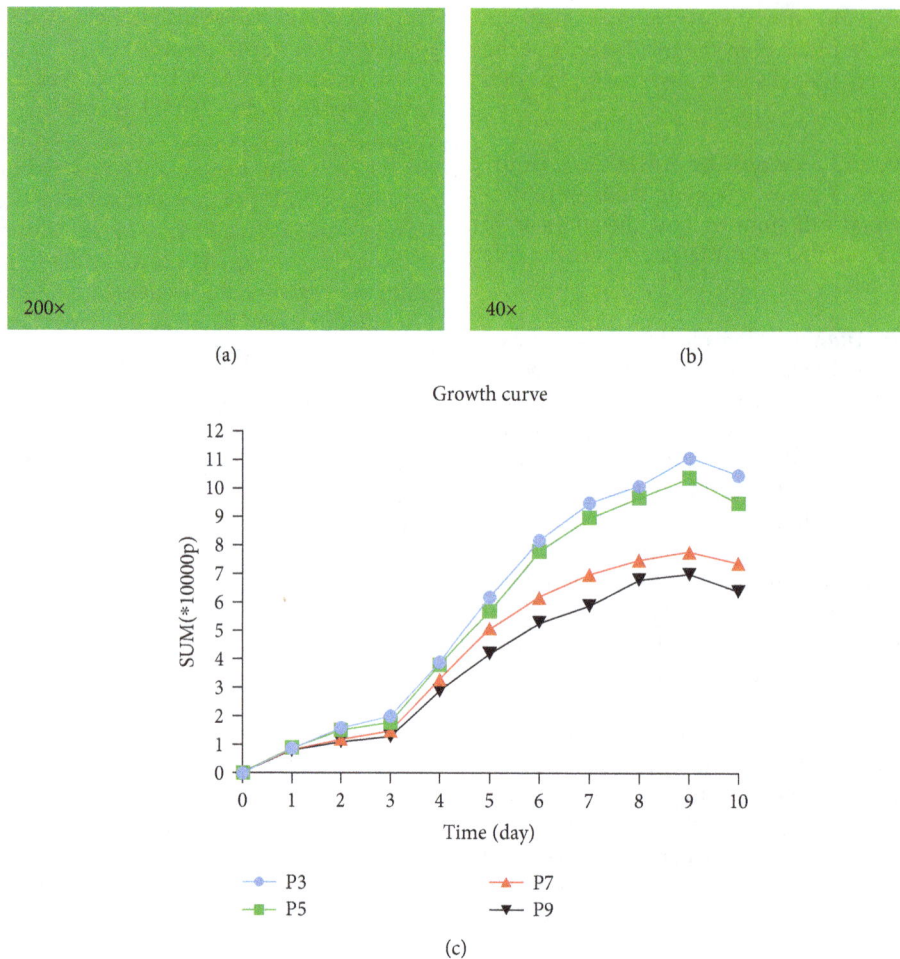

FIGURE 1: (a) (200x) Cells were elongated or long fusiform. (b) (40x) The cells were spirally divergent. (c) The growth curve of the 3rd, 5th, 7th, and 9th passage cells.

showing the spiral divergent growth around the center, and the local density was increased (Figure 1(b)). The cells were cultured until the ninth passage, and the cell homogeneity and growth were good. Because of the relatively small number of the 1st and 2nd passage (P1 and P2) cells and the good growth condition of the 3rd passage (P3) cells, we selected the 3rd passage hUMSCs with good growth status. The growth curve is plotted in Figure 1(c).

3.2. Cellular Phenotype of hUMSCs. We detected the cell phenotype of the 2nd, 5th, and 10th passages of hUMSCs by flow cytometry and found that all generations of cells tested coexpressed CD105, CD90, and CD73 but not CD11b, CD34, CD19, CD45, and histocompatibility antigen HLA-DR (MHC-II) (Figure 2).

3.3. Morphological and Quantitative Changes of Neuron-like Cells in Each Group. The hUMSC incubation with Edaravone showed the morphological properties of neuron-like cells. After 1 h incubation with low dose of Edaravone, the hUMSCs were presented with the sporadic cell body contraction, the enhanced refraction, and the cell morphology which turned into a long oval or round and out of one or more elongated processes (Figure 3(a)). After 4 h, the number of protrusions increased, and the length of protrusions and the number of bifurcations increased. 12 h later, about 50% of the cells had the above changes; adjacent cells protruding protuberances will gradually intertwine connected into a network. The percentage of neuron-like cells reached the peak at 24 hours. The hUMSCs in the MD group were presented with obvious changes after adding Edaravone for 1 hour. In the MD group at 12 hours, the percentage of neuron-like cells reached the peak, which was much earlier than the LD group. In the HD group, a large number of cells became neuron-like cells at 1 hour; neuron-like cells reached a peak at 4 hours (Figure 3(b)) and remained at high rates of change until 24 hours. Blank group was the control group. There was no significant change in 24 h after continuous observation. Under the inverted microscope, 3 nonoverlapping visual fields were randomly selected; the total number of cells and the number of neuron-like cells were counted, and the rate of neuron-like cells was calculated. The result was expressed by mean ± s.e. The curve of the rate of neuron-like cells in each group is shown in Figure 4. There was significant difference in the positive rate between each group, $P < 0.01$. The cells in the HD group

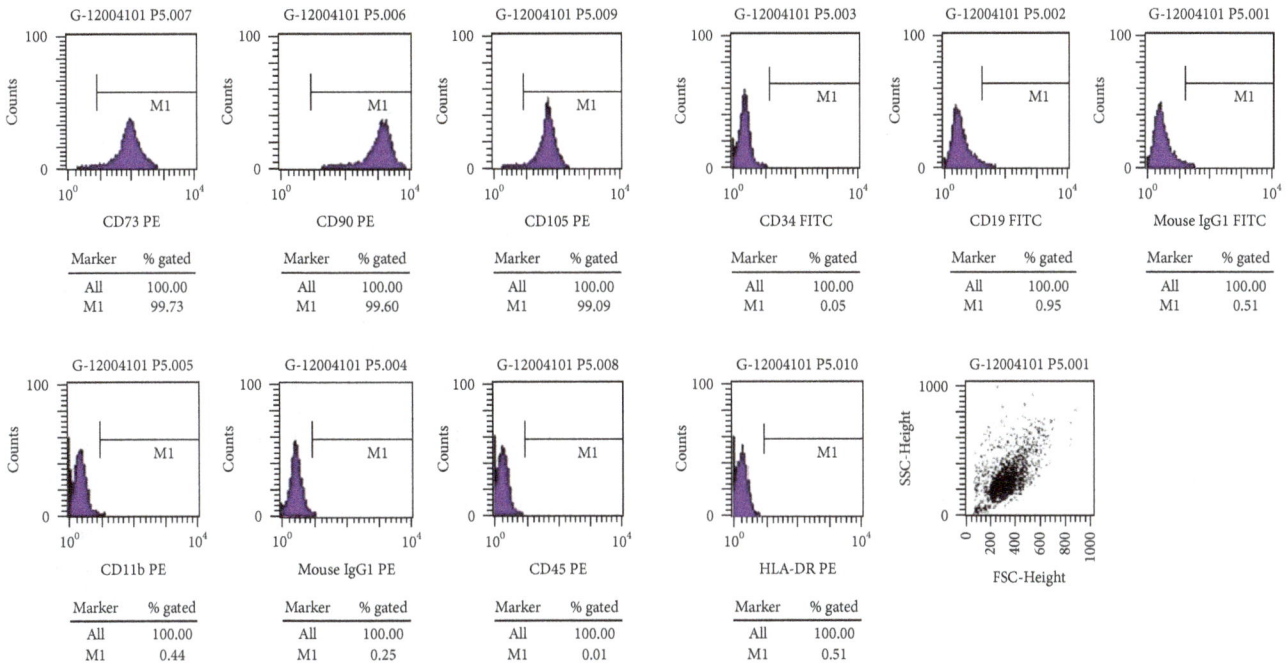

FIGURE 2: Cellular phenotype of hUMSCs detected by flow cytometry.

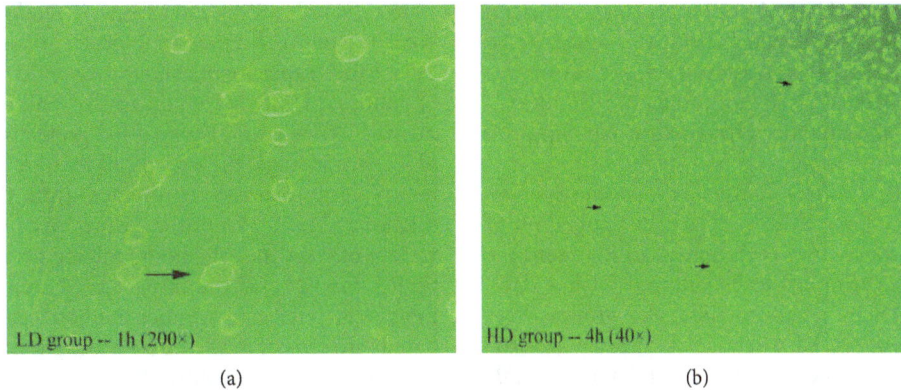

FIGURE 3: (a) (200x) Arrowheads show neuron-like cells. (b) (40x) A large number of neuron-like cells, arrowheads show neuron-like cells.

changed the most rapidly and maintained at a relatively high positive rate.

3.4. Result of Immunochemistry Analysis.

The neurological markers were detected after different concentrations of Edaravone incubation for 12 hours. As shown in Figure 5, brown cell bodies and the purple nucleus were nestin, NSE, or GFAP-positive cells. By contrast, no cells positively expressed these markers in the control group. Under the inverted microscope, 3 nonoverlapping visual fields were randomly selected; the total number of cells and the number of neuron-like cells were counted, and the rate of neuron-like cells was calculated. After 12 hours of induction, the positive rate of neuronal markers in each group is shown in Figure 6. The result was expressed by mean $\pm$ s.e. Differences in expression levels of nestin, GFAP, and NSE between any two groups were significant ($P < 0.05$). The results showed

that the expression of nerve markers in the HD group was the most.

3.5. RT-PCR Analysis Results of the HD Group.

The highest positive rate and stable expression of each nerve cell marker were detected in the HD group (2.62 mg/ml). Therefore, we use semiquantitative RT-PCR to detect the expression of mRNA in the HD group. According to the induction time, the groups were divided into blank, 2 h, 4 h, 6 h, 12 h, and 24 h. Through statistical neural marker expression amount and reference, to calculate the neural marker expression level, the result was expressed by mean $\pm$ s.e. RT-PCR results of NSE, nestin, GFAP, and GAPDH at each time point are shown in (Figure 7).

3.6. Western Blot Analysis Results of the HD Group.

We use Western blot analysis to detect the expression of protein in the HD group. According to the induction time, the groups

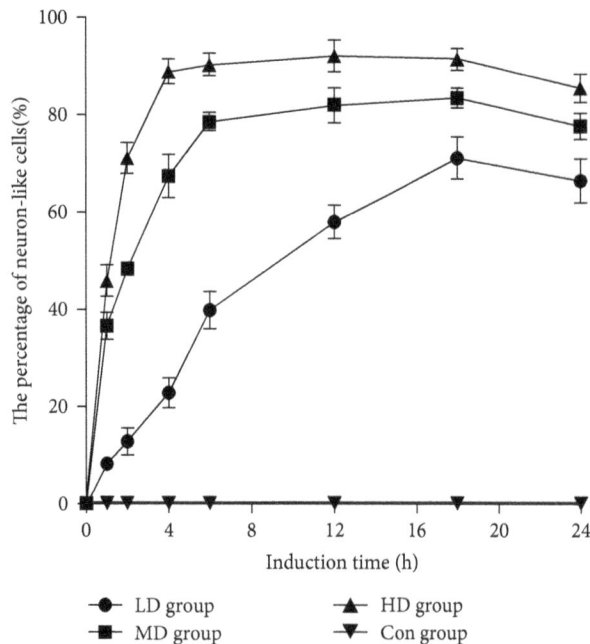

FIGURE 4: The percentage of neuron-like cells in each group was changed with the induction time.

were divided into blank, 2 h, 4 h, 6 h, 12 h, and 24 h. Through statistical neural marker expression amount and reference, to calculate the neural marker expression level, the result was expressed by mean ± s.e. Western blot results of NSE, nestin, GFAP, and GAPDH at each time point are shown in Figure 8.

3.7. Real-Time PCR Analysis Results of Specific Synapse Marker. We use Real-Time PCR to detect the expression of mRNA in the HD group. After replacement of maintenance fluid, nerve-like cells continued to be cultured for five days. According to maintenance culture time, the groups were divided into blank, 1 d, 2 d, 3 d, 4 d, and 5 d. Through statistical synaptic marker expression amount and reference, to calculate the synaptic markers expression level, the result was expressed by mean ± s.e. SYN, PSD95, and GAP43 at each time point are shown in Figure 9.

4. Discussion

With the rapid development of stem cell therapy research, stem cell transplantation is considered to be a potential treatment. At the same time, mesenchymal stem cells as a new source of cell therapy are of concern to a large number of scholars and researchers [17, 18]. In theory, pluripotent embryonic stem cells and the inner layer of blastocysts are the ideal cell transplantation option. However, the application of these cells is ethically restricted and has teratogenicity and tumorigenicity. MSC can have in vitro long-term survival and constantly amplify and induce differentiation into nerve, vascular endothelium, myocardial, corneal endothelium, cartilage, islet, and other functional cells [5]. The nervous system has little ability to repair itself after being damaged, so the nerve cells that are targeted by neural tissue engineering may be able to repair the damaged nerve tissue.

Previous studies have shown that bone marrow MSCs, neural stem cells, adipose MSC, umbilical cord MSC, umbilical cord blood MSC, and placental stem cells from different species and sources can be used for the treatment of neurological diseases. Shen et al. [19] report the treatment of ischemic or some degenerative disease caused by nervous system dysfunction; mesenchymal stem cells can provide a stable source of nutrition and reflect its multidirectional differentiation potential. At the same time, MSC do not appear to decrease with the number of passages, and there is no risk of differentiation with time [20]. This conclusion has been demonstrated in models of intracerebral hemorrhage and Parkinson's disease in rats and spinal cord injury in primates [21, 22]. Previous adult stem cell research mostly focused on bone marrow-derived mesenchymal stem cells. There are limitations and defects in bone marrow MSC because of limited number and difficulty in obtaining. The number and differentiation potential of bone marrow mesenchymal stem cells will decrease with age. At present, human umbilical cord mesenchymal stem cells (hUMSCs) are popular cells in cell culture. hUMSCs have the advantages of strong proliferative ability, low immunogenicity, stable amplification in vitro, wide source, without any ethical restriction, and can be divided into multiple germ layers. At present, there is no study on the differentiation of human umbilical cord mesenchymal stem cells induced by Edaravone. Therefore, we used Edaravone to induce human umbilical cord mesenchymal stem cells. More experiments show that under certain conditions of culture, hUMSCs spontaneously tend to differentiate into neuron-like cells and have a good protective effect of neurons [23]. At this stage, the use of cell therapy in the treatment of neurological diseases is divided into the following two methods [24, 25]. One is the purpose of the cells through a variety of ways into the body, relying on its own differentiation potential, and the impact of the environment plays a therapeutic effect. In another method, cells are first differentiated into cells of interest by various means and then into the body to play a therapeutic effect.

The most reported method of induction into nerve cells is divided into three kinds: cell nutrition factor, antioxidant, and nerve cell coculture method. In general, the main factors of cell nutrition are bFGF, transforming growth factor-β, and BDNF. Antioxidants are mainly DMSO, compound or single herb, or active ingredients of traditional Chinese medicine. The neural cell coculture method is to coculture MSCs with neural cells. There are also reports that microRNA-124 can also regulate the directional differentiation of MSCs to neurons [26]. These neuron-like cells can express a variety of neurological markers, such as nesin, GFAP, NSE, NF-H, and MAP-2. In this study, different concentrations of Edaravone were used to induce hUMSCs. It was found that the astigmatism of hUMSCs became stronger, and the cells protruded elongated protrusions, which had the morphological characteristics of neuron-like cells. The results of immunocytochemistry showed that NSE, GFAP, and nestin were positive, and the induction efficiency of 2.62 mg/ml group was significant. The results of RT-PCR and Western blot showed that the expressions of NSE, GFAP, and nestin in the induced group were significantly higher than those in the blank

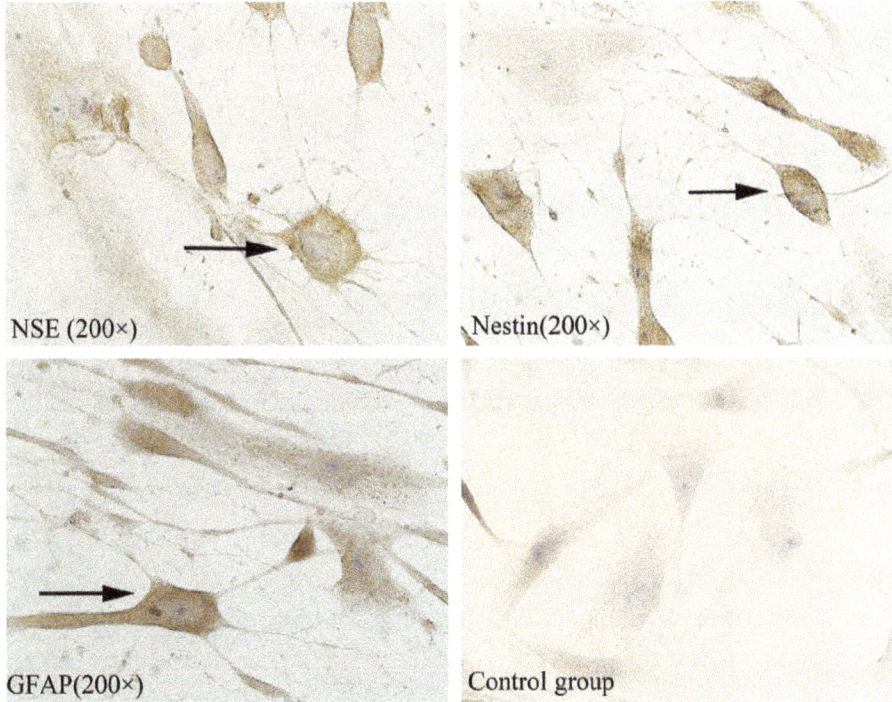

FIGURE 5: Immunohistochemical staining of neuron-like cells in treatment groups for NSE, nestin, and GFAP, respectively. The arrows in figures indicate neuron-like cells.

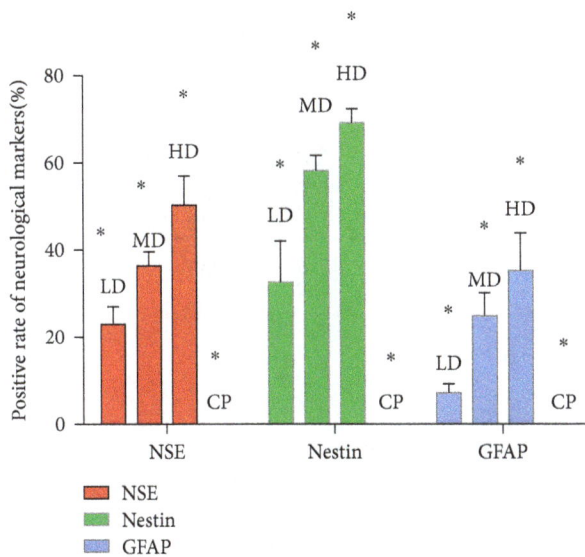

FIGURE 6: After 12 hours of induction, the positive rate of neuronal markers in each group.

control group. And 2.62 mg/ml is the higher concentration available, close to its maximum solubility in L-DMEM [27]. This study demonstrates that Edaravone can effectively induce hUMSCs to differentiate into neuron-like cells and the concentration of 2.62 mg/ml for the appropriate induction concentration.

The mechanism of each induction method is also different, such as bFGF induction mechanism as a neurotrophic factor in promoting cell mitosis in the process of simulation of embryonic neural cell growth microenvironment, thus leading to hUMSC differentiation into nerve cells. The induction mechanism of coculture may be related to the secretion of various nerve growth factors from various nerve cells. In this growing microenvironment, hUMSCs tend to differentiate into neuron-like cells, also providing the conditions for axonal development [28, 29]. Tetramethylpyrazine can promote the differentiation of hUMSCs into neuron-like cells by inhibiting the expression of Ca2+ signaling, promoting the increase of cAMP content in the second messenger and changing the expression of MEK-ERK signaling pathway [30]. Chemical antioxidant β-mercaptoethanol is also regulating the second messenger cAMP content, thus initiating the PKA pathway to promote MSC differentiation [31]. In recent years, with the development of biological tissue engineering technology, some scholars have proposed that using certain cell scaffold compounds can promote the differentiation of MSCs [32]. Edaravone is widely used in the treatment of ischemic stroke and a variety of spinal cord injury. Edaravone has the effect of reducing cerebral edema, improving cerebral ischemic symptoms, protecting brain tissue, and so on. It is a kind of oxygen free radical scavenger with good curative effect. Edaravone has antioxidant, anti-ischemia and reperfusion injury, antifibrosis, inhibition of nerve cell damage, and other effects; it can inhibit the peroxidation to protect the brain cells [33]. Edaravone is a kind of brain protective agent, which can reduce the death of nerve cells. In brain hemorrhage and cerebral infarction experiments, it can inhibit the decrease of local cerebral blood flow around the infarct. We hope to use cell transplantation to

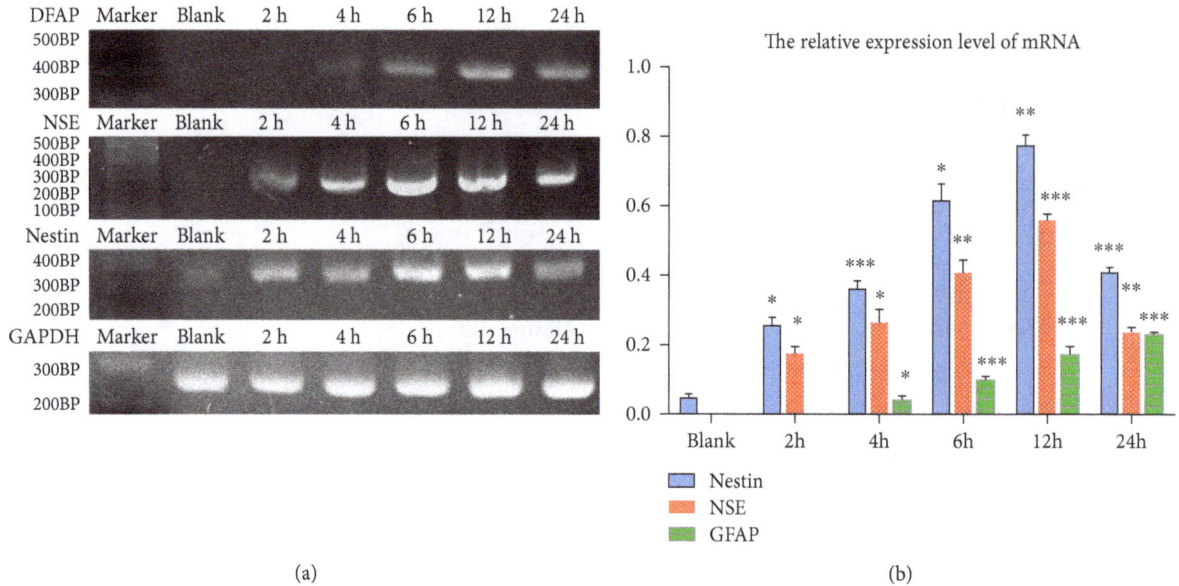

(a)   (b)

FIGURE 7: (a) Result of semiquantitative RT-PCR. (b) Relative expression level of mRNA.

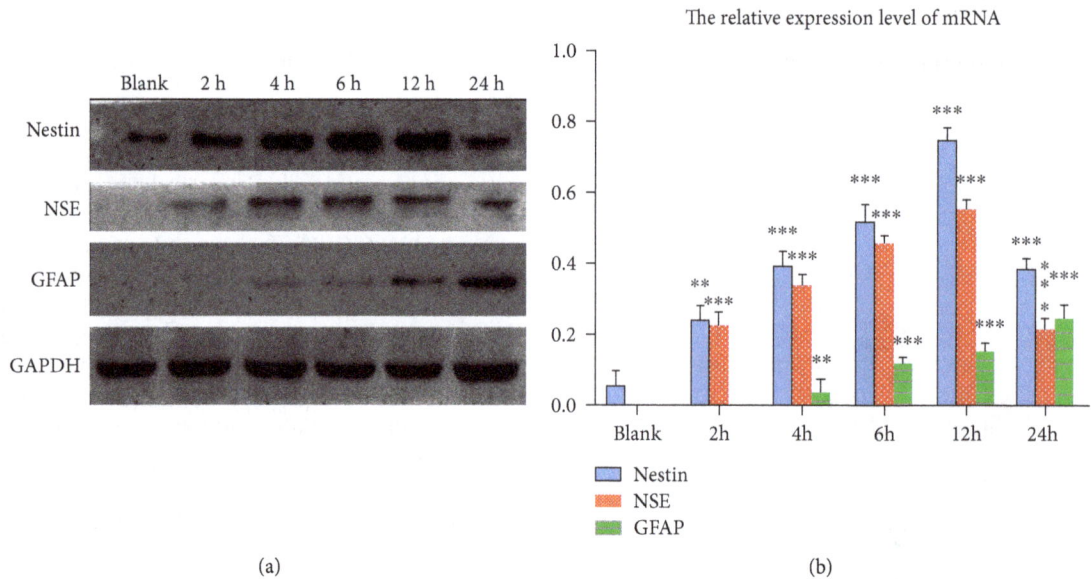

(a)   (b)

FIGURE 8: (a) Result of Western blot. (b) Relative expression level of protein.

improve the neuron injury caused by brain injury, bleeding, infarction, and the adverse effects of Parkinson's disease, amyotrophic lateral sclerosis, and other degenerative diseases. We look forward that cells derived from Edaravone can also play a role in brain protection, providing cell support for the next further experiments. Therefore, in this study, we used Edaravone to induce hUMSCs to differentiate into neuron-like cells. At the same time, it was found that those neuron-like cells induced by Edaravone had the electrophysiological basis for neuronal cells [34]. However, the induction mechanism of Edaravone is still unclear at this stage. Weissmann et al. [35] and other studies have shown that in the growth and development of nerve cells, the cytoskeleton played a key role. Doherty [36] and other

studies have pointed out that in the development of nerve cells, Shh signaling pathway has an important role; it can be conducive to the survival of nerve cells in the microenvironment. The next research direction is whether the Shh signaling pathway and cytoskeleton play an important role in the induction of hUMSCs into neuron-like cells by Edaravone.

Synaptic plasticity has long been recognized as the basis of neurocognitive biology. Many studies have found that memory can be preserved for a long time by the brain at the synapse level [37]. The existing proteins are modified to give signals to the nucleus. So a specific gene is expressed. Gene products are transported to synapses, and new proteins are synthesized locally, thus establishing new synapses and forming new information transfer functions [38]. This

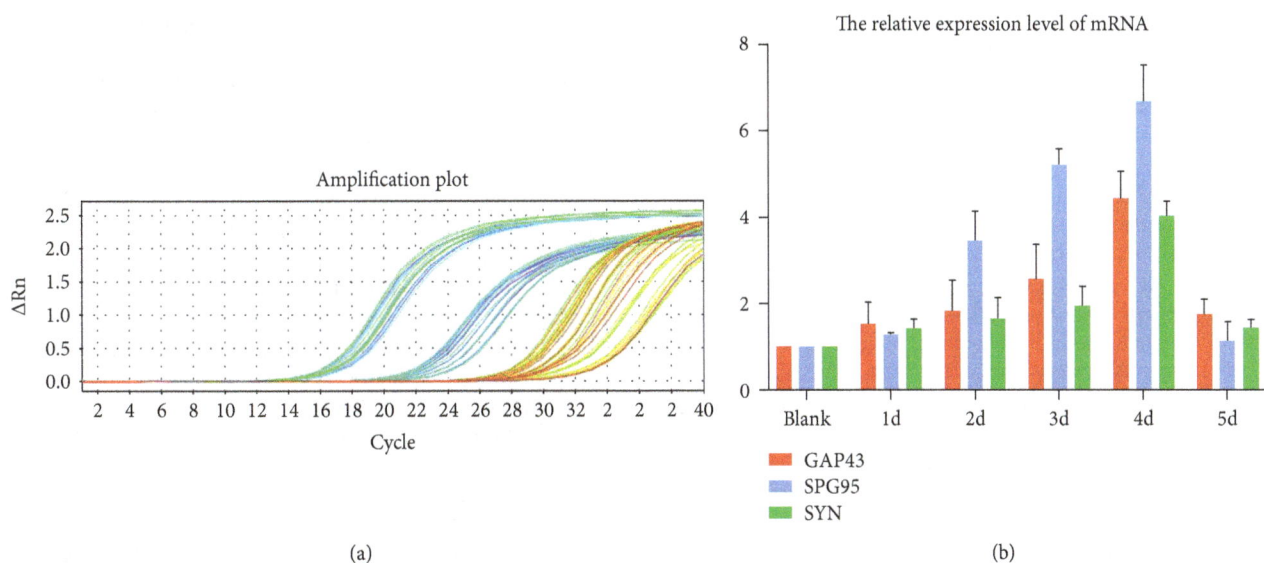

FIGURE 9: (a) Result of Real-Time PCR. (b) Relative expression level of mRNA.

process is called synaptic plasticity. Changes in synaptic markers can reflect changes in morphological plasticity. Synaptophysin (SYN), as one of the most important markers of synaptogenesis, plays an important role in the process of synaptogenesis and differentiation [39]. Postsynaptic density 95 is mainly involved in maintaining synaptic structure and plays an important role in the regulation of synapse morphology [40]. Growth-associated protein 43 (GAP43), as a specific phosphorylated protein, is mainly located in the presynaptic membrane of neurons. It is widely involved in the development, differentiation, and regeneration of the nervous system and is closely related to the formation and plasticity of synapses [41]. Therefore, we examined the expression levels of SYN, GAP43, and postsynaptic density 95. However, whether the obtained neuron-like cells have synapses capable of transmitting information needs further neuro-electrophysiological studies.

At the same time, hUMSCs cannot only directly inhibit the growth of some tumors in vivo and in vitro but also easily accept foreign gene modification and have the characteristics of target migration to tumor tissue, damaged tissue, and chronic inflammatory response sites. We would like to discuss whether the cells can also have the characteristics of nerve cell protection and tumor cell apoptosis by using eukaryotic cell transfection. There are also many difficulties in introducing nerve cells which are differentiated into cells into the body and have a therapeutic effect. In the next days, we still need to continue efforts.

Acknowledgments

This research was supported by the National Natural Science Foundation of China (81870984, 81401032) and the Hebei Provincial Natural Science Foundation (H2015206309).

References

[1] A. Bongso, C. Y. Fong, and K. Gauthaman, "Taking stem cells to the clinic: major challenges," *Journal of Cellular Biochemistry*, vol. 105, no. 6, pp. 1352–1360, 2008.

[2] M. L. Weiss and D. L. Troyer, "Stem cells in the umbilical cord," *Stem Cell Reviews*, vol. 2, no. 2, pp. 155–162, 2006.

[3] T. J. Sun, R. Tao, Y. Q. Han, G. Xu, J. Liu, and Y. F. Han, "Wnt3a promotes human umbilical cord mesenchymal stem cells to differentiate into epidermal-like cells," *European Review for Medical and Pharmacological Sciences*, vol. 19, no. 1, pp. 86–91, 2015.

[4] M. Makridakis, M. G. Roubelakis, and A. Vlahou, "Stem cells: insights into the secretome," *Biochimica et Biophysica Acta (BBA) - Proteins and Proteomics*, vol. 1834, no. 11, pp. 2380–2384, 2013.

[5] A. J. Friedenstein, J. F. Gorskaja, and N. N. Kulagina, "Fibroblast precursors in normal and irradiated mouse hematopoietic organs," *Experimental Hematology*, vol. 4, no. 5, pp. 267–274, 1976.

[6] J. Li-shan, Z. Yun, Z. Ya, Z. Jian, Z. Ting, and Y. Xiangming, "In vitro induced differentiation of mesenchymal stem cells from bone marrow mesenchymal stem cells into vascular endothelial cells," *Chinese Journal of Tissue Engineering Research*, vol. 13, no. 19, pp. 3698–3702, 2009.

[7] W. Jin, Y. P. Xu, A. H. Yang, and Y. Q. Xing, "In vitro induction and differentiation of umbilical cord mesenchymal stem cells into neuron-like cells by all-trans retinoic acid," *International Journal of Ophthalmology*, vol. 8, no. 2, pp. 250–256, 2015.

[8] L. Guo, L. Wang, L. Wang et al., "Resveratrol induces differentiation of human umbilical cord mesenchymal stem cells into neuron-like cells," *Stem Cells International*, vol. 2017, Article ID 1651325, 7 pages, 2017.

[9] N. C. Joyce, D. L. Harris, V. Markov, Z. Zhang, and B. Saitta, "Potential of human umbilical cord blood mesenchymal stem cells to heal damaged corneal endothelium," *Molecular Vision*, vol. 18, pp. 547–564, 2012.

[10] Y. Sun, F. Duan, and X. Chen, "Inducing differentiation of human umbilical cord blood mesenchymal stem cells into hepatocyte-like cells in vitro," *Chinese Journal of Gastroenterology and Hepatology*, vol. 13, pp. 239–243, 2004.

[11] D. Kong, J. Zhu, Q. Liu et al., "Mesenchymal stem cells protect neurons against hypoxic-ischemic injury via inhibiting parthanatos, necroptosis, and apoptosis, but not autophagy," *Cellular and Molecular Neurobiology*, vol. 37, no. 2, pp. 303–313, 2017.

[12] Z. Yin, H. Xu, and N. Yuan, "Clinical evaluation of edaravone in removal of free redicals and treatment for brain edema after intracerebral hemorrhage," *Journal of Apoplexy and Nervous Diseases*, vol. 25, no. 3, pp. 313–315, 2008.

[13] K. Abe, M. Aoki, S. Tsuji et al., "Safety and efficacy of edaravone in well defined patients with amyotrophic lateral sclerosis: a randomised, double-blind, placebo-controlled trial," *The Lancet Neurology*, vol. 16, no. 7, pp. 505–512, 2017.

[14] G. W. Zhang, T. X. Gu, X. J. Sun et al., "Edaravone promotes activation of resident cardiac stem cells by transplanted mesenchymal stem cells in a rat myocardial infarction model," *The Journal of Thoracic and Cardiovascular Surgery*, vol. 152, no. 2, pp. 570–582, 2016.

[15] L. Siyu, W. Fengchang, X. Haixiong et al., "Biological features and differentiation of human umbilical cord mesenchymal stem cells at different passages," *Chinese Journal of Tissue Engineering Research*, vol. 21, no. 13, pp. 2015–2022, 2017.

[16] M. L. Weiss, S. Medicetty, A. R. Bledsoe et al., "Human umbilical cord matrix stem cells: preliminary characterization and effect of transplantation in a rodent model of Parkinson's disease," *Stem Cells*, vol. 24, no. 3, pp. 781–792, 2006.

[17] N. K. Satija, V. K. Singh, Y. K. Verma et al., "Mesenchymal stem cell-based therapy: a new paradigm in regenerative medicine," *Journal of Cellular and Molecular Medicine*, vol. 13, no. 11-12, pp. 4385–4402, 2009.

[18] E. Syková, P. Jendelová, L. Urdzíková, P. Lesný, and A. Hejcl, "Bone marrow stem cells and polymer hydrogels—two strategies for spinal cord injury repair," *Cellular and Molecular Neurobiology*, vol. 26, no. 7-8, pp. 1113–1129, 2006.

[19] J. Shen, A. Nair, R. Saxena, C. C. Zhang, J. Borrelli, and L. Tang, "Tissue engineering bone using autologous progenitor cells in the peritoneum," *PLoS One*, vol. 9, no. 3, article e93514, 2014.

[20] Z. Li, W. Zhao, W. Liu, Y. Zhou, J. Jia, and L. Yang, "Transplantation of placenta-derived mesenchymal stem cell-induced neural stem cells to treat spinal cord injury," *Neural Regeneration Research*, vol. 9, no. 24, pp. 2197–2204, 2014.

[21] A. Gugliandolo, P. Bramanti, and E. Mazzon, "Mesenchymal stem cell therapy in Parkinson's disease animal models," *Current Research in Translational Medicine*, vol. 65, no. 2, pp. 51–60, 2017.

[22] G. Ping, S. Zhan-sheng, W. Bo-min, L. Lian-xin, W. Fu, and M. Le-ming, "Transplantation of neuron-like cells from bone marrow mesenchymal stem cells for treatment of spinal cord injury," *Journal of Clinical Rehabilitative Tissue Engineering Research*, vol. 17, no. 23, pp. 4256–4263, 2013.

[23] Y. J. Zheng, L. Y. Hai, and L. Meng, "Differentiation and application of umbilical cord blood mesenchymal stem cells to neurons," *Chongqing Medicine*, vol. 43, no. 3, pp. 366–368, 2014.

[24] S. R. Cho, M. S. Yang, S. H. Yim et al., "Neurally induced umbilical cord blood cells modestly repair injured spinal cords," *NeuroReport*, vol. 19, no. 13, pp. 1259–1263, 2008.

[25] V. R. Dasari, K. K. Veeravalli, A. J. Tsung et al., "Neuronal apoptosis is inhibited by cord blood stem cells after spinal cord injury," *Journal of Neurotrauma*, vol. 26, no. 11, pp. 2057–2069, 2009.

[26] M. Mondanizadeh, E. Arefian, G. Mosayebi, M. Saidijam, B. Khansarinejad, and S. M. Hashemi, "MicroRNA-124 regulates neuronal differentiation of mesenchymal stem cells by targeting Sp1 mRNA," *Journal of Cellular Biochemistry*, vol. 116, no. 6, pp. 943–953, 2015.

[27] Z. Jian, *The Research of Supramolecular Complexes of Edaravone and Cyclodextrins*, Nanjing Normal University, 2011.

[28] R. J. Tolwani, P. S. Buckmaster, S. Varma et al., "BDNF overexpression increases dendrite complexity in hippocampal dentate gyrus," *Neuroscience*, vol. 114, no. 3, pp. 795–805, 2002.

[29] K. A. Trzaska, C. C. King, K. Y. Li et al., "Brain-derived neurotrophic factor facilitates maturation of mesenchymal stem cell-derived dopamine progenitors to functional neurons," *Journal of Neurochemistry*, vol. 110, no. 3, pp. 1058–1069, 2009.

[30] Y. Y. Liu, X. X. Zhao, H. B. Zhao, B. F. Ge, X. Y. Liu, and K. M. Chen, "Tetramethylpyrazine induces the differentiation of mouse bone marrow-derived mesenchymal stem cells into nerve cells mediated by Ca~(2+) signaling," *Journal of Gansu Agricultural University*, vol. 45, no. 2, pp. 1–5, 2010.

[31] W. Deng, M. Obrocka, I. Fischer, and D. J. Prockop, "In vitro differentiation of human marrow stromal cells into early progenitors of neural cells by conditions that increase intracellular cyclic AMP," *Biochemical and Biophysical Research Communications*, vol. 282, no. 1, pp. 148–152, 2001.

[32] W. Yue, F. Yan, Y. L. Zhang et al., "Differentiation of rat bone marrow mesenchymal stem cells into neuron-like cells in vitro and co-cultured with biological scaffold as transplantation carrier," *Medical Science Monitor*, vol. 22, pp. 1766–1772, 2016.

[33] N. Nakamoto, S. Tada, K. Kameyama et al., "A free radical scavenger, edaravone, attenuates steatosis and cell death via reducing inflammatory cytokine production in rat acute liver injury," *Free Radical Research*, vol. 37, no. 8, pp. 849–859, 2003.

[34] R. Zeng, Z. Hu, and W. Guo, "Electrophysiology study on differentiation of rat bone marrow stromal stem cells into neuron-like cells in vitro by edaravone," *Modern Practical Medicine*, vol. 21, no. 3, pp. 197–200, 2009.

[35] C. Weissmann, H. J. Reyher, A. Gauthier, H. J. Steinhoff, W. Junge, and R. Brandt, "Microtubule binding and trapping at the tip of neurites regulate tau motion in living neurons," *Traffic*, vol. 10, no. 11, pp. 1655–1668, 2009.

[36] D. Doherty, "Joubert syndrome: insights into brain development, cilium biology, and complex disease," *Seminars in Pediatric Neurology*, vol. 16, no. 3, pp. 143–154, 2009.

[37] C. H. Bailey, E. R. Kandel, and K. M. Harris, "Structural components of synaptic plasticity and memory consolidation," *Cold Spring Harbor Perspectives in Biology*, vol. 7, no. 7, article a021758, 2015.

[38] J. N. Bourne and K. M. Harris, "Nanoscale analysis of structural synaptic plasticity," *Current Opinion in Neurobiology*, vol. 22, no. 3, pp. 372–382, 2012.

[39] H. D. Guo, J. X. Tian, J. Zhu et al., "Electroacupuncture suppressed neuronal apoptosis and improved cognitive impairment in the AD model rats possibly via downregulation of notch signaling pathway," *Evidence-Based Complementary and Alternative Medicine*, vol. 2015, Article ID 393569, 9 pages, 2015.

9

Bioprocessing of Mesenchymal Stem Cells and their Derivatives: Toward Cell-Free Therapeutics

Jolene Phelps,[1,2] Amir Sanati-Nezhad,[2,3,4] Mark Ungrin,[2,4,5] Neil A. Duncan,[2,4,6] and Arindom Sen [1,2,4]

[1]Pharmaceutical Production Research Facility, Department of Chemical and Petroleum Engineering, Schulich School of Engineering, University of Calgary, 2500 University Drive N.W., Calgary, AB, Canada T2N 1N4
[2]Biomedical Engineering Graduate Program, University of Calgary, 2500 University Drive N.W., Calgary, AB, Canada T2N 1N4
[3]BioMEMS and Bioinspired Microfluidic Laboratory, Department of Mechanical and Manufacturing Engineering, Schulich School of Engineering, University of Calgary, 2500 University Drive N.W., Calgary, AB, Canada T2N 1N4
[4]Center for Bioengineering Research and Education, Schulich School of Engineering, University of Calgary, 2500 University Drive N.W., Calgary, AB, Canada T2N 1N4
[5]Faculty of Veterinary Medicine, Heritage Medical Research Building, University of Calgary, 3330 Hospital Drive N.W., Calgary, AB, Canada T2N 4N1
[6]Musculoskeletal Mechanobiology and Multiscale Mechanics Bioengineering Lab, Department of Civil Engineering, Schulich School of Engineering, University of Calgary, 2500 University Drive N.W., Calgary, AB, Canada T2N 1N4

Correspondence should be addressed to Arindom Sen; asen@ucalgary.ca

Academic Editor: Elias T. Zambidis

Mesenchymal stem cells (MSCs) have attracted tremendous research interest due to their ability to repair tissues and reduce inflammation when implanted into a damaged or diseased site. These therapeutic effects have been largely attributed to the collection of biomolecules they secrete (i.e., their secretome). Recent studies have provided evidence that similar effects may be produced by utilizing only the secretome fraction containing extracellular vesicles (EVs). EVs are cell-derived, membrane-bound vesicles that contain various biomolecules. Due to their small size and relative mobility, they provide a stable mechanism to deliver biomolecules (i.e., biological signals) throughout an organism. The use of the MSC secretome, or its components, has advantages over the implantation of the MSCs themselves: (i) signals can be bioengineered and scaled to specific dosages, and (ii) the nonliving nature of the secretome enables it to be efficiently stored and transported. However, since the composition and therapeutic benefit of the secretome can be influenced by cell source, culture conditions, isolation methods, and storage conditions, there is a need for standardization of bioprocessing parameters. This review focuses on key parameters within the MSC culture environment that affect the nature and functionality of the secretome. This information is pertinent to the development of bioprocesses aimed at scaling up the production of secretome-derived products for their use as therapeutics.

1. Introduction

Mesenchymal stem cells (MSCs) are unspecialized cells that can be isolated from various tissues within the body including bone marrow, adipose, dermal, umbilical cord blood, and synovial fluid [1–3]. A cell population isolated from these tissues is considered to contain primarily MSCs if it meets the following minimum criteria defined by the International Society for Cellular Therapy: (i) the cell population must be plastic-adherent; (ii) ≥95% of the cell population needs to express the surface antigens CD105, CD73, and CD90 and ≤2% may express CD45, CD34, CD14 or CD11b, CD79α or CD19, and HLA-DR; and (iii) the cells need to be able to differentiate to bone, fat, and cartilage fates in vitro [4].

MSCs have attracted great research interest for the treatment of medical disorders due to their ability to repair tissues and reduce inflammation when implanted into a damaged or diseased site. Numerous clinical trials have now demonstrated the safety and feasibility of MSC implantation therapies in applications of tissue repair, as well as in disease mitigation through immunomodulation [5]. However, despite moderate successes, many concerns remain regarding the therapeutic efficacy of MSCs due to the high degree of variability in clinical outcomes [6]. There is a clear need to find methods that can consistently yield positive results. MSC therapies also face challenges in having to immunologically match donors and recipients to minimize the possibility of rejection, as well as technical considerations around the storage and transport of viable cells. Furthermore, in many cases it has been found that there is very limited retention of MSCs within an injury site. Despite reports of therapeutic benefits, often less than 1% of the transplanted MSCs are retained long-term within the target tissue [7, 8].

Whereas it was initially believed that these cells contribute to tissue repair by differentiating into the specialized cell types required to replace the dead and damaged cells native to that tissue, there is increasing evidence to suggest that much of the observed therapeutic benefit associated with MSC therapy may be attributed to the bioactivity of factors and molecules secreted by these cells. In fact, the focus of many clinical trials has been to evaluate the therapeutic effects of the factors and molecules produced by mesenchymal stem cells, rather than integration of the cells themselves. These secreted factors and molecules, collectively referred to as the MSC "secretome," are hypothesized to upregulate endogenous repair and immunomodulation mechanisms [9]. It has even been proposed that MSCs now be referred to as medicinal signalling cells to more accurately reflect their mode of action [10]. This raises the possibility of administering MSC-derived products as therapeutics rather than implanting the cells themselves, which would address some of the key challenges for the clinical translation of MSC-based therapies.

Registered clinical trials are currently underway to evaluate the effectiveness of extracellular vesicles derived from the MSC secretome, including one involving patients with ischemic stroke (December 2017), a second for the healing of macular holes (February 2018), and a third involving the maintenance of β-cell mass in type I diabetes mellitus (T1DM) (2014) [11]. Prior studies utilizing MSC-derived extracellular vesicles in human patients for graft versus host disease (GvHD) [12] and chronic kidney disease (CKD) [13], demonstrated improved outcomes and immunosuppressive effects. The exclusion of implanted cells in this approach means products can be bioengineered to enhance therapeutic potential and improve quality control, can be scaled to specific dosages, and benefits from reduced immunogenicity [14]. In addition, the nonliving nature of the secretome means that it can be characterized, stored, packaged, and transported significantly more easily than viable cells—a critical consideration for the economic viability of new therapies.

Several challenges need to be overcome to make this technology clinically available and to utilize the MSC secretome as a cell-free therapeutic. The MSC secretome differs depending on the tissue from which the MSCs are isolated, and there is substantial variation between donors and in response to differing culture conditions [15, 16]. While much work has been done to understand how the cells themselves change in response to environmental factors such as oxygenation, mechanical forces, and chemical stimuli, considerably less work has focused on the effect of these factors on resultant secretome profiles. Such studies would not only enable secretome optimization for specific applications but also provide an essential foundation for larger-scale production. Though it is simple and cost-effective to study MSCs in static monolayer cultures, such conditions are not conducive to large-scale production. This review outlines the therapeutic products that can be obtained from MSCs and important culture parameters that need to be considered for the scalable production and clinical translation of the MSC secretome.

2. The Composition of the MSC Secretome

The MSC secretome contains many cell signalling molecules, including growth factors and cytokines that modulate cell behaviours such as proliferation, differentiation, and extracellular matrix production or provide pro- and anti-inflammatory effects. Recent studies have provided evidence that MSCs also secrete small membrane-bound extracellular vesicles (EVs) that contain a number of biomolecules, including not only growth factors and cytokines but also various forms of RNA capable of triggering a variety of biological responses throughout an organism [17]. Notably, it has recently been reported that EVs alone may provide similar or enhanced therapeutic benefit to their cellular counterparts [18].

During a culture period, the MSC secretome can be recovered from the expended medium. The term "conditioned medium" (CM) is used to describe an expended medium, or a combination of fresh medium and expended medium from prior cell cultures. CM is primarily prepared by centrifuging expended medium to remove cell debris and then using the resulting supernatant directly, or by adding a concentrated or fractionated form of it to fresh medium. By fractionating the CM, it is possible to correlate a particular molecular subset with a specific measured effect. Studies spanning a wide array of physiological applications have demonstrated the benefits of the MSC secretome through the utilization of CM. Table 1 outlines the biological effects identified from the MSC secretome or MSC secretome-derived products, in various disease models.

2.1. Cytokines and Growth Factors. MSCs secrete a wide variety of cell signalling cytokines and growth factors. These bioactive molecules can stimulate endogenous cell populations to undergo responses which may contribute to healing in a variety of tissues. Some of the most physiologically relevant biomolecules secreted by MSCs include hepatocyte growth factor (HGF), which has been reported to be involved in immunomodulation, cell migration, development, wound healing and antiapoptosis; transforming growth factor-

TABLE 1: Biological effect of MSC secretome-derived products on disease models.

MSC source	Paracrine factors	Biological effect	Ref.
		Skin wounds and radiation	
Human adipose tissue	Supernatant of cell lysate	(i) Faster wound closure when applied topically on cutaneous wound (ii) Upregulation of dermal fibroblast proliferation, migration, and ECM production	[25]
Human adipose tissue	Hypoxic conditioned medium	(i) Protected epithelial, endothelial, and myoepithelial cells from radiation damage and tissue remodelling	[92]
Adipose tissue	Exosomes	(i) Stimulated fibroblast migration, proliferation, and collagen synthesis (ii) Recruited to soft tissue wound in mouse skin incision model and accelerated cutaneous wound healing	[137]
Human and murine bone marrow	Exosomes and microvesicles	(i) Mitigated radiation injury to marrow stem cells (ii) Restoration of marrow stem cell engraftment and partial recovery of peripheral blood counts postirradiation	[41]
Human amniotic epithelial cells	Exosomes	(i) Promoted migration and proliferation of fibroblasts (ii) Deposition of ECM partly abolished (iii) In rat model, improved skin wound healing with well-organized collagen fibers	[138]
Human umbilical cord blood	Exosomes	(i) Promoted cell migration and collagen synthesis of human dermal fibroblasts (ii) Increased expressions of collagen I and elastin 3 days posttreatment on human skin	[139]
		Bone and cartilage	
Human fetal MSCs	Conditioned medium	(i) Increased expression of ALP and osteogenic marker genes and increased calcium deposits in rat BM-MSCs (ii) Improved bone consolidation in a rat osteogenesis model	[26]
Human synovial membrane	Exosomes	(i) Enhance proliferation and antiapoptotic abilities of bone marrow-derived stromal cells (ii) Prevented GC-induced trabecular bone loss, bone marrow necrosis, and fatty cells accumulation in rat model	[140]
Human embryo	Exosomes	(i) Enhanced gross appearance and histological scores of osteochondral defects in adult rats with complete restoration of cartilage and subchondral bone	[141]
Human bone marrow	Exosomes compared to exosome-free conditioned medium	(i) Exosomes, but not exosome-free conditioned medium, rescued retardation of fracture healing in $CD9^{-/-}$ mice	[31]
Human iPS-MSCs	Exosomes	(i) In a rat osteonecrosis model, exosomes prevented bone loss and increased microvessel density (ii) Enhanced proliferation, migration, and tube-forming capacities of endothelial cells in vitro	[142]
Human bone marrow	Exosomes, miR-21	(i) Suppressed TNF-α-induced nucleus pulposus cell apoptosis	[46]
		Kidneys	
SD rat bone marrow	Conditioned media compared to MSCs	(i) In an acute kidney injury model, MSCs and their CM equally ameliorated kidney function deterioration, Kim-1 shedding in urine, renal tissue damage, and tubular cell apoptosis (ii) Both reduced interstitial fibrosis	[27]
Bone marrow	Conditioned medium, MSCs, and microvesicles	(i) Ameliorated induced acute kidney injury in rats with little differences in effectiveness between CM, microvesicles, and MSCs	[143]
		Diabetes mellitus	
Murine bone marrow	miR-106b-5p, miR-222-3p	(i) Promoted postinjury β-cell proliferation (ii) Improved hyperglycemia in STZ-treated mice	[47]
Human adipose tissue	Conditioned media compared to MSCs	(i) Reversed mechanical, thermal allodynia, and thermal hyperalgesia (ii) Restored correct pro/anti-inflammatory cytokine balance and prevented skin innervation loss (iii) Reestablished Th1/Th2 balance in spleens of STZ-treated mice (iv) Recovered kidney morphology	[144]

TABLE 1: Continued.

MSC source	Paracrine factors	Biological effect	Ref.
Human bone marrow	Extracellular vesicles	(i) Prevented onset of T1DM and experimental autoimmune uveoretinitis in a murine model (ii) Inhibited activation of antigen-presenting cells and suppressed development of Th1 and Th17 cells	[145]
		Cardiovascular system	
Human embryonic MSCs	Exosomes	(i) Reduced infarct size in a mouse model of myocardial ischemia/reperfusion injury	[39]
SD rat bone marrow	Exosomes compared to MSCs	(i) Exosomes reduced inflammation, inhibited fibrosis, and improved cardiac function in rat myocardial infarction model (significantly superior to MSCs) (ii) Exosomes stimulated cardiomyocyte H9C2 cell proliferation, inhibited apoptosis, and inhibited fibroblast differentiation to myofibroblast	[18]
SD rat bone marrow overexpressing Akt	Hypoxic conditioned medium	(i) Suppressed hypoxia-induced apoptosis and triggered contraction of adult rat cardiomyocytes (ii) Upregulation of VEGF, FGF-2, HGF, IGF-1, and TB4 in Akt-MSCs	[146]
Human bone marrow	Conditioned medium—products >1000 kDa (100–220 nm)	(i) Cardioprotection in a mouse model of ischemia and reperfusion injury with a 60% reduction in infarct size (ii) Reduced myocardial nuclear oxidative stress (iii) Reduced TGF-β signalling and apoptosis (iv) Improved systolic and diastolic cardiac performance	[38]
huES9.E1	Exosomes	(i) Alleviated features of reperfusion injury (ii) Preservation of left ventricular geometry and contractile performance (iii) Increased levels of ATP and NADH and decreased oxidative stress (iv) Reduced local and systemic inflammation (v) Reduced infarct size by 45%	[34]
Murine bone marrow	Exosomes enriched in miR-22 from ischemic preconditioned MSCs	(i) Reduced cardiac fibrosis in a myocardial infarction mouse model (ii) Mobilized to cardiomyocytes where they reduced apoptosis due to ischemia	[91]
Human umbilical cord	Exosomes	(i) Improved cardiac systolic function and reduced cardiac fibrosis after litigation of LAD coronary artery in a rat model (ii) Protected myocardial cells from apoptosis and promoted tube formation	[147]
SD rat bone marrow	Exosomes from GATA-4-overexpressing MSCs, miR-19a	(i) Restored cardiac contractile function and reduced infarct size following ligation of coronary artery in rat heart (ii) Increased cardiomyocyte survival and preserved mitochondrial membrane potential	[148]
Murine bone marrow	Extracellular vesicles, miR-210	(i) Improved angiogenesis and exerted a therapeutic effect on myocardial infarction in a mouse model (ii) miR-210 necessary for proangiogenic effect	[45]
SD rat bone marrow	Exosomes	(i) Enhanced tube formation of human umbilical vein endothelial cells (ii) Impaired T cell function by inhibiting proliferation in vitro (iii) Reduced infarct size, preserved cardiac systolic and diastolic performance, and enhanced density of new capillaries in a rat myocardial infarction model	[149]
SD rat bone marrow	Exosomes	(i) Reduced H_2O_2-induced ROS production and cell apoptosis of rat H9C2 cardiomyocytes	[150]
Human bone marrow	Exosomes from ischemic MSC culture conditions	(i) Induced angiogenesis via NFκB pathway in HUVECs	[88]
Human Wharton jelly	Microvesicles	(i) Improved survival rate and renal function in renal ischemia-reperfusion injury after cardiac death (ii) Decreased number of CD68$^+$ macrophages in kidney (iii) Decreased protein levels of α-SMA and TGF-β1 and increased HGF levels	[151]

TABLE 1: Continued.

MSC source	Paracrine factors	Biological effect	Ref.
Murine bone marrow	Extracellular vesicles	(i) Increased blood reperfusion and formation of new blood vessels in a hindlimb ischemia model	[134]
		Cancer	
Human embryonic kidney cell line 293	GE11-positive exosomes containing miR-let-7a	(i) Suppressed tumour growth and development in tumour-bearing mice (ii) Delivered miRNA to EGFR-expressing xenograft breast cancer tissue	[152]
		Muscle injury	
Human bone marrow	Conditioned media compared to exosomes	(i) Promoted myogenesis and angiogenesis in vitro (ii) Exosomes promoted muscle regeneration in a mouse muscle injury model	[30]
Human adipose tissue	Extracellular vesicles	(i) Modulated anti-inflammatory effects inducing macrophage polarization (ii) Mitigated inflammatory milieu within injured tissues in CTX injury of mouse TA muscle (iii) Accelerated muscle regeneration process	[89]
		Immunomodulatory	
Human umbilical cord blood	Microvesicles	(i) Decreased chemotactic index of CD14$^+$ cells (enhanced immunomodulatory effect)	[83]
Human bone marrow	Conditioned medium, PGE2	(i) CM from spheroids inhibited LPS-stimulated macrophages from secreting proinflammatory cytokines and increased their production of anti-inflammatory cytokines	[28]
		CNS	
Human bone marrow	Exosomes	(i) Promoted survival of retinal ganglion cells (RGCs) and regeneration of their axons (ii) Partially prevented RGC axonal loss and dysfunction	[153]
Human bone marrow	Exosomes from hypoxic MSCs	(i) Intravitreal exosome treatment in a oxygen-induced retinopathy murine model partially preserved retinal vascular flow in vivo and reduced retina thinning	[154]
Bone marrow	Exosomes	(i) In T2DM rats, stroke treatment 3 days poststroke improved functional outcome and reduced blood brain barrier leakage and haemorrhage (ii) Increased axon and myelin density and oligodendrocyte and oligodendrocyte progenitor cell number (iii) Increased expression of ABCA1 and IGFR1	[155]
Human adipose tissue	Conditioned medium	(i) Protected SH-SY5Y neuron-like cells against H_2O_2-induced neurotoxicity (ii) Promoted recovery of normal axonal morphology, electrophysiological features, and cell viability	[156]
SD rat bone marrow	Extracellular vesicles	(i) Promoted functional recovery and nerve regeneration of crush-injured sciatic nerves in rats	[157]
Wistar rat bone marrow	Conditioned medium	(i) Enhanced motor functional recovery, increased spared spinal cord tissue, enhanced GAP-43 expression, and attenuated inflammation after spinal cord injury in a rat model	[158]
		Pulmonary	
Bone marrow	Exosomes	(i) Reduced levels of white blood cells and neutrophils to bronchoalveolar lavage fluid in endotoxin-injured mice	[94]
Human bone marrow	Microvesicles	(i) Reduced symptoms of idiopathic pulmonary fibrosis such as reduced collagen deposition and inflammation in mouse fibrosis model	[159]
Human Wharton jelly, bone marrow	Exosomes	(i) Ameliorated alveolar simplification, fibrosis, and pulmonary vascular remodelling in a hyperoxia-exposed mouse model (ii) Suppressed proinflammatory macrophage M1 state and augmented anti-inflammatory M2 state	[160]

TABLE 1: Continued.

MSC source	Paracrine factors	Biological effect	Ref.
SD rat bone marrow	Microvesicles	(i) Alleviated PAH in a rat model by regulating the angiotensin system (ii) Relieved pulmonary artery pressure, pulmonary vessel wall thickness and lumen area, right ventricular hypertrophy, inflammation, and collagen fiber volume	[161]
		Liver	
Human umbilical cord	Exosomes	(i) Reduced surface fibrous capsules and alleviated hepatic inflammation and collagen deposition in a mouse model of CCl4-induced liver fibrosis	[162]

(TGF-) β potentiated in immunomodulation, cell growth, proliferation and differentiation, and wound healing; vascular endothelial growth factor (VEGF), playing a large role in angiogenesis but also in immunomodulation and cell survival; and molecules such as tumor necrosis factor-stimulated gene- (TSG-) 6, prostaglandin E2 (PGE2), and galectins 1 and 9 which are all reported to play a large role in immunomodulation [19, 20]. For a more detailed examination, see the thorough review by Bai et al. [19] that describes the function of bioactive molecules secreted by umbilical cord-derived MSCs.

Various clinical trials have injected individual biomolecular species in an effort to elicit a positive therapeutic response [21–23]. The injection of vascular endothelial growth factor (VEGF) was effective in improving angiogenesis in coronary heart disease patients; however, such trials have not been able to match the therapeutic efficacy of MSCs [24]. Similarly, high-dose bolus interleukin-2 (IL-2) has FDA approval for metastatic melanoma and renal cell carcinoma, but is challenged by low response rates and notorious toxicities [23].

CM derived from MSC cultures has shown promising benefits in a wide range of therapeutic and immunomodulatory applications, including the treatment of skin wounds, distraction osteogenesis, and kidney injury [25–28]. Despite the wide array of bioactive molecules released by MSCs, their use as a therapeutic is limited by their stability. Under physiological conditions, the functional stability of cytokines and growth factors can decay within minutes [29]. It has been shown that many of these same bioactive molecules can also be found within the EVs secreted by MSCs, albeit in much lower amounts [30, 31]. Remarkably, it has been demonstrated that EVs, but not EV-depleted CM, can elicit therapeutic benefits such as rescuing the retardation of fracture healing in a CD9$^{-/-}$ mouse model [31]. This suggests that the bioactivity possessed by EVs may give clinical value to such secreted structures.

2.2. Extracellular Vesicles. EVs are phospholipid membrane-bound particles secreted from cells that contain biological materials including DNA, RNA, bioactive lipids, and proteins. The internal components, or "cargo," are specific to cell source (i.e., the individual, as well as the particular tissue from which the MSCs were derived) and the pathological state of the cells. EVs can be targeted to local cells or transported to cells in distant tissues via biological fluids. After binding to recipient cells, EVs may remain stably associated with the plasma membrane, dissociate, directly fuse with the membrane, or be internalized through endocytic pathways [32]. EVs provide the advantages of a stable delivery system well tolerated in biological fluids, the ability to home to target cells or tissues, and are thought to possess negligible immunogenicity *in vivo* [33]. The importance of the EV delivery system was demonstrated where intact, but not lysed, EVs enhanced myocardial viability in a myocardial ischemia/reperfusion mouse injury model [34]. Some studies have demonstrated immunosuppressive behaviour which may be owing to soluble or surface expressed HLA-G, thoroughly reviewed by Rebmann et al. [35].

EVs is an umbrella term for different types of vesicles secreted by MSCs: exosomes, microvesicles (also referred to as ectosomes), and apoptotic bodies. Explorations of the therapeutic value of EVs are currently focused primarily on exosomes and microvesicles. Each type of vesicle is characterized by its origin, size, and unique identifying markers (Figure 1). The term EVs has been recommended as an inclusive term by the International Society for Extracellular Vesicles (ISEV) as the commonly used methods for isolation of each individual type of EV are not able to exclusively sort one from the other [36].

A majority of research in EVs has focused on the exosome-rich fraction. Exosomes have been described as a relatively homogeneous population in terms of size and are the best characterized among all EVs [37]. The first studies by Timmers et al. [38] provided evidence that MSC-derived CM could provide therapeutic benefits without the use of cells. Different fractionations of conditioned medium were injected into a mouse model of cardiac ischemia and reperfusion injury where it was determined that CM-containing products greater than 1000 kDa were effective in cardioprotection and reduction of infarct size. This size range suggests the involvement of exosomes, which were isolated and tested successfully in a follow-up study [39]. A number of studies have compared such exosome-rich fractions to CM and described comparable results, further indicating that exosomes may be responsible for the therapeutic effects of MSC-derived CM [18, 30, 31]. More recently, exosomes have been compared to microvesicles with variable results. In a model of acute kidney injury, only the exosome-enriched fraction induced an improvement of renal function and morphology [40] while the best formulation to reduce radiation damage to bone marrow stem cells included both types of EVs [41]. Regardless, the beneficial properties of EVs have been attributed to not only their stable delivery of cytokines and growth factors, but also their enclosed RNAs, which play

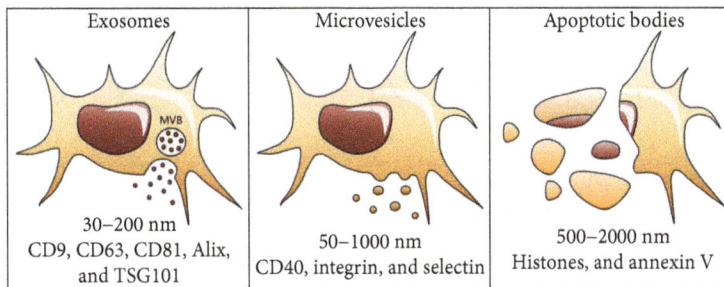

FIGURE 1: Types of extracellular vesicles and their identifying characteristics. Exosomes, with diameters ranging from 30 to 200 nm, are formed by the inward budding of multivesicular bodies (MVBs), which then fuse with the plasma membrane to be released into the extracellular environment. Exosomes are classified by tetraspanins CD9, CD63, and CD81 and the proteins Alix and TSG101 involved in MVB biogenesis. Microvesicles, also referred to as ectosomes, are larger with diameters from 50 to 1000 nm and bud directly from the plasma membrane. Microvesicles encompass identifying markers CD40, integrin, and selectin. Apoptotic bodies range from 500 to 2000 nm and encompass fragments of dead or dying cells. These are characterized by the presence of histones and annexin V.

a large role in regulating gene expression to control cell function [30, 31, 42].

2.3. Coding and Noncoding RNAs. MSCs secrete protein-coding messenger RNAs (mRNAs) and noncoding RNAs such as microRNAs (miRNAs), long noncoding RNAs (lncRNAs), and circular RNAs (circRNAs) via their extracellular vesicles (EVs). Such components are potentially capable of eliciting changes in function via protein translation or the alteration of gene expression in recipient cells. Recent developments in RNA sequencing and RT-qPCR techniques have enabled the detection of RNAs even in low amounts [42]. Additionally, evidence that mRNAs residing in EVs can be transported into a recipient cell and then translated to contribute to protein expression has had a large impact on the field. For example, kidney tubular cells lacking IL-10 expression exposed to MSC-derived EVs acquired IL-10 mRNA and translated it to the corresponding protein [43].

miRNAs are small noncoding, highly conserved, single-stranded RNAs with function in RNA silencing but are also capable of regulating gene expression through posttranscriptional modifications. miRNAs typically degrade more quickly than do mRNAs. However, they are able to become more stable by associating with RNA-binding proteins (RBPs) or high- and low-density lipoproteins or through EV encapsulation [42]. miRNAs have been shown to be associated with a wide range of biological processes including cell apoptosis, stem cell differentiation, cardiac and skeletal muscle development, hematopoiesis, neurogenesis, insulin secretion, and immune response [44–47]. With such an importance in physiology, miRNA dysfunction can be correlated to disease [48], and consequently it is intensely studied as a diagnostic and prognostic biomarker.

LncRNAs and circRNAs are two more subsets of small RNAs enclosed within EVs. LncRNAs are involved in cellular processes such as chromatic organization, gene transcription, mRNA turnover, protein translation, and the assembly of macromolecular complexes [42]. They have been identified in EVs with differing expression patterns to their parent cells and present specific motifs that appear to complement those of certain miRNAs [42]. Thus, it has been proposed that lncRNAs may capture miRNA subsets and target them into

EVs. circRNAs are highly abundant with a long half-life due to their lack of free ends which prevent degradation by exonucleases. Such circRNAs may enable critical transcriptional and posttranscriptional modifications and control miRNA function as regulators of mRNA stability and/or translation [42].

3. Bioprocess Development for Secretome-Derived Products

To properly characterize and assess the therapeutic potential of the MSC secretome and the associated EVs, there is a requirement for the standardization of protocols for the expansion of MSC cultures, collection of the secretome, and isolation of defined components. To meet clinical needs for MSC secretome-derived products, isolated MSC populations need to be expanded *in vitro* using defined culture conditions that are reproducible, scalable, and well-controlled to limit heterogeneity and enhance predictability in the composition and function of secretome-derived products. Methods to expand populations of these cells have been developed [49], but have not taken into account the effects on the secretome—now an area of growing importance, particularly in relation to therapeutic efficacy.

Key factors in the development of a cell-based production system include the medium in which the cells are grown, cell source, and culture conditions (Figure 2). Also pertinent are the timing and method of secretome collection, as the secretome is highly dynamic [16]. It is also important to evaluate and develop protocols for the storage, transport, and delivery of secretome-derived products to enable researchers to properly compare and reproduce studies and further the development of therapies and drugs utilizing the MSC secretome. No reliable assay currently exists to test EV membrane integrity, which may impact the therapeutic benefit of the EVs and/or the level of reproducibility after administration [50]. There is also no standard list of biomolecules or RNAs to be quantified, which has resulted in a range of studies that selected their own molecule(s) of interest while disregarding others. Furthermore, there is a need to look at active molecules that may be oncogenic, as the MSC secretome contains proteins and RNAs capable of altering the genome of recipient cells

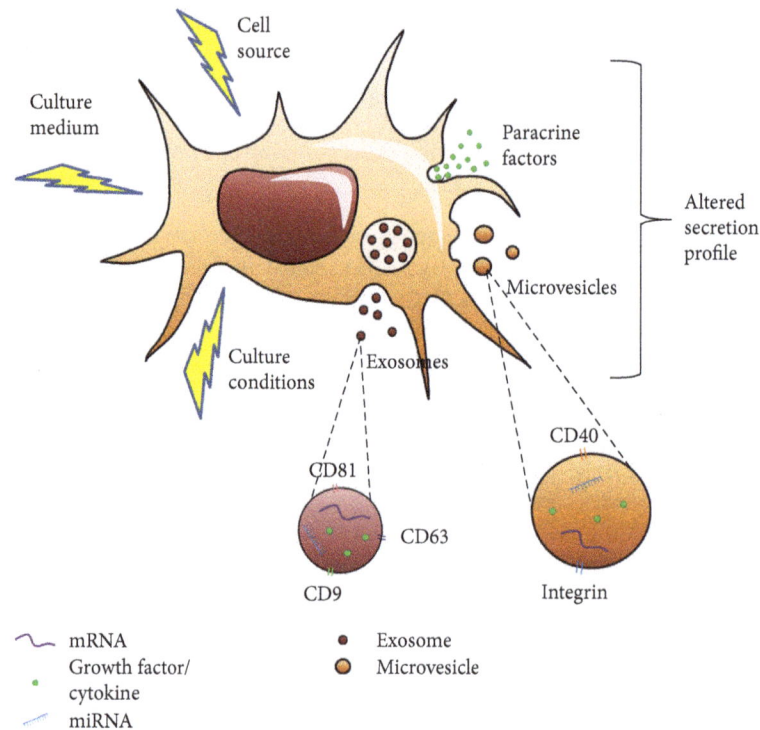

FIGURE 2: The secretion profile of MSCs may be altered by several factors including culture medium, cell source (i.e., bone marrow and adipose) and culture conditions (i.e., 3D cultures, hypoxia, and mechanical stimuli). The therapeutic portion of the secretion profile includes the amount and composition of paracrine factors and EVs (microvesicles and exosomes). The composition within EVs is also altered which includes RNAs such as mRNAs and miRNAs, growth factors, and cytokines.

[50]. Despite MSCs having demonstrated therapeutic effects in the treatment of various cancers, there is evidence that certain MSC phenotypes may promote tumor progression and metastasis [51, 52]. The specific mechanisms for cross-talk between MSCs and cancer cells is currently poorly understood, and thus, the oncogenic potential of MSCs and the MSC secretome remains controversial [51, 52].

3.1. Culture Medium. A well-defined culture medium is critical to translating MSC secretome-derived products to the clinic. For characterization and analysis of the secretome, a thorough understanding of what is already contained within the medium is required. The majority of studies that culture MSCs report utilizing fetal bovine serum (FBS) in the medium due to the relatively low level of antibodies and high amounts of growth factors that it contains [53, 54]. However, FBS presents high variability in composition depending on where, when, and how it was collected and can also be contaminated with animal-derived infectious agents [55]. Furthermore, when human MSCs are cultured in a medium containing animal proteins, the proteins are retained within the cells and may elicit an immunologic response when the cells or cell products are transplanted [53, 56]. Serum also contains its own exosomes, which must first be removed in exosome and EV-based studies to prevent co-isolation with those derived from the MSCs [57].

Alternatives to FBS include human platelet lysate (HPL) supplementation in media and a variety of chemically defined serum-free media (SFM). Compared to FBS, HPL reduces immunological reactions and enhances the proliferation of MSCs [57]. HPL has a high fibrinogen content that promotes the formation of fibrin gels in calcium-containing media, although this effect can be alleviated by utilizing a recently developed fibrinogen depletion method [57]. Although HPL may represent a cost-effective alternative to FBS for MSC expansion, it has been reported that HPL-expanded MSCs exhibited highly compromised immunosuppressive properties [58]; thus, it is important to fully analyze its effects on the therapeutic properties of MSCs.

A wide variety of chemically defined SFM have been developed for the expansion of human MSCs (hMSCs) that hold more promise, albeit at a higher price tag. Compared to MSCs expanded in serum-containing medium, the defined nature of SFM limits the heterogeneity between batches of cells and enhances MSC proliferation while generating smaller-diameter cells with stable surface marker expression [58, 60]. The difference in therapeutic benefits of secretome-derived products from cells grown in serum-free formulations compared to FBS still needs to be studied. Commercially available serum-free media that have been shown to successfully expand hMSC cultures include StemPro MSC SFM (Invitrogen), MesenCult-SF/XF (Stem-cell Technologies), and Becton Dickinson Mosaic hMSC SFM [53, 59, 60]. Of the commercially available SFMs, Stem-Pro MSC SFM is the only FDA-approved serum-free formulation [61]. Additionally, many research labs have developed their own xeno- or serum-free media. PPRF-msc6 is a serum-free medium developed by our laboratory group with a published component list to encourage further research and standardization [62].

3.2. Cell Source.

MSCs are very broadly defined. For this reason, populations of cells which adhere to this definition can still vary from one another. This variability may be evident when comparing MSC populations sourced from different individuals or even from different tissues within an individual. MSCs also vary in function depending on the tissue from which they are isolated within the body, displaying distinct secretome profiles specific to their native tissue. Further, MSCs can be genetically engineered to enhance the therapeutic benefit of their derived products, as detailed by Hodgkinson et al. [63]. It will be important to match donor characteristics and tissue source to secretome functionality in specific disease models.

3.2.1. Donor-to-Donor Variability.

It is well known that inherent variability exists between MSCs derived from different donors/patients, related to factors such as the age and health of the individual [64]. For example, Heathman et al. [65] showed substantial differences in metabolite consumption and production, growth characteristics, and immunoregulation abilities *in vivo* between five different bone marrow-derived MSC lines. Similarly, Paladino et al. [66] described unique behaviour of Wharton jelly-derived MSCs derived from different individuals, exhibiting differing cytokine profiles and immunomodulatory capacities. Phenotype, donor age, and gender have all been found to be contributing factors in the function of MSCs [67].

The metabolic state of the individual is another large factor found to influence MSCs and their secretome-derived products, with exosomes in particular being associated with metabolic organ crosstalk [68]. Between adipose-derived MSCs from lean and obese patients, distinct expression patterns of stem cell markers and varied lncRNA expression levels within exosomes were found [69]. Obesity was further found to reduce the proangiogenic potential of adipose MSC-derived EVs, showing reduced amounts of VEGF, MMP-2, and miR-126 within the EV cargo [70]. Interestingly, it has been found that MSCs derived from type 2 diabetes mellitus (T2DM) patients display no difference in cell surface marker phenotype, morphology, or multilineage potential compared to healthy individuals, but have decreased potency, oxidative stress-dependent dysfunctions, and a dysfunctional secretome composition that enhances proangiogenic function [71].

In comparing MSCs derived from healthy individuals to those from diseased states, it is not surprising that those from diseased states exhibit reduced function. For example, compared to a healthy control, CM obtained from MSC cultures using cells derived from multiple sclerosis (MS) patients eliminated the neuroprotective effect of MSC-CM when used in a model of progressive MS [72]. In some cases, such as in MSCs derived from T1DM patients, the MSCs show no differences in terms of morphology, immune-suppressive activity, and migration capacity, but had gene expression differences that could have impacted their *in vivo* function [71]. The mechanisms by which donor characteristics such as age

and gender, metabolic state, and disease alter MSC function and their corresponding secretome are currently not well understood. Further understanding the impact of these factors will be crucial to the development and application of secretome-derived products.

3.2.2. Tissue Source.

Proteomic comparisons of the secretomes of MSCs derived from different tissue sources have revealed differing secretome profiles. Between bone marrow, adipose tissue, and dental pulp-derived MSCs, only 124 of 1533 identified proteins were common across all three sources [73]. These commonly secreted proteins are factors with functions linked to MSC-related biological effects. A different comparative analysis among bone marrow, adipose tissue, and umbilical cord perivascular cells revealed differing secretome profiles of neuroregenerative factors [1]. One study showed Wharton's jelly-derived MSCs secrete greater amounts of cytokines, proinflammatory proteins, and growth factors, while those derived from adipose tissue have an enhanced angiogenic profile and secrete greater amounts of extracellular matrix (ECM) proteins and metalloproteinases [74]. The enhanced angiogenic profile of adipose-derived MSCs was also confirmed by Hsiao et al. [2]. Within the literature, the profiles secreted by different source-derived MSCs are relatively consistent, with embryonic or umbilical-derived stem cells showing enhanced proliferative and developmental molecules, and those from adult sources, such as bone marrow and adipose tissue, secreting higher amounts of ECM maintenance-related proteins [15].

In terms of EVs, fewer studies have compared profiles of different MSC sources to date. Bone marrow- and adipose tissue-derived MSCs secrete exosomes with highly similar RNA expression profiles, but with distinctive enrichments in specific tRNAs [75]. Compared to bone marrow, umbilical cord, and chorion-derived stem cells, exosomes secreted by menstrual-derived MSCs were shown to enhance neurite outgrowth response, relevant to recovery from neurodegenerative disorders such as Parkinson's disease [76]. Cell source is clearly an important aspect of process development which needs to be tailored towards specific therapeutic targets. Further studies need to be done to correlate the impact of different cell sources towards the therapeutic benefit for various disease models.

3.3. Culture Conditions.

The characteristics of MSCs are impacted by environmental parameters including temperature, pH, cell density at which they are seeded, oxygen level, and any mechanical, electromagnetic, or biochemical stimuli to which they are exposed. Culture conditions may function as a regulator to generate a certain MSC population with characteristics suitable for a particular application. Consequently, it is important to match culture conditions to the specific intended application. Similarly, culture conditions also impact the composition and bioactivity of the MSC secretome in culture. Therefore, steps need to be taken to ensure that a particular set of culture conditions results in secretome-derived products valuable for a specific application.

One way to alter the culture environment is to change the platform on which the cells are grown. Tissue culture flasks (T-flasks) provide a simple means of cell population expansion and are commonly used in small-scale research studies. In T-flasks, MSCs adhere to the surface and grow under static conditions as a 2D monolayer. However, when considering scalability towards clinical applications, the large number of T-flasks needed can lead to flask-to-flask variability, increases the chance of contamination, and can be labour-intensive [53]. Another common platform for expanding large populations of cells is a stirred suspension bioreactor, where the cells are grown in suspension in the presence of mechanical agitation. MSCs are traditionally grown in suspension bioreactors as an adherent monolayer by adding small beads called microcarriers on which the cells can attach and grow [56]. Suspension bioreactors offer a higher level of homogeneity and process control which serve to reduce both batch-to-batch and within-batch variability of cell cultures. Furthermore, stirred suspension bioreactors are highly scalable and several variables such as dissolved oxygen, pH, and temperature can be computer-controlled to provide a high level of process control and thus more uniform batches of products. The use of bioreactor technology has been thoroughly reviewed by Schnitzler et al. [56].

A wide variety of platforms and methods are available to grow MSCs. The differing effects of these platforms and methods should be realized in early stages of development to ensure scalable and effective clinical translation. It is important to further consider the implications of differing culture conditions within the chosen culture platform to effectively optimize product development. The MSC secretome can be tailored through altering culture conditions such as forced cell-cell interactions, oxygen level, and exposure to mechanical forces or biochemical factors (Figure 3), as described below [24, 77]. Advances in understanding the effect of differing culture conditions on the MSC secretome and/or its enclosed EVs are summarized in Table 2.

3.3.1. Three-Dimensional Spheroid Culture. MSCs can be induced to grow as three-dimensional (3D) aggregates (spheroids) where the cells attach to each other instead of a surface. The most common method to create spheroids is the hanging drop method, in which small droplets of cell suspension are placed on a static tissue culture flask and cultured upside down over a bath of buffer solution such as phosphate-buffered saline (PBS). Spheroids have also been created spontaneously in low attachment plates, in microwell-based systems such as AggreWells, and in suspension bioreactors by inoculating the cells at a high density [77–79]. Compared to traditional 2D adherent monolayer cultures, growth as 3D spheroids is considered more physiologically relevant [80]. MSCs within 3D aggregates have been shown to exhibit enhanced anti-inflammatory, angiogenic, and tissue reparative/regenerative properties [80]. The mechano-physical properties in MSC spheroids are drastically different, with cytoskeletal reorganization and changes in cell morphology which create relatively smaller cells with a spherical shape. MSCs grown within spheroids also have significant differences in gene expression and enhanced stem cell

properties (i.e., stemness) including improved multidifferentiation potential [81].

Similarly, it has been demonstrated that CM derived from spheroid MSC cultures is more effective than MSCs grown as a monolayer in suppressing an inflammatory response in stimulated macrophages in coculture and in a mouse model [28, 82]. This effect has been attributed to significantly higher expression levels of anti-inflammatory factors TSG-6, STC-1, and CXCR4 and increased secretion of PGE2 as the principal mediator of inflammation. CM from spheroid MSCs inhibited macrophages from secreting proinflammatory cytokines TNF-α, CXCL2, IL-12p40, and IL-23 and increased their secretion of anti-inflammatory cytokines IL-10 and IL-2Rα. Another study revealed a significant decrease in the chemotactic index of CD14$^+$ cells when incubated with 3D MSC spheroid-derived microvesicles compared to 2D MSC-derived microvesicles. This suggests that MSC culture mode can impact the immunomodulatory characteristics of the resulting microvesicle population [83].

MSCs cultured as 3D spheroids also exhibited an increased level of certain proteins and cytokines with more than purely immunomodulatory effects, such as antioncogenic proteins IL-24, TNF-α, CD82, vasculogenesis and angiogenesis promoter VEGF, and proteins involved in cell differentiation and survival such as TGF-β3 [82, 83]. Furthermore, MSCs grown in 3D spheroids cocultured with osteoarthritic chondrocytes exhibited higher potential for cartilage repair compared to those grown as a 2D monolayer [84]. Although there is limited research on the effect of spheroid culture on many aspects of the secretome, one would expect the increase in cell-cell interaction, altered cell morphology, and the potentially hypoxic nature of the spheroid's internal microenvironment to have a large effect on the composition of the resulting MSC secretome.

3.3.2. Hypoxia/Anoxia. The majority of *in vitro* cultures are exposed to headspace oxygen levels of 21%. Since MSCs are typically not exposed to such high levels of oxygen in their native environment, this oxygen level can be considered to be hyperoxic, a culture condition that has been reported to contribute to oxidative stress and genetic instability resulting in DNA damage and reduced lifespan [85]. Anoxia on the other hand, defined as a headspace oxygen level of <1%, is used to simulate ischemic injury conditions *in vitro*. Whereas MSC survival rates decrease with increased exposure times to anoxia, the lack of oxygen can upregulate the release of chemotactic and angiogenic mediators of crucial importance for tissue regeneration and repair applications [86]. While not necessarily directly reflective of the oxygen levels to which the cells are exposed, conditioning of MSCs at headspace oxygen concentrations of 1–5%, often referred to as hypoxic culture conditions, is employed as a less extreme method than anoxia to induce the activation of survival pathways and the secretion of products that may adapt the cells to their stressed environment [24]. This has resulted in populations that exhibit increased growth kinetics, greater differentiation capacity, and therapeutically desirable characteristics via the activation of hypoxia-inducible factor- (HIF-) 1α [87].

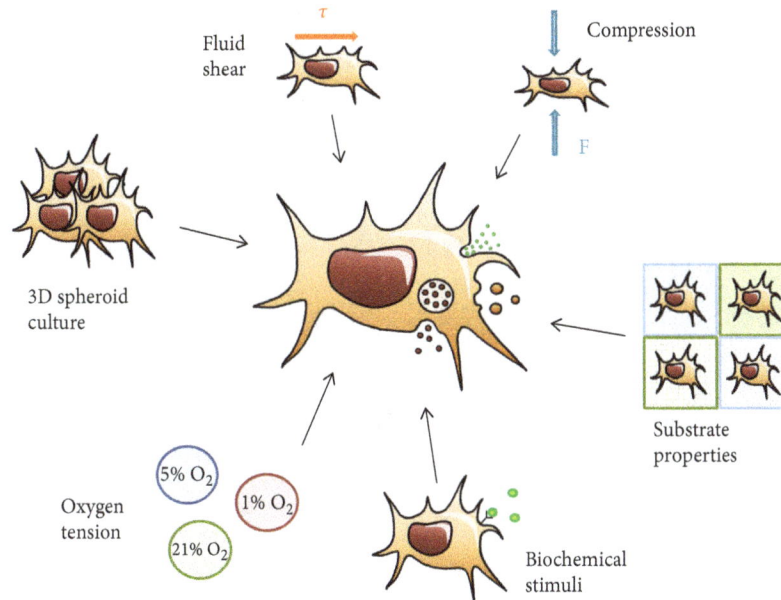

FIGURE 3: Alterations to MSC cultures reported to have an influence on the MSC secretome profile. 3D spheroid culture (i.e., forced cell-cell interactions), fluid shear, compression forces, the properties of the cells' residing substrate (i.e., stiffness and topography), biochemical stimuli (i.e., exposure to inflammatory factors), and the amount of oxygen cells are exposed to influence the amount and types of biomolecules secreted by MSCs.

Hypoxia has been reported to enhance both the secretion profile of MSCs and the quantity of exosomes released [88–90]. An overexpression of miRNAs involved in inflammatory, proliferative, and differentiative phases has been observed, including miR-223, -146b, -126, -199a, -11, -22, -24, and -210 [89, 91]. This is consistent with an upregulation of factors involved in cellular proliferation, differentiation, survival, angiogenesis, immunomodulation, and/or neuroregulation including VEGF, GM-CSF, IGF-1, IL-6, EGF, FGF, PDGF, and GCSF [88, 90, 92, 93]. Furthermore, *in vivo* studies have demonstrated enhanced muscle regeneration and an elevated protective effect on endotoxin-induced acute lung injury with injection of hypoxia-preconditioned MSC-derived EVs [89, 94].

There are some discrepancies between studies in terms of the upregulation or downregulation of factors resulting from differing oxygen concentrations, exposure times, cell source, or culture environment. Paquet et al. [86] reported that CM from anoxic conditions (0.1% O_2 headspace) had enhanced chemotactic and proangiogenic properties, along with a reduced inflammatory mediator content, while it showed no substantial differences between hypoxic (5% O_2 headspace) and normoxic (21% O_2 headspace) conditions, contrary to other studies. TGF-β1 was reported to be upregulated at a headspace concentration of 1% O_2 [93] but downregulated at 5% O_2 [92]. Hung et al. [93] also showed upregulated osteogenic and adipogenic factors, but a decrease in chondrogenic factors, contrary to several studies that demonstrated enhanced chondrogenesis in hypoxia-induced MSCs [95–97]. Li et al. [94] demonstrated the importance of exposure time in a study where they exposed MSCs to a hypoxic environment for 30, 60, or 90 minutes with differing resultant secretome profiles.

The MSC secretome is highly dynamic, and there is a clear need for accurate reporting in oxygen tension studies. Although studies report the oxygen concentration in the air, the dissolved oxygen levels to which cells are exposed in culture may differ depending on parameters such as depth of medium, cell density and oxygen consumption rate. The issue of exposure time is also often overlooked. There are differences between cells exposed to short-term hypoxic preconditioning and those that have undergone long-term expansion in low oxygen environments. Cells exposed to hypoxia from passage 0 to passage 2 were reported to be able to proliferate faster compared to those cultured in normoxia, and displayed enhanced expression of genes involved in ECM assembly, neural and muscle development, and epithelial development [98]. With MSCs exhibiting altered growth characteristics and gene expression, it is likely that the secretome profile would also be altered in such circumstances. It is clear that hypoxic conditions heavily affect the therapeutic properties of MSCs, but standardization of hypoxia-related protocols is needed to properly compare and reproduce results.

3.3.3. Mechanical Stimuli. MSCs have been shown to be highly mechanosensitive [99]. Cell behaviours such as proliferation and differentiation, as well as their secretome profile, have been shown to be strongly influenced by mechanical stimuli such as fluid shear stress and compression [24, 100]. MSCs transfer mechanical stimuli from their surrounding microenvironment into biochemical signals via mechanotransduction [100]. While the majority of publications in this area have focused on mechanical stimulation as a means of impacting cellular differentiation [99, 101], it is increasingly evident that the paracrine factors generated by the cells

TABLE 2: Effects of differing culture conditions on the MSC secretome. The results shown are in comparison to the secretome of control cells cultured as a 2D monolayer in static tissue culture flasks under normoxic (21% O_2) conditions. The medium listed does not include antibiotics or antimycotics.

MSC source	Culture mode	Medium	Results	Ref.
		3D spheroid cultures		
Human femoral heads	3D spheroid culture in spinner flasks and rotating wall vessels	αMEM + 15% FBS	(i) Decrease in surface marker expression levels (ii) Decreased cell size (iii) Enhanced osteogenic and adipogenic differentiation (iv) Differing gene expression profile	[77]
Human umbilical cord blood	Spheroids (hanging drop method)	DMEM + 10% FBS, 1% L-glutamine	(i) IL-2Rα, IL-7, IL-16, MCP-3, TGF-β3, and VEGF detected only in spheroid CM (ii) Significant increase in IL-6, MCP-1, LIF, G-CSF, and SDF-1α (iii) Decrease in TGF-β1 and TGF-β2 levels (iv) Decreased chemotactic index of CD14$^+$ cells (v) Enhanced capability to promote signal factors secretion	[83]
Human bone marrow	3D spheroids (hanging drop method)	CCM + 17% FBS	(i) More effective in suppressing inflammatory responses in the coculture system with LPS-activated macrophages (ii) Maximally expressed TSG-6 (iii) Expressed high levels of stanniocalcin-1, IL-24, TNF-α-related apoptosis inducing ligand, and CD82 (iv) 1/4 of the volume of monolayer cells	[82]
Human bone marrow	3D spheroids (hanging drop method)	CCM + 17% FBS	(i) Inhibited LPS-stimulated macrophages from secreting proinflammatory cytokines TNF-α, CXCL2, IL-12p40, and IL-23 (ii) Increased secretion of anti-inflammatory cytokines IL-10 and IL-1rα	[28]
Human adipose tissue	3D spheroids in suspension using ultra low attachment plates	αMEM + 10% FBS	(i) Enhanced production of VEGF, SDF, and HGF (ii) Lowered expression of proapoptotic markers	[78]
		Oxygen tension (hypoxia/anoxia)		
Human adipose tissue	Hypoxia (1% O_2)	DMEM	(i) Higher HIF-1α expression (ii) Increased release of EVs (iii) Induced overexpression of miRNAs implicated in inflammatory (miR-223, -146b), proliferative, and differentiative phases (miR-126, -199a) of the healing process (iv) Enhanced muscle regeneration process	[89]
Human	Anoxia (0.1% O_2), hypoxia (5% O_2)	αMEM +5 g/L glucose	(i) CM from anoxic conditions enhanced chemotactic and proangiogenic properties and reduced inflammatory mediator content (ii) Enhanced expression of VEGF-A, VEGF-C, IL-8, RANTES, and monocyte chemoattractant protein 1	[86]
Human adipose tissue	Hypoxia (5% O_2)	RKCM	(i) Promoted antiapoptotic effects (ii) Higher levels of GM-CSF, VEGF, IL-6, and IGF-1 (iii) Lower levels of TGF-β1	[92]
Human umbilical cord Wharton jelly	Hypoxia (5% O_2)	PPRF-msc6	(i) Increased secretion profile (ii) Upregulated thymosin-beta and EF-2 significantly (iii) Enhanced neuroregulatory secretome profile	[90]

TABLE 2: Continued.

MSC source	Culture mode	Medium	Results	Ref.
Human bone marrow	Hypoxia (1% O_2)	DMEM + 10% FBS + 2 mM L-glutamine	(i) Upregulated protein level of vimentin, fibronectin, and N-cadherin (ii) Enhanced stemness genes Oct4, Nanog, Sall4, and Klf4 (iii) Higher levels of osteocalcin and osteopontin (iv) Reduced levels of COL2A1, COMP, and aggrecan (v) Lower expression of adipsin, FASN, and FABP4 (vi) Upregulated IGFs, VEGF, EGF, GCSF, GM-CSF, TGF-β1, and TGF-β2	[93]
Human bone marrow	Hypoxia (1% O_2) with serum starvation	Opti-MEM + 1% L-glutamine	(i) Significant increases in rate-limiting proteins of glycolysis and the NRF2/glutathione pathway (ii) Upregulated angiogenic associated pathways of PDGF, EGF, and FGF (iii) Microvesicle secretion decreased, exosome secretion substantially increased	[88]
Murine bone marrow	Repeated cycles of anoxia	StemPro MSC SFM	(i) miR-11, miR-22, miR-24, miR-199a-3p, and miR-210 upregulated in exosomes	[91]
Human bone marrow	Hypoxia for 30, 60, or 90 min	Unknown	(i) The 60 min group had the greatest protective effect on endotoxin-induced acute lung injury model	[94]
Mechanical stimuli				
Human bone marrow	TGF-β1 stimulation (1 ng/mL) or mechanical load (multiaxial shear and compression) in fibrin-poly(ester-urethane) scaffolds	αMEM + 10% FBS + 5 ng/mL bFGF	(i) TGF-β1 stimulation and load had distinct effects, both enhanced chondrogenic profile compared to control (ii) Nitrite content in media higher in loaded groups (iii) TGF-β1 enhanced expression of leptin, leptin receptor, and MDC (iv) Load enhanced expression of uPAR, LAP, MIP3α, angiogenin, ALCAM, angiopoietin 2, osteoprotegerin, and DR6; reduced expression of GRO (v) Both TGF-β1 and load enhanced the expression of BLC, MCP3, MIF, VEGF, MMP13, and PDGFaa	[100]
Human bone marrow	Computer-controlled bioreactors, on Cytodex 3 microcarriers (2 g/L)	PPRF-msc6	(i) Enhanced the neuroregulatory profile of secretome (ii) Increased the secretion of Cys C, GDN, Gal-1, and PEDF (iii) Upregulation of miR-16 (iv) Number of CNS regulators only detected in CM of bioreactor cultured MSCs (v) Upregulation of classical trophic factors BDNF, VEGF, and IGF-1	[16]
Human bone marrow	Bioreactors	DMEM + 10% FBS	(i) Enhanced angiogenesis by CM from mechanically stimulated MSCs via FGFR and VEGFR signalling cascades (ii) Enrichment of MMP-2, TGF-β1, and bFGF	[102]
Human	PAM hydrogels of various rigidity	DMEM-low glucose + 10% FBS	(i) VEGF, angiogenin, and IGF upregulated with increasing elastic modulus (ii) EGF, IL-6, and IL-8 were not stiffness-dependent	[103]

TABLE 2: Continued.

MSC source	Culture mode	Medium	Results	Ref.
Adipose tissue	Fibrous scaffolds of variously aligned fibers	α-MEM + 10% FBS	(i) Higher levels of anti-inflammatory and proangiogenic cytokines were produced from cells seeded on electrospun scaffolds (ii) CM from scaffold cultures accelerated wound closure and macrophage recruitment in wound bed	[163]
		Electromagnetic stimuli		
Equine adipose tissue	Static magnetic field (0.5 T)	DMEM/F12 + 10% FBS	(i) Reached doubling time earlier, colony-forming potential higher (ii) Considerable increase in the number of secreted microvesicles (iii) Release of BMP-2, VEGF, and p53 increased (iv) Reduced release of TNF-α	[113]
		Biochemical stimuli		
Human bone marrow	IFN-γ and TNF-α stimulation	DMEM-low glucose	(i) Elevated secretion levels of IL-6, HGF, VEGF, and TGF-β	[119]
Murine bone marrow	IFN-γ and either TNF-α, IL-1α, or IL-1β stimulation	α-MEM+ 10% FBS + 2 mM glutamine	(i) Provoked the expression of CXCL-9 and CXCL-10 and inducible nitric oxide synthase	[118]
Human adipose tissue	TGF-β1 stimulation	DMEM + 0.1% BSA + 1% glutamine	(i) Upregulated secretion of PlGF, IGFBP-3, LIF, OSM, IL-4, IL-7, IL-13, CXCL9, CCL26, and OPN (ii) Downregulated secretion of CCL7, CCL11, CXCL6, OPG, IL-5, IL-10, CCL8, CXCL1, CXCL10, HGF, leptin, FGF-7, and GM-CSF	[123]
Adipose tissue	TNF-α stimulation	MesenPRO RS Basal Medium + 2 mM L-glutamine + MesenPRO RS Growth Supplement	(i) TNF-α-preconditioned ASCs secreted exosomes with elevated Wnt-3a content (ii) Enhanced proliferation and osteogenic differentiation in human primary osteoblastic cells	[120]
Human umbilical cord	LPS preconditioning	DMEM-low glucose + 10% FBS and sigma serum-free medium	(i) Improved regulatory abilities for macrophage polarization and resolution of chronic inflammation (ii) Unique expression of miR-let7b	[115]
Human adipose tissue	LPS preconditioning	DMEM-low glucose	(i) Enhanced mRNA expression of IL-6, TNF-α, HGF, and VEGF (ii) Enhanced liver regeneration in partially hepatectomized mice	[116]
Human adipose tissue	H$_2$O$_2$ stimulation	α-MEM + 10% exo-free FBS	(i) Exosomes that had been H$_2$O$_2$-stimulated enhanced skin flap recovery and capillary density	[121]

are highly influenced by their mechanical environment [16, 100, 102, 103]. For example, culturing MSCs on microcarriers within stirred suspension bioreactors, where cells are exposed to fluid shear forces, was found to enhance the neuroregulatory profile of the secretome, including a number of CNS regulators only detected in the CM of bioreactor-cultured MSCs and not in the CM of cells grown in static tissue culture plates [16]. Classic trophic factors BDNF, VEGF, and IGF-1 were also upregulated in dynamic bioreactor culture [16]. MSC constructs exposed to physiological compression had an enhanced angiogenic profile within the CM, which was also enriched with the soluble regulators MMP-2, TGF-β1, and bFGF [102]. Further, the exposure of MSCs to multiaxial shear and compression enhanced their chondrogenic profile similarly, but

distinctly, to that caused by TGF-β1 stimulation [100]. Nitric oxide (NO) production was significantly higher in loaded groups, with NO playing an effective role in MSC immunomodulation through the suppression of T cell response [100].

MSCs also respond to the mechanical properties of their substrate (i.e., the surface on which they are attached) including rigidity [99]. Matrix stiffness can guide differentiation of cells towards specific lineages [99], and as such, changes to cell state alter the secretome [100]. VEGF, angiogenin, and IGF are upregulated with increasing elastic moduli, whereas EGF, IL-6, and IL-8 levels are not responsive to the change of stiffness [103]. It is apparent that mechanical stimulation plays a significant role in determining the composition and function of the secretome, and further research should explore ways to take advantage of dynamic cultures and the mechanical properties of cell culture substrates.

3.3.4. Electromagnetic Stimuli.

Exposure of MSCs to electromagnetic fields (EMFs) is another strategy to influence cell behaviour as cells communicate with each other through sending and receiving electromagnetic signals [104]. In collagen-rich tissues, such as bone and cartilage, small, endogenous electric fields are produced during applied mechanical stresses [105]. Therefore, most research involving MSCs in this area to date has focused on osteogenic and chondrogenic differentiation through EMF stimulation [106]. For example, exposure of Wharton jelly-derived MSCs to EMF (1.8 mT, 75 Hz, 8 h/day for 21 days) increased cell division and cell densities, induced early chondrogenic differentiation, and increased collagen II expression levels [107]. Similarly, though dependent on intensity, time of exposure, and frequency of EMF, EMF exposure has been used to enhance osteogenic and neural differentiation [108–110], impact cell metabolism and structure [111], and increase cell viability [112].

Very little work has focused on the effect of EMF on MSC secretions. Marędziak et al. [113] reported that under static magnetic field (0.5 T), adipose-derived MSCs secreted a considerably higher number of microvesicles compared to a control with no magnetic stimulation. In addition, microvesicles collected from the magnetically stimulated MSCs contained higher amounts of BMP-2, VEGF, and p53 and lower amounts of TNF-α. Thus, controlling EMF exposure, along with mechanical, electrical, and biochemical stimuli, may provide a significant opportunity to enhance and optimize bioprocesses for MSC secretome-derived products.

3.3.5. Biochemical Stimuli.

MSCs are also highly influenced by direct biochemical signals elicited by various biomolecules. Much of the research involving the MSC secretome in terms of biochemical signalling is based around the fact that stimulated MSCs release molecules and EVs to counteract such biological signals and, thus, produce higher amounts of supportive proteins, miRNA, lipids, and other metabolites [114]. One way to induce a proinflammatory stressed phenotype is to precondition MSCs with lipopolysaccharide (LPS) [115, 116]. In traditional 2D monolayer cultures, compared to a control of MSCs cultured without LPS, LPS preconditioning induced MSCs to release proinflammatory cytokines IL-1β, IL-6, IL-8, IL-12, IFNs, and TNF-α, which, in turn, lowered the secretion of proinflammatory cytokines from other cell types [115, 116]. LPS-preconditioned MSC-derived exosomes were injected in a cutaneous wound model in streptozotocin-induced diabetic rats and were able to upregulate the expression of anti-inflammatory cytokines and promote M2 macrophage activation [115]. In partially hepatectomized mice, intravenously administered CM from LPS-preconditioned MSCs lowered the secretion of proinflammatory cytokines IL-6 and TNF-α and enhanced liver regeneration [116].

MSCs also produce immunomodulatory and regenerative factors in response to inflammatory stimuli such as interferon gamma (IFN-γ) and TNF-α. IFN-γ exposure has been shown to enhance immunosuppressive properties of MSCs by enhancing or inducing MSC inhibitory factors, downregulating T cell activation, enhancing T cell negative signalling, altering T cells from a proinflammatory to an anti-inflammatory phenotype, interacting with antigen-presenting cells, and increasing or inducing regulatory cells [117]. It was, however, shown that IFN-γ alone did not induce immunosuppression, and only when combined with either TNF-α, IL-1α, or IL-1β did immunosuppression by MSCs occur to inhibit the proliferation of T cells [118]. With any one of these combinations, MSCs produced several chemokines including CXCL-9 and CXCL-10 in large amounts [118]. Also, for MSCs treated with both IFN-γ and TNF-α, the secretion levels of IL-6, HGF, VEGF, and TGF-β were significantly increased, and the secretion levels with the combination of the two were significantly higher than that of either IFN-γ or TNF-α on their own [119]. From a different perspective, TNF-α-preconditioned exosomes promoted the proliferation and osteogenic differentiation of human primary osteoblastic cells [120].

Hydrogen peroxide (H_2O_2) can be used to induce an ischemia-mimicking microenvironment. Though high concentrations of H_2O_2 can induce cell death or damage, low concentrations may trigger processes that provide protective effects against stressful conditions. Stimulation with H_2O_2 has been shown to increase the expression of proangiogenic proteins such as VEGF and HGF [121], as well as the secretion of IL-6 [122]. Bai et al. demonstrated that MSCs stimulated with H_2O_2 enhanced their angiogenic effect on HUVECs and increased skin flap survival in an in vivo model [121].

Transforming growth factor- (TGF-) β1 has links to cellular proliferation, differentiation, and both anti- and proinflammatory effects. TGF-β1 exposure modulates the MSC secretome by altering the secretion of cytokines and chemokines (listed in Table 2) involved in immunosuppression, allergic response, and bone resorption [123]. Such studies provide evidence that the secretome can be modulated by biochemical factors, but a significant amount of research still needs be done to evaluate how exposure time and dose of biochemical stimulation impact the resulting paracrine factor profile for MSCs.

3.4. Isolation.

The isolation of MSC secretome-derived products is an important consideration in bioprocess development because of the highly dynamic nature of the secretome. The type and amount of products secreted depend on the culture period, or culture growth phase, from which the secretome is isolated. The method of isolation of specific products, primarily of EVs within the medium, also needs to be considered. Many challenges exist with current methods for EV isolation, as recently reviewed by Li et al. [124] and Gholizadeh et al. [125]. Ultracentrifugation, while able to deal with relatively large volumes, and currently considered to be the gold standard for separating these structures, only sees recovery rates of up to 25% and is a long cumbersome process [126]. There is also evidence that the high forces involved (typically

100,000g) can affect the bioactivity of the EVs themselves [127]. Size exclusion and antibody-based capture mechanisms are limited by a low throughput and the need for a final concentration step [128]. Furthermore, the use of antibody-based mechanisms is limited in many applications due to high cost. Microfluidics approaches enable simultaneous isolation and characterization of EVs, but EV recovery from such devices remains challenging [125]. More recently, anion-exchange chromatography has been used to isolate EVs in a single step with high purity, which exploits the negative charge of EVs [129]. There is a great need for EV isolation technologies that enable high throughput, maintain EV integrity and bioactivity, and are not cost prohibitive for clinical applications. It will be important to take advantage of the intrinsic properties of EVs to develop cost-effective isolation methods going forward.

3.5. Storage. For the storage and transport of MSC secretome-derived products, it is important to consider the effects of freeze-thaw, stability at various temperatures, and the effects of freeze-drying components. CM can reportedly be stored at −20°C for several months without experiencing functional deterioration [130]. For EVs, it has been shown that freeze-thaw does not affect the size of exosomes or impair the membrane integrity, but there is 60% reduction in size after 2 days at a physiological temperature of 37°C as well as a reduction after 3–4 days at 4°C [131]. When frozen at −20°C, exosomes are stable for periods as long as 6 months without a loss in their biochemical activity [9]. However, a study by Zhou et al. [132] demonstrated that protease inhibitors were essential for proper preservation, and freezing urinary exosomes at −20°C resulted in major losses, while freezing at −80°C enabled almost complete recovery after up to 7 months of storage. Further, extensive vortexing (i.e., 90 seconds) enabled maximum recovery of thawed exosome samples. These studies demonstrate that exosomes can undergo long-term storage with high recovery without a loss in bioactivity. Compared to cells, which exhibit impaired therapeutic properties as a result of freeze-thaw and require the use of preservatives for proper cryostorage, secretome-derived products are more amenable to storage, a key consideration from a translational perspective [53].

3.6. Delivery. *In vivo* delivery of secretome-derived products offers similar limitations to cell therapies. The majority of studies utilize simple intravenous injection of culture media or EVs in PBS into the site of injury. Despite the ability of exosomes to home to target tissues, there is limited retention in these areas, and repeated injections need to be performed for effective treatment [133]. One publication outlined the use of a photoinduced imine-cross-linking hydrogel which could be embedded with exosomes and used as a hydrogel tissue patch [133]. Cells were able to migrate into the hydrogel and internalize the encapsulated exosomes. Gangadaran et al. [134] also demonstrated enhanced EV retention within an injury site when mixed and injected with a Matrigel scaffold. Such a system prevents migration of cell-derived products, such as exosomes, from the target site and enables better integration for tissue repair. Depending on the application of such cell-derived therapeutics, hydrogel systems may enable more effective treatments via the slow release of products to prevent rapid site clearance or premature degradation.

MSC-derived exosomes have also been successfully delivered via integration into tissue-engineered bone [135] and within a fibrin surgical mesh [136]. The exosomes were added to enhance healing and to encourage migration of cells into the scaffolds. While the primary goals of these studies were to improve the outcomes of such constructs, the success of EV integration and retention offers an additional perspective for the use of cell-free therapeutics.

4. Conclusions

With recent reports attributing the main therapeutic benefits of MSCs to their paracrine effects, the secretome and its constituent exosomes may represent a novel and safer approach for the treatment of medical conditions compared to direct cell-based therapies. The fact that the secretome and its components are nonliving will facilitate the development of therapeutic strategies that can ensure higher sterility, lower immune response, and the ease of transport and storage. Understanding how cell source, media, and culture conditions interact to determine the quantity, quality, and types of biomolecules secreted is essential to the development of bioprocesses aimed at scaling up the production of secretome-derived products. Furthermore, standardization of protocols for isolation, characterization, storage, and delivery are needed to properly compare studies and ensure effective quality control.

Abbreviations

Akt:	Protein kinase B
ALCAM:	Activated leukocyte cell adhesion molecule
αMEM:	Alpha minimal essential medium
ALP:	Alkaline phosphatase
ATP:	Adenosine triphosphate
bFGF:	Basic fibroblast growth factor
BLC:	B lymphocyte chemoattractant
BMP-2:	Bone morphogenetic protein-2
CCL:	Chemokine (C-C motif) ligand
CCM:	Complete culture medium
CD:	Cluster of differentiation
CKD:	Chronic kidney disease
CM:	Conditioned medium
CNS:	Central nervous system
COMP:	Cartilage oligomeric matrix protein
CTX:	Cardiotoxin
CXCL:	Chemokine (C-X-C motif) ligand
Cys:	Cystatin
DMEM:	Dulbecco's modified Eagle's medium
DR6:	Death receptor 6
ECM:	Extracellular matrix
EGF:	Epidermal growth factor
EGFR:	Epidermal growth factor receptor
EMF:	Electromagnetic field
EV:	Extracellular vesicle

FABP:	Fatty acid binding protein
FASN:	Fatty acid synthase
FBS:	Fetal bovine serum
FGF:	Fibroblast growth factor
Gal:	Galactosidase
GAP:	Growth-associated protein
GC:	Glucocorticoid
G-CSF:	Granulocyte colony-stimulating factor
GDN:	Glia-derived nexin
GM-CSF:	Granulocyte macrophage colony-stimulating factor
GRO:	Growth-related oncogene
GvHD:	Graft versus host disease
H_2O_2:	Hydrogen peroxide
HGF:	Hepatocyte growth factor
HIF:	Hypoxia-inducible factor
HPL:	Human platelet lysate
HUVEC:	Human umbilical vein endothelial cell
IFN:	Interferon
IGF:	Insulin-like growth factor
IGFBP:	Insulin-like growth factor binding protein
IGFR:	Insulin-like growth factor receptor
IL:	Interleukin
LAP:	Latency-associated peptide
LIF:	Leukemia inhibitory factor
LPS:	Lipopolysaccharide
MCP:	Monocyte chemotactic protein
MDC:	Macrophage-derived chemokine
MIF:	Macrophage migration inhibitory factor
MIP:	Macrophage inflammatory protein
MMP:	Matrix metalloproteinase
MS:	Multiple sclerosis
MSC:	Mesenchymal stem cell
MVB:	Multivesicular body
NADH:	Nicotinamide adenine dinucleotide
NO:	Nitric oxide
OPG:	Osteoprotegerin
OPN:	Osteopontin
OSM:	Oncostatin M
P53:	Tumor suppressor 53
PAH:	Pulmonary arterial hypertension
PDGF:	Platelet-derived growth factor
PEDF:	Pigment epithelium-derived factor
PIGF:	Placental growth factor
RANTES:	Regulated on activation, normal T cell expressed and secreted
RGC:	Retinal ganglion cell
ROS:	Reactive oxygen species
RNA:	Ribonucleic acid
RT-qPCR:	Quantitative reverse transcription
SD:	Sprague Dawley
SDF:	Stromal cell-derived factor
SF:	Serum-free
SFM:	Serum-free media
STC:	Stanniocalcin
STZ:	Streptozocin
T1DM:	Type 1 diabetes mellitus
T2DM:	Type 2 diabetes mellitus
TB:	Thymosin beta

TGF:	Transforming growth factor
Th:	T helper
TNF:	Tumor necrosis factor
TSG:	Tumor necrosis factor-inducible gene protein
uPAR:	Urokinase-type plasminogen activator receptor
VEGF:	Vascular endothelial growth factor
XF:	Xeno-free.

Conflicts of Interest

Under a licensing agreement between Stemcell Technologies Inc. and Dr. Ungrin/University of Toronto, Dr. Ungrin is entitled to a share of royalties on sales of the AggreWell technology. This did not in any way affect the neutrality or objectivity of this article and does not alter the authors' adherence to the journal's policies on sharing data and materials.

References

[1] A. O. Pires, B. Mendes-Pinheiro, F. G. Teixeira et al., "Unveiling the differences of secretome of human bone marrow mesenchymal stem cells, adipose tissue derived stem cells and human umbilical cord perivascular cells: a proteomic analysis," *Stem Cells and Development*, vol. 25, no. 14, pp. 1073–1083, 2016.

[2] S. T.-F. Hsiao, A. Asgari, Z. Lokmic et al., "Comparative analysis of paracrine factor expression in human adult mesenchymal stem cells derived from bone marrow, adipose, and dermal tissue," *Stem Cells and Development*, vol. 21, no. 12, pp. 2189–2203, 2012.

[3] E. A. Jones, A. English, K. Henshaw et al., "Enumeration and phenotypic characterization of synovial fluid multipotential mesenchymal progenitor cells in inflammatory and degenerative arthritis," *Arthritis and Rheumatism*, vol. 50, no. 3, pp. 817–827, 2004.

[4] M. Dominici, K. le Blanc, I. Mueller et al., "Minimal criteria for defining multipotent mesenchymal stromal cells. The International Society for Cellular Therapy position statement," *Cytotherapy*, vol. 8, no. 4, pp. 315–317, 2006.

[5] N. Kim and S.-G. Cho, "Clinical applications of mesenchymal stem cells," *The Korean Journal of Internal Medicine*, vol. 28, no. 4, pp. 387–402, 2013.

[6] N. Kim and S.-G. Cho, "New strategies for overcoming limitations of mesenchymal stem cell-based immune modulation," *International Journal of Stem Cells*, vol. 8, no. 1, pp. 54–68, 2015.

[7] F. Tögel, Z. Hu, K. Weiss, J. Isaac, C. Lange, and C. Westenfelder, "Administered mesenchymal stem cells protect against ischemic acute renal failure through differentiation-independent mechanisms," *American Journal of Physiology-Renal Physiology*, vol. 289, no. 1, pp. F31–F42, 2005.

[8] R. W. Y. Yeo, R. C. Lai, B. Zhang et al., "Mesenchymal stem cell: an efficient mass producer of exosomes for drug delivery," *Advanced Drug Delivery Reviews*, vol. 65, no. 3, pp. 336–341, 2013.

[9] V. B. R. Konala, M. K. Mamidi, R. Bhonde, A. K. Das, R. Pochampally, and R. Pal, "The current landscape of the mesenchymal stromal cell secretome: a new paradigm for cell-free regeneration," *Cytotherapy*, vol. 18, no. 1, pp. 13–24, 2016.

[10] A. I. Caplan, "Mesenchymal stem cells: time to change the name!," *Stem Cells Translational Medicine*, vol. 6, no. 6, pp. 1445–1451, 2017.

[11] US National Institutes of Health, http://ClinicalTrials.gov. Retrieved March 6, 2017, https://www.clinicaltrials.gov/.

[12] L. Kordelas, V. Rebmann, A. K. Ludwig et al., "MSC-derived exosomes: a novel tool to treat therapy-refractory graft-versus-host disease," *Leukemia*, vol. 28, no. 4, pp. 970–973, 2014.

[13] W. Nassar, M. el-Ansary, D. Sabry et al., "Umbilical cord mesenchymal stem cells derived extracellular vesicles can safely ameliorate the progression of chronic kidney diseases," *Biomaterials Research*, vol. 20, no. 1, p. 21, 2016.

[14] K. I. Mentkowski, J. D. Snitzer, S. Rusnak, and J. K. Lang, "Therapeutic potential of engineered extracellular vesicles," *The AAPS Journal*, vol. 20, no. 3, p. 50, 2018.

[15] A. M. Billing, H. Ben Hamidane, S. S. Dib et al., "Comprehensive transcriptomic and proteomic characterization of human mesenchymal stem cells reveals source specific cellular markers," *Scientific Reports*, vol. 6, no. 1, article 21507, 2016.

[16] F. G. Teixeira, K. M. Panchalingam, R. Assunção-Silva et al., "Modulation of the mesenchymal stem cell secretome using computer-controlled bioreactors: impact on neuronal cell proliferation, survival and differentiation," *Scientific Reports*, vol. 6, no. 1, 2016.

[17] S. Rani, A. E. Ryan, M. D. Griffin, and T. Ritter, "Mesenchymal stem cell-derived extracellular vesicles: toward cell-free therapeutic applications," *Molecular Therapy*, vol. 23, no. 5, pp. 812–823, 2015.

[18] L. Shao, Y. Zhang, B. Lan et al., "MiRNA-sequence indicates that mesenchymal stem cells and exosomes have similar mechanism to enhance cardiac repair," *BioMed Research International*, vol. 2017, 9 pages, 2017.

[19] L. Bai, D. Li, J. Li et al., "Bioactive molecules derived from umbilical cord mesenchymal stem cells," *Acta Histochemica*, vol. 118, no. 8, pp. 761–769, 2016.

[20] M. Madrigal, K. S. Rao, and N. H. Riordan, "A review of therapeutic effects of mesenchymal stem cell secretions and induction of secretory modification by different culture methods," *Journal of Translational Medicine*, vol. 12, no. 1, p. 260, 2014.

[21] N. Beohar, J. Rapp, S. Pandya, and D. W. Losordo, "Rebuilding the damaged heart: the potential of cytokines and growth factors in the treatment of ischemic heart disease," *Journal of the American College of Cardiology*, vol. 56, no. 16, pp. 1287–1297, 2010.

[22] C. Nicholas and G. B. Lesinski, "Immunomodulatory cytokines as therapeutic agents for melanoma," *Immunotherapy*, vol. 3, no. 5, pp. 673–690, 2011.

[23] S. Lee and K. Margolin, "Cytokines in cancer immunotherapy," *Cancer*, vol. 3, no. 4, pp. 3856–3893, 2011.

[24] S. H. Ranganath, O. Levy, M. S. Inamdar, and J. M. Karp, "Harnessing the mesenchymal stem cell secretome for the treatment of cardiovascular disease," *Cell Stem Cell*, vol. 10, no. 3, pp. 244–258, 2012.

[25] Y. K. Na, J.-J. Ban, M. Lee, W. Im, and M. Kim, "Wound healing potential of adipose tissue stem cell extract," *Biochemical and Biophysical Research Communications*, vol. 485, no. 1, pp. 30–34, 2017.

[26] J. Xu, B. Wang, Y. Sun et al., "Human fetal mesenchymal stem cell secretome enhances bone consolidation in distraction osteogenesis," *Stem Cell Research & Therapy*, vol. 7, no. 1, p. 134, 2016.

[27] M. Abouelkheir, D. A. ElTantawy, M.-A. Saad et al., "Mesenchymal stem cells versus their conditioned medium in the treatment of cisplatin-induced acute kidney injury: evaluation of efficacy and cellular side effects," *International Journal of Clinical and Experimental Medicine*, vol. 9, no. 12, pp. 23222–23234, 2016.

[28] J. H. Ylöstalo, T. J. Bartosh, K. Coble, and D. J. Prockop, "Human mesenchymal stem/stromal cells cultured as spheroids are self-activated to produce prostaglandin E2 that directs stimulated macrophages into an anti-inflammatory phenotype," *Stem Cells*, vol. 30, no. 10, pp. 2283–2296, 2012.

[29] A. Kelso, "Cytokines: principles and prospects," *Immunology and Cell Biology*, vol. 76, no. 4, pp. 300–317, 1998.

[30] Y. Nakamura, S. Miyaki, H. Ishitobi et al., "Mesenchymal-stem-cell-derived exosomes accelerate skeletal muscle regeneration," *FEBS Letters*, vol. 589, no. 11, pp. 1257–1265, 2015.

[31] T. Furuta, S. Miyaki, H. Ishitobi et al., "Mesenchymal stem cell-derived exosomes promote fracture healing in a mouse model," *Stem Cells Translational Medicine*, vol. 5, no. 12, pp. 1620–1630, 2016.

[32] G. Raposo and W. Stoorvogel, "Extracellular vesicles: exosomes, microvesicles, and friends," *Journal of Cell Biology*, vol. 200, no. 4, pp. 373–383, 2013.

[33] S.-M. Kim and H.-S. Kim, "Engineering of extracellular vesicles as drug delivery vehicles," *Stem Cell Investigation*, vol. 4, no. 9, pp. 74–74, 2017.

[34] F. Arslan, R. C. Lai, M. B. Smeets et al., "Mesenchymal stem cell-derived exosomes increase ATP levels, decrease oxidative stress and activate PI3K/Akt pathway to enhance myocardial viability and prevent adverse remodeling after myocardial ischemia/reperfusion injury," *Stem Cell Research*, vol. 10, no. 3, pp. 301–312, 2013.

[35] V. Rebmann, L. König, F. . S. Nardi, B. Wagner, L. F. S. Manvailer, and P. A. Horn, "The potential of HLA-G-bearing extracellular vesicles as a future element in HLA-G immune biology," *Frontiers in Immunology*, vol. 7, 2016.

[36] J. Lötvall, A. F. Hill, F. Hochberg et al., "Minimal experimental requirements for definition of extracellular vesicles and their functions: a position statement from the International Society for Extracellular Vesicles," *Journal of Extracellular Vesicles*, vol. 3, no. 1, article 26913, 2014.

[37] A. Marote, F. G. Teixeira, B. Mendes-Pinheiro, and A. J. Salgado, "MSCs-derived exosomes: cell-secreted nanovesicles with regenerative potential," *Frontiers in Pharmacology*, vol. 7, 2016.

[38] L. Timmers, S. K. Lim, F. Arslan et al., "Reduction of myocardial infarct size by human mesenchymal stem cell conditioned medium," *Stem Cell Research*, vol. 1, no. 2, pp. 129–137, 2008.

[39] R. C. Lai, F. Arslan, M. M. Lee et al., "Exosome secreted by MSC reduces myocardial ischemia/reperfusion injury," *Stem Cell Research*, vol. 4, no. 3, pp. 214–222, 2010.

[40] S. Bruno, M. Tapparo, F. Collino et al., "Renal regenerative potential of different extra-cellular vesicle populations derived from bone marrow mesenchymal stromal cells," *Tissue Engineering Part A*, vol. 23, no. 21-22, pp. 1262–1273, 2017.

[41] S. Wen, M. Dooner, Y. Cheng et al., "Mesenchymal stromal cell-derived extracellular vesicles rescue radiation damage to

murine marrow hematopoietic cells," *Leukemia*, vol. 30, no. 11, pp. 2221–2231, 2016.

[42] K. M. Kim, K. Abdelmohsen, M. Mustapic, D. Kapogiannis, and M. Gorospe, "RNA in extracellular vesicles," *WIREs RNA*, vol. 8, no. 4, article e1413, 2017.

[43] E. Ragni, F. Banfi, M. Barilani et al., "Extracellular vesicle-shuttled mRNA in mesenchymal stem cell communication," *Stem Cells*, vol. 35, no. 4, pp. 1093–1105, 2017.

[44] Y. Zhang, X. Huang, and Y. Yuan, "MicroRNA-410 promotes chondrogenic differentiation of human bone marrow mesenchymal stem cells through down-regulating Wnt3a," *American Journal of Translational Research*, vol. 9, no. 1, pp. 136–145, 2017.

[45] N. Wang, C. Chen, D. Yang et al., "Mesenchymal stem cells-derived extracellular vesicles, via miR-210, improve infarcted cardiac function by promotion of angiogenesis," *Biochimica et Biophysica Acta (BBA) - Molecular Basis of Disease*, vol. 1863, no. 8, pp. 2085–2092, 2017.

[46] X. Cheng, G. Zhang, L. Zhang et al., "Mesenchymal stem cells deliver exogenous miR-21 via exosomes to inhibit nucleus pulposus cell apoptosis and reduce intervertebral disc degeneration," *Journal of Cellular and Molecular Medicine*, vol. 22, no. 1, pp. 261–276, 2018.

[47] S. Tsukita, T. Yamada, K. Takahashi et al., "MicroRNAs 106b and 222 improve hyperglycemia in a mouse model of insulin-deficient diabetes via pancreatic β-cell proliferation," *eBioMedicine*, vol. 15, pp. 163–172, 2017.

[48] A. M. Ardekani and M. M. Naeini, "The role of microRNAs in human diseases," *Avicenna Journal of Medical Biotechnology*, vol. 2, no. 4, pp. 161–179, 2010.

[49] Y. Yuan, M. S. Kallos, C. Hunter, and A. Sen, "Improved expansion of human bone marrow-derived mesenchymal stem cells in microcarrier-based suspension culture," *Journal of Tissue Engineering and Regenerative Medicine*, vol. 8, no. 3, pp. 210–225, 2014.

[50] S. Taverna, M. Pucci, and R. Alessandro, "Extracellular vesicles: small bricks for tissue repair/regeneration," *Annals of Translational Medicine*, vol. 5, no. 4, p. 83, 2017.

[51] E. N. Momin, G. Vela, H. A. Zaidi, and A. Quinones-Hinojosa, "The oncogenic potential of mesenchymal stem cells in the treatment of cancer: directions for future research," *Current Immunology Reviews*, vol. 6, no. 2, pp. 137–148, 2010.

[52] L. Zimmerlin, T. S. Park, E. T. Zambidis, V. S. Donnenberg, and A. D. Donnenberg, "Mesenchymal stem cell secretome and regenerative therapy after cancer," *Biochimie*, vol. 95, no. 12, pp. 2235–2245, 2013.

[53] K. M. Panchalingam, S. Jung, L. Rosenberg, and L. A. Behie, "Bioprocessing strategies for the large-scale production of human mesenchymal stem cells: a review," *Stem Cell Research & Therapy*, vol. 6, no. 1, p. 225, 2015.

[54] M. R. Placzek, I. M. Chung, H. M. Macedo et al., "Stem cell bioprocessing: fundamentals and principles," *Journal of the Royal Society, Interface*, vol. 6, no. 32, pp. 209–32, 2009.

[55] R. Versteegen, "Serum: what, when, and where?," *Bioprocessing Journal*, vol. 15, no. 1, pp. 18–21, 2016.

[56] A. C. Schnitzler, A. Verma, D. E. Kehoe et al., "Bioprocessing of human mesenchymal stem/stromal cells for therapeutic use: current technologies and challenges," *Biochemical Engineering Journal*, vol. 108, pp. 3–13, 2016.

[57] K. Pachler, T. Lener, D. Streif et al., "A Good Manufacturing Practice–grade standard protocol for exclusively human

[58] A. Oikonomopoulos, W. K. van Deen, A.-R. Manansala et al., "Optimization of human mesenchymal stem cell manufacturing: the effects of animal/xeno-free media," *Scientific Reports*, vol. 5, no. 1, article 16570, 2015.

[59] H. Agata, N. Watanabe, Y. Ishii et al., "Feasibility and efficacy of bone tissue engineering using human bone marrow stromal cells cultivated in serum-free conditions," *Biochemical and Biophysical Research Communications*, vol. 382, no. 2, pp. 353–358, 2009.

[60] H. Miwa, Y. Hashimoto, K. Tensho, S. Wakitani, and M. Takagi, "Xeno-free proliferation of human bone marrow mesenchymal stem cells," *Cytotechnology*, vol. 64, no. 3, pp. 301–308, 2012.

[61] C. Ikebe and K. Suzuki, "Mesenchymal stem cells for regenerative therapy: optimization of cell preparation protocols," *BioMed Research International*, vol. 2014, Article ID 951512, 11 pages, 2014.

[62] S. Jung, A. Sen, L. Rosenberg, and L. A. Behie, "Human mesenchymal stem cell culture: rapid and efficient isolation and expansion in a defined serum-free medium," *Journal of Tissue Engineering and Regenerative Medicine*, vol. 6, no. 5, pp. 391–403, 2012.

[63] C. P. Hodgkinson, J. A. Gomez, M. Mirotsou, and V. J. Dzau, "Genetic engineering of mesenchymal stem cells and its application in human disease therapy," *Human Gene Therapy*, vol. 21, no. 11, pp. 1513–1526, 2010.

[64] M. Mendicino, A. M. Bailey, K. Wonnacott, R. K. Puri, and S. R. Bauer, "MSC-based product characterization for clinical trials: an FDA perspective," *Cell Stem Cell*, vol. 14, no. 2, pp. 141–145, 2014.

[65] T. R. J. Heathman, Q. A. Rafiq, A. K. C. Chan et al., "Characterization of human mesenchymal stem cells from multiple donors and the implications for large scale bioprocess development," *Biochemical Engineering Journal*, vol. 108, pp. 14–23, 2016.

[66] F. V. Paladino, L. R. Sardinha, C. A. Piccinato, and A. C. Goldberg, "Intrinsic variability present in Wharton's jelly mesenchymal stem cells and T cell responses may impact cell therapy," *Stem Cells International*, vol. 2017, Article ID 8492797, 12 pages, 2017.

[67] G. Siegel, T. Kluba, U. Hermanutz-Klein, K. Bieback, H. Northoff, and R. Schäfer, "Phenotype, donor age and gender affect function of human bone marrow-derived mesenchymal stromal cells," *BMC Medicine*, vol. 11, no. 1, 2013.

[68] C. Guay and R. Regazzi, "Exosomes as new players in metabolic organ cross-talk," *Diabetes, Obesity and Metabolism*, vol. 19, pp. 137–146, 2017.

[69] R. S. Patel, G. Carter, G. el Bassit et al., "Adipose-derived stem cells from lean and obese humans show depot specific differences in their stem cell markers, exosome contents and senescence: role of protein kinase C delta (PKCδ) in adipose stem cell niche," *Stem Cell Investigation*, vol. 3, p. 2, 2016.

[70] G. Togliatto, P. Dentelli, M. Gili et al., "Obesity reduces the pro-angiogenic potential of adipose tissue stem cell-derived extracellular vesicles (EVs) by impairing miR-126 content: impact on clinical applications," *International Journal of Obesity*, vol. 40, no. 1, pp. 102–111, 2016.

[71] L. Zazzeroni, G. Lanzoni, G. Pasquinelli, and C. Ricordi, "Considerations on the harvesting site and donor derivation

for mesenchymal stem cells-based strategies for diabetes," *CellR⁴*, vol. 5, no. 5, article e2435, 2017.

[72] P. Sarkar, J. Redondo, K. Kemp et al., "Reduced neuroprotective potential of the mesenchymal stromal cell secretome with *ex vivo* expansion, age and progressive multiple sclerosis," *Cytotherapy*, vol. 20, no. 1, pp. 21–28, 2018.

[73] Y. Tachida, H. Sakurai, and J. Okutsu, "Proteomic comparison of the secreted factors of mesenchymal stem cells from bone marrow, adipose tissue and dental pulp," *Journal of Proteomics & Bioinformatics*, vol. 8, no. 12, pp. 266–273, 2015.

[74] P. R. Amable, M. V. T. Teixeira, R. B. V. Carias, J. M. Granjeiro, and R. Borojevic, "Protein synthesis and secretion in human mesenchymal cells derived from bone marrow, adipose tissue and Wharton's jelly," *Stem Cell Research & Therapy*, vol. 5, no. 2, p. 53, 2014.

[75] S. R. Baglio, K. Rooijers, D. Koppers-Lalic et al., "Human bone marrow- and adipose-mesenchymal stem cells secrete exosomes enriched in distinctive miRNA and tRNA species," *Stem Cell Research & Therapy*, vol. 6, no. 1, p. 127, 2015.

[76] M. A. Lopez-Verrilli, A. Caviedes, A. Cabrera, S. Sandoval, U. Wyneken, and M. Khoury, "Mesenchymal stem cell-derived exosomes from different sources selectively promote neuritic outgrowth," *Neuroscience*, vol. 320, pp. 129–139, 2016.

[77] J. E. Frith, B. Thomson, and P. G. Genever, "Dynamic three-dimensional culture methods enhance mesenchymal stem cell properties and increase therapeutic potential," *Tissue Engineering Part C, Methods*, vol. 16, no. 4, pp. 735–749, 2010.

[78] J. H. Lee, Y. S. Han, and S. H. Lee, "Long-duration three-dimensional spheroid culture promotes angiogenic activities of adipose-derived mesenchymal stem cells," *Biomolecules & Therapeutics*, vol. 24, no. 3, pp. 260–267, 2016.

[79] P. R. Baraniak and T. C. McDevitt, "Scaffold-free culture of mesenchymal stem cell spheroids in suspension preserves multilineage potential," *Cell and Tissue Research*, vol. 347, no. 3, pp. 701–711, 2012.

[80] Z. Cesarz and K. Tamama, "Spheroid culture of mesenchymal stem cells," *Stem Cells International*, vol. 2016, Article ID 9176357, 11 pages, 2016.

[81] Y. Petrenko, E. Syková, and Š. Kubinová, "The therapeutic potential of three-dimensional multipotent mesenchymal stromal cell spheroids," *Stem Cell Research & Therapy*, vol. 8, no. 1, p. 94, 2017.

[82] T. J. Bartosh, J. H. Ylostalo, A. Mohammadipoor et al., "Aggregation of human mesenchymal stromal cells (MSCs) into 3D spheroids enhances their antiinflammatory properties," *Proceedings of the National Academy of Sciences of the United States of America*, vol. 107, no. 31, pp. 13724–13729, 2010.

[83] L. Xie, M. Mao, L. Zhou, L. Zhang, and B. Jiang, "Signal factors secreted by 2D and spheroid mesenchymal stem cells and by cocultures of mesenchymal stem cells derived microvesicles and retinal photoreceptor neurons," *Stem Cells International*, vol. 2017, Article ID 2730472, 13 pages, 2017.

[84] M. Khurshid, A. Mulet-Sierra, A. Adesida, and A. Sen, "Osteoarthritic human chondrocytes proliferate in 3d co-culture with mesenchymal stem cells in suspension bioreactors," *Journal of Tissue Engineering and Regenerative Medicine*, vol. 12, no. 3, pp. e1418–e1432, 2018.

[85] J. C. Estrada, C. Albo, A. Benguría et al., "Culture of human mesenchymal stem cells at low oxygen tension improves growth and genetic stability by activating glycolysis," *Cell Death and Differentiation*, vol. 19, no. 5, pp. 743–755, 2012.

[86] J. Paquet, M. Deschepper, A. Moya, D. Logeart-Avramoglou, C. Boisson-Vidal, and H. Petite, "Oxygen tension regulates human mesenchymal stem cell paracrine functions," *Stem Cells Translational Medicine*, vol. 4, no. 7, pp. 809–821, 2015.

[87] M. Ejtehadifar, K. Shamsasenjan, A. Movassaghpour et al., "The effect of hypoxia on mesenchymal stem cell biology," *Advanced Pharmaceutical Bulletin*, vol. 5, no. 2, pp. 141–149, 2015.

[88] J. D. Anderson, H. J. Johansson, C. S. Graham et al., "Comprehensive proteomic analysis of mesenchymal stem cell exosomes reveals modulation of angiogenesis via nuclear factor-kappaB signaling," *Stem Cells*, vol. 34, no. 3, pp. 601–613, 2016.

[89] C. Lo Sicco, D. Reverberi, C. Balbi et al., "Mesenchymal stem cell-derived extracellular vesicles as mediators of anti-inflammatory effects: endorsement of macrophage polarization," *Stem Cells Translational Medicine*, vol. 6, no. 3, pp. 1018–1028, 2017.

[90] F. G. Teixeira, K. M. Panchalingam, S. I. Anjo et al., "Do hypoxia/normoxia culturing conditions change the neuroregulatory profile of Wharton jelly mesenchymal stem cell secretome?," *Stem Cell Research & Therapy*, vol. 6, no. 1, p. 133, 2015.

[91] Y. Feng, W. Huang, M. Wani, X. Yu, and M. Ashraf, "Ischemic preconditioning potentiates the protective effect of stem cells through secretion of exosomes by targeting Mecp2 via miR-22," *PLoS One*, vol. 9, no. 2, article e88685, 2014.

[92] H. Y. An, H. S. Shin, J. S. Choi, H. J. Kim, J. Y. Lim, and Y. M. Kim, "Adipose mesenchymal stem cell secretome modulated in hypoxia for remodeling of radiation-induced salivary gland damage," *PLoS One*, vol. 10, no. 11, p. e0141862, 2015.

[93] S.-P. Hung, J. H. Ho, Y.-R. V. Shih, T. Lo, and O. K. Lee, "Hypoxia promotes proliferation and osteogenic differentiation potentials of human mesenchymal stem cells," *Journal of Orthopaedic Research*, vol. 30, no. 2, pp. 260–266, 2012.

[94] L. Li, S. Jin, and Y. Zhang, "Ischemic preconditioning potentiates the protective effect of mesenchymal stem cells on endotoxin-induced acute lung injury in mice through secretion of exosome," *International Journal of Clinical and Experimental Medicine*, vol. 8, no. 3, pp. 3825–3832, 2015.

[95] M. Kanichai, D. Ferguson, P. J. Prendergast, and V. A. Campbell, "Hypoxia promotes chondrogenesis in rat mesenchymal stem cells: a role for AKT and hypoxia-inducible factor (HIF)-1α," *Journal of Cellular Physiology*, vol. 216, no. 3, pp. 708–715, 2008.

[96] H.-H. Lee, C.-C. Chang, M.-J. Shieh et al., "Hypoxia enhances chondrogenesis and prevents terminal differentiation through PI3K/Akt/FoxO dependent anti-apoptotic effect," *Scientific Reports*, vol. 3, no. 1, article 2683, 2013.

[97] E. Duval, C. Baugé, R. Andriamanalijaona et al., "Molecular mechanism of hypoxia-induced chondrogenesis and its application in in vivo cartilage tissue engineering," *Biomaterials*, vol. 33, no. 26, pp. 6042–6051, 2012.

[98] L. Basciano, C. Nemos, B. Foliguet et al., "Long term culture of mesenchymal stem cells in hypoxia promotes a genetic program maintaining their undifferentiated and multipotent status," *BMC Cell Biology*, vol. 12, no. 1, p. 12, 2011.

[99] L. MacQueen, Y. Sun, and C. A. Simmons, "Mesenchymal stem cell mechanobiology and emerging experimental platforms," *Journal of the Royal Society, Interface*, vol. 10, no. 84, article 20130179, 2013.

[100] O. F. W. Gardner, N. Fahy, M. Alini, and M. J. Stoddart, "Differences in human mesenchymal stem cell secretomes during chondrogenic induction," *European Cells & Materials*, vol. 31, pp. 221–235, 2016.

[101] J. Hao, Y. Zhang, D. Jing et al., "Mechanobiology of mesenchymal stem cells: perspective into mechanical induction of MSC fate," *Acta Biomaterialia*, vol. 20, pp. 1–9, 2015.

[102] G. Kasper, N. Dankert, J. Tuischer et al., "Mesenchymal stem cells regulate angiogenesis according to their mechanical environment," *Stem Cells*, vol. 25, no. 4, pp. 903–910, 2007.

[103] A. A. Abdeen, J. B. Weiss, J. Lee, and K. A. Kilian, "Matrix composition and mechanics direct proangiogenic signaling from mesenchymal stem cells," *Tissue Engineering Part A*, vol. 20, no. 19-20, pp. 2737–2745, 2014.

[104] S. H. Tamrin, F. S. Majedi, M. Tondar, A. Sanati-Nezhad, and M. M. Hasani-Sadrabadi, "Electromagnetic fields and stem cell fate: when physics meets biology," *Reviews of Physiology, Biochemistry and Pharmacology*, vol. 171, pp. 63–97, 2016.

[105] T. A. Banks, P. S. B. Luckman, J. E. Frith, and J. J. Cooper-White, "Effects of electric fields on human mesenchymal stem cell behaviour and morphology using a novel multichannel device," *Integrative Biology*, vol. 7, no. 6, pp. 693–712, 2015.

[106] A. Maziarz, B. Kocan, M. Bester et al., "How electromagnetic fields can influence adult stem cells: positive and negative impacts," *Stem Cell Research & Therapy*, vol. 7, no. 1, p. 54, 2016.

[107] M. Esposito, A. Lucariello, C. Costanzo et al., "Differentiation of human umbilical cord-derived mesenchymal stem cells, WJ-MSCs, into chondrogenic cells in the presence of pulsed electromagnetic fields," *In Vivo*, vol. 27, no. 4, pp. 495–500, 2013.

[108] J.-E. Park, Y.-K. Seo, H.-H. Yoon, C.-W. Kim, J.-K. Park, and S. Jeon, "Electromagnetic fields induce neural differentiation of human bone marrow derived mesenchymal stem cells via ROS mediated EGFR activation," *Neurochemistry International*, vol. 62, no. 4, pp. 418–424, 2013.

[109] K. S. Kang, J. M. Hong, J. A. Kang, J.-W. Rhie, Y. H. Jeong, and D.-W. Cho, "Regulation of osteogenic differentiation of human adipose-derived stem cells by controlling electromagnetic field conditions," *Experimental & Molecular Medicine*, vol. 45, no. 1, article e6, 2013.

[110] S. Hassanpour-Tamrin, H. Taheri, M. Mahdi Hasani-Sadrabadi et al., "Nanoscale optoregulation of neural stem cell differentiation by intracellular alteration of redox balance," *Advanced Functional Materials*, vol. 27, no. 38, 2017.

[111] M. Walther, F. Mayer, W. Kafka, and N. Schütze, "Effects of weak, low-frequency pulsed electromagnetic fields (BEMER type) on gene expression of human mesenchymal stem cells and chondrocytes: an in vitro study," *Electromagnetic Biology and Medicine*, vol. 26, no. 3, pp. 179–190, 2007.

[112] E. Kaivosoja, V. Sariola, Y. Chen, and Y. T. Konttinen, "The effect of pulsed electromagnetic fields and dehydroepiandrosterone on viability and osteo-induction of human mesenchymal stem cells," *Journal of Tissue Engineering and Regenerative Medicine*, vol. 9, no. 1, pp. 31–40, 2015.

[113] M. Marędziak, K. Marycz, D. Lewandowski, A. Siudzińska, and A. Śmieszek, "Static magnetic field enhances synthesis and secretion of membrane-derived microvesicles (MVs) rich in VEGF and BMP-2 in equine adipose-derived stromal cells (EqASCs)—a new approach in veterinary regenerative medicine," *In Vitro Cellular & Developmental Biology - Animal*, vol. 51, no. 3, pp. 230–240, 2015.

[114] C. Merino-González, F. A. Zuñiga, C. Escudero et al., "Mesenchymal stem cell-derived extracellular vesicles promote angiogenesis: potential clinical application," *Frontiers in Physiology*, vol. 7, 2016.

[115] D. Ti, H. Hao, C. Tong et al., "LPS-preconditioned mesenchymal stromal cells modify macrophage polarization for resolution of chronic inflammation via exosome-shuttled let-7b," *Journal of Translational Medicine*, vol. 13, no. 1, p. 308, 2015.

[116] S. C. Lee, H. J. Jeong, S. K. Lee, and S.-J. Kim, "Lipopolysaccharide preconditioning of adipose-derived stem cells improves liver-regenerating activity of the secretome," *Stem Cell Research & Therapy*, vol. 6, no. 1, p. 75, 2015.

[117] K. N. Sivanathan, S. Gronthos, D. Rojas-Canales, B. Thierry, and P. T. Coates, "Interferon-gamma modification of mesenchymal stem cells: implications of autologous and allogeneic mesenchymal stem cell therapy in allotransplantation," *Stem Cell Reviews*, vol. 10, no. 3, pp. 351–375, 2014.

[118] G. Ren, L. Zhang, X. Zhao et al., "Mesenchymal stem cell-mediated immunosuppression occurs via concerted action of chemokines and nitric oxide," *Cell Stem Cell*, vol. 2, no. 2, pp. 141–150, 2008.

[119] C. Li, G. Li, M. Liu, T. Zhou, and H. Zhou, "Paracrine effect of inflammatory cytokine-activated bone marrow mesenchymal stem cells and its role in osteoblast function," *Journal of Bioscience and Bioengineering*, vol. 121, no. 2, pp. 213–219, 2016.

[120] Z. Lu, Y. J. Chen, C. Dunstan, S. Roohani-Esfahani, and H. Zreiqat, "Priming adipose stem cells with tumor necrosis factor-alpha preconditioning potentiates their exosome efficacy for bone regeneration," *Tissue Engineering Part A*, vol. 23, no. 21-22, pp. 1212–1220, 2017.

[121] Y. Bai, Y. D. Han, X. L. Yan et al., "Adipose mesenchymal stem cell-derived exosomes stimulated by hydrogen peroxide enhanced skin flap recovery in ischemia- reperfusion injury," *Biochemical and Biophysical Research Communications*, vol. 500, no. 2, pp. 310–317, 2018.

[122] J. Zhang, G. H. Chen, Y. W. Wang et al., "Hydrogen peroxide preconditioning enhances the therapeutic efficacy of Wharton's jelly mesenchymal stem cells after myocardial infarction," *Chinese Medical Journal*, vol. 125, no. 19, pp. 3472–3478, 2012.

[123] T. M. Rodríguez, A. Saldías, M. Irigo, J. V. Zamora, M. J. Perone, and R. A. Dewey, "Effect of TGF-β1 stimulation on the secretome of human adipose-derived mesenchymal stromal cells," *Stem Cells Translational Medicine*, vol. 4, no. 8, pp. 894–898, 2015.

[124] P. Li, M. Kaslan, S. H. Lee, J. Yao, and Z. Gao, "Progress in exosome isolation techniques," *Theranostics*, vol. 7, no. 3, pp. 789–804, 2017.

[125] S. Gholizadeh, M. Shehata Draz, M. Zarghooni et al., "Microfluidic approaches for isolation, detection, and characterization of extracellular vesicles: current status and future directions," *Biosensors and Bioelectronics*, vol. 91, pp. 588–605, 2017.

[126] M. He, J. Crow, M. Roth, Y. Zeng, and A. K. Godwin, "Integrated immunoisolation and protein analysis of circulating

exosomes using microfluidic technology," *Lab on a Chip*, vol. 14, no. 19, pp. 3773–3780, 2014.

[127] I. Helwa, J. Cai, M. D. Drewry et al., "A comparative study of serum exosome isolation using differential ultra-centrifugation and three commercial reagents," *PLoS One*, vol. 12, no. 1, p. e0170628, 2017.

[128] R. J. Lobb, M. Becker, S. Wen Wen et al., "Optimized exosome isolation protocol for cell culture supernatant and human plasma," *Journal of Extracellular Vesicles*, vol. 4, no. 1, pp. 1–11, 2015.

[129] N. Heath, L. Grant, T. M. de Oliveira et al., "Rapid isolation and enrichment of extracellular vesicle preparations using anion exchange chromatography," *Scientific Reports*, vol. 8, no. 1, p. 5730, 2018.

[130] T. Kursad, "Human embryonic stem cell protocols," *Methods in Molecular Biology*, vol. 331, 2006.

[131] B. Yu, X. Zhang, and X. Li, "Exosomes derived from mesenchymal stem cells," *International Journal of Molecular Sciences*, vol. 15, no. 3, pp. 4142–4157, 2014.

[132] H. Zhou, P. S. T. Yuen, T. Pisitkun et al., "Collection, storage, preservation, and normalization of human urinary exosomes for biomarker discovery," *Kidney International*, vol. 69, no. 8, pp. 1471–1476, 2006.

[133] X. Liu, Y. Yang, Y. Li et al., "Integration of stem cell-derived exosomes with in situ hydrogel glue as a promising tissue patch for articular cartilage regeneration," *Nanoscale*, vol. 9, no. 13, pp. 4430–4438, 2017.

[134] P. Gangadaran, R. L. Rajendran, H. W. Lee et al., "Extracellular vesicles from mesenchymal stem cells activates VEGF receptors and accelerates recovery of hindlimb ischemia," *Journal of Controlled Release*, vol. 264, pp. 112–126, 2017.

[135] W. Li, Y. Liu, P. Zhang et al., "Tissue-engineered bone immobilized with human adipose stem cells-derived exosomes promotes bone regeneration," *ACS Applied Materials and Interfaces*, vol. 10, no. 6, pp. 5240–5254, 2018.

[136] R. Blázquez, F. M. Sánchez-Margallo, V. Álvarez, A. Usón, F. Marinaro, and J. G. Casado, "Fibrin glue mesh fixation combined with mesenchymal stem cells or exosomes modulates the inflammatory reaction in a murine model of incisional hernia," *Acta Biomaterialia*, vol. 71, pp. 318–329, 2018.

[137] L. Hu, J. Wang, X. Zhou et al., "Exosomes derived from human adipose mensenchymal stem cells accelerates cutaneous wound healing via optimizing the characteristics of fibroblasts," *Scientific Reports*, vol. 6, no. 1, article 32993, 2016.

[138] B. Zhao, Y. Zhang, S. Han et al., "Exosomes derived from human amniotic epithelial cells accelerate wound healing and inhibit scar formation," *Journal of Molecular Histology*, vol. 48, no. 2, pp. 121–132, 2017.

[139] Y.-J. Kim, S. . Yoo, H. H. Park et al., "Exosomes derived from human umbilical cord blood mesenchymal stem cells stimulates rejuvenation of human skin," *Biochemical and Biophysical Research Communications*, vol. 493, no. 2, pp. 1102–1108, 2017.

[140] S. C. Guo, S. C. Tao, W. J. Yin, X. Qi, J. G. Sheng, and C. Q. Zhang, "Exosomes from human synovial-derived mesenchymal stem cells prevent glucocorticoid-induced osteonecrosis of the femoral head in the rat," *International Journal of Biological Sciences*, vol. 12, no. 10, pp. 1262–1272, 2016.

[141] S. Zhang, W. C. Chu, R. C. Lai, S. K. Lim, J. H. P. Hui, and W. S. Toh, "Exosomes derived from human embryonic mesenchymal stem cells promote osteochondral regeneration," *Osteoarthritis and Cartilage*, vol. 24, no. 12, pp. 2135–2140, 2016.

[142] X. Liu, Q. Li, X. Niu et al., "Exosomes secreted from human-induced pluripotent stem cell-derived mesenchymal stem cells prevent osteonecrosis of the femoral head by promoting angiogenesis," *International Journal of Biological Sciences*, vol. 13, no. 2, pp. 232–244, 2017.

[143] M. Salem, O. Helal, H. Metwaly, A. HadyEl, and S. Ahmed, "Histological and immunohistochemical study of the role of stem cells, conditioned medium and microvesicles in treatment of experimentally induced acute kidney injury in rats," *Journal of Medical Histology*, vol. 1, no. 1, pp. 69–83, 2017.

[144] A. T. Brini, G. Amodeo, L. M. Ferreira et al., "Therapeutic effect of human adipose-derived stem cells and their secretome in experimental diabetic pain," *Scientific Reports*, vol. 7, no. 1, p. 9904, 2017.

[145] T. Shigemoto-Kuroda, J. Y. Oh, D. K. Kim et al., "MSC-derived extracellular vesicles attenuate immune responses in two autoimmune murine models: type 1 diabetes and uveoretinitis," *Stem Cell Reports*, vol. 8, no. 5, pp. 1214–1225, 2017.

[146] M. Gnecchi, H. He, N. Noiseux et al., "Evidence supporting paracrine hypothesis for Akt-modified mesenchymal stem cell-mediated cardiac protection and functional improvement," *The FASEB Journal*, vol. 20, no. 6, pp. 661–669, 2006.

[147] Y. Zhao, X. Sun, W. Cao et al., "Exosomes derived from human umbilical cord mesenchymal stem cells relieve acute myocardial ischemic injury," *Stem Cells International*, vol. 2015, Article ID 761643, 12 pages, 2015.

[148] B. Yu, H. W. Kim, M. Gong et al., "Exosomes secreted from GATA-4 overexpressing mesenchymal stem cells serve as a reservoir of anti-apoptotic microRNAs for cardioprotection," *International Journal of Cardiology*, vol. 182, no. C, pp. 349–360, 2015.

[149] X. Teng, L. Chen, W. Chen, J. Yang, Z. Yang, and Z. Shen, "Mesenchymal stem cell-derived exosomes improve the microenvironment of infarcted myocardium contributing to angiogenesis and anti-inflammation," *Cellular Physiology and Biochemistry*, vol. 37, no. 6, pp. 2415–2424, 2015.

[150] L. Liu, X. Jin, C. F. Hu, R. Li, Z. Zhou, and C.-X. Shen, "Exosomes derived from mesenchymal stem cells rescue myocardial ischaemia/reperfusion injury by inducing cardiomyocyte autophagy via AMPK and Akt pathways," *Cellular Physiology and Biochemistry*, vol. 43, pp. 52–68, 2017.

[151] X. Wu, T. Yan, Z. Wang et al., "Micro-vesicles derived from human Wharton's jelly mesenchymal stromal cells mitigate renal ischemia-reperfusion injury in rats after cardiac death renal transplantation," *Journal of Cellular Biochemistry*, vol. 119, no. 2, pp. 1879–1888, 2018.

[152] S. Ohno, M. Takanashi, K. Sudo et al., "Systemically injected exosomes targeted to EGFR deliver antitumor microRNA to breast cancer cells," *Molecular Therapy*, vol. 21, no. 1, pp. 185–191, 2013.

[153] B. Mead and S. Tomarev, "Bone marrow-derived mesenchymal stem cells-derived exosomes promote survival of retinal ganglion cells through miRNA-dependent mechanisms," *Stem Cells Translational Medicine*, vol. 6, no. 4, pp. 1273–1285, 2017.

[154] E. Moisseiev, J. D. Anderson, S. Oltjen et al., "Protective effect of intravitreal administration of exosomes derived from mesenchymal stem cells on retinal ischemia," *Current Eye Research*, vol. 42, no. 10, pp. 1358–1367, 2017.

[155] P. Venkat, M. Chopp, A. Zacharek, and J. Chen, "Abstract WMP46: exosomes derived from bone marrow mesenchymal stem cells of type two diabetes rats promotes neurorestoration after stroke in type two diabetic rats," *Stroke*, vol. 48, article AWMP46, Supplement 1, 2017.

[156] T. Palomares, M. Cordero, C. Bruzos-Cidon, M. Torrecilla, L. Ugedo, and A. Alonso-Varona, "The neuroprotective effect of conditioned medium from human adipose-derived mesenchymal stem cells is impaired by N-acetyl cysteine supplementation," *Molecular Neurobiology*, vol. 55, no. 1, pp. 13–25, 2018.

[157] Y. Ma, S. Ge, J. Zhang, D. Zhou, X. Wang, and J. Su, "Mesenchymal stem cell-derived extracellular vesicles promote nerve regeneration after sciatic nerve crush injury in rats," *International Journal of Clinical and Experimental Pathology*, vol. 10, no. 9, pp. 10032–10039, 2017.

[158] D. Cizkova, V. Cubinkova, T. Smolek et al., "Localized intrathecal delivery of mesenchymal stromal cells conditioned medium improves functional recovery in a rat model of spinal cord injury," *International Journal of Molecular Sciences*, vol. 19, no. 3, pp. 1–13, 2018.

[159] M. Choi, T. Ban, and T. Rhim, "Therapeutic use of stem cell transplantation for cell replacement or cytoprotective effect of microvesicle released from mesenchymal stem cell," *Molecules and Cells*, vol. 37, no. 2, pp. 133–139, 2014.

[160] G. R. Willis, A. Fernandez-Gonzalez, J. Anastas et al., "Mesenchymal stromal cell exosomes ameliorate experimental bronchopulmonary dysplasia and restore lung function through macrophage immunomodulation," *American Journal of Respiratory and Critical Care Medicine*, vol. 197, no. 1, pp. 104–116, 2018.

[161] Z. Liu, J. Liu, M. Xiao et al., "Mesenchymal stem cell–derived microvesicles alleviate pulmonary arterial hypertension by regulating renin-angiotensin system," *Journal of the American Society of Hypertension*, vol. 12, no. 6, pp. 470–478, 2018.

[162] T. Li, Y. Yan, B. Wang et al., "Exosomes derived from human umbilical cord mesenchymal stem cells alleviate liver fibrosis," *Stem Cells and Development*, vol. 22, no. 6, pp. 845–854, 2013.

[163] N. Su, P. L. Gao, K. Wang, J. Y. Wang, Y. Zhong, and Y. Luo, "Fibrous scaffolds potentiate the paracrine function of mesenchymal stem cells: a new dimension in cell-material interaction," *Biomaterials*, vol. 141, pp. 74–85, 2017.

10

GM1 Ganglioside Promotes Osteogenic Differentiation of Human Tendon Stem Cells

Sonia Bergante,[1] Pasquale Creo,[1] Marco Piccoli ⓘ,[1] Andrea Ghiroldi,[1] Alessandra Menon ⓘ,[1] Federica Cirillo,[1] Paola Rota,[1] Michelle M. Monasky,[2] Giuseppe Ciconte,[2] Carlo Pappone,[2] Pietro Randelli ⓘ,[3,4] and Luigi Anastasia ⓘ[1,4]

[1]Laboratory of Stem Cells for Tissue Engineering, Scientific Institute for Research, Hospitalization, and Health Care (IRCCS) Policlinico San Donato, San Donato 20097, Italy
[2]Arrhythmology Department, Scientific Institute for Research, Hospitalization, and Health Care (IRCCS) Policlinico San Donato, San Donato Milanese, Italy
[3]Azienda Socio Sanitaria Territoriale Centro Specialistico Ortopedico Traumatologico Gaetano Pini-CTO, Milano 20122, Italy
[4]Department of Biomedical Sciences for Health (L.I.T.A.), Università degli Studi di Milano, Segrate 20090, Italy

Correspondence should be addressed to Pietro Randelli; pietro.randelli@unimi.it and Luigi Anastasia; luigi.anastasia@unimi.it

Academic Editor: Salvatore Scacco

Gangliosides, the sialic acid-conjugated glycosphingolipids present in the lipid rafts, have been recognized as important regulators of cell proliferation, migration, and apoptosis. Due to their peculiar localization in the cell membrane, they modulate the activity of several key cell receptors, and increasing evidence supports their involvement also in stem cell differentiation. In this context, herein we report the role played by the ganglioside GM1 in the osteogenic differentiation of human tendon stem cells (hTSCs). In particular, we found an increase of GM1 levels during osteogenesis that is instrumental for driving the process. In fact, supplementation of the ganglioside in the medium significantly increased the osteogenic differentiation capability of hTSCs. Mechanistically, we found that GM1 supplementation caused a reduction in the phosphorylation of the platelet-derived growth factor receptor-β (PDGFR-β), which is a known inhibitor of osteogenic commitment. These results were further corroborated by the observation that GM1 supplementation was able to revert the inhibitory effects on osteogenesis when the process was inhibited with exogenous PDGF.

1. Introduction

Injuries to the tendon-to-bone enthesis are common in the field of orthopedic medicine, and high failure rates are often associated with their repair [1]. The use of biologic adjuvants that promote tissue regeneration, such as growth factors, platelet-rich plasma, and stem cells, have shown great potential for improving healing rates and function after surgery [2]. Accordingly, the use of tendon stem cells to improve tendon-bone junction repair has been considered advantageous, as tendon stem cells already belong to the tendon environment and possess the plasticity to potentially recover the different tissues found in the tendon-to-bone enthesis [3]. Along these lines, we reported the first isolation of human tendon stem cells from the supraspinatus and long head of the biceps tendons, and we demonstrated that they can be induced to differentiate toward osteoblasts, adipocytes, and muscle cells [4]. Nonetheless, an open issue in the stem cell field is to perfect the differentiation strategies in order to drive the process toward a specific phenotype and to avoid undesired cell commitment or, even more detrimental, the uncontrolled proliferation of undifferentiated progenitor cells. In this context, herein we investigated the role of gangliosides, which are sialic acid-containing glycosphingolipids (GSLs) ubiquitously distributed in cell membranes [5], in the osteogenic differentiation of hTSCs. Numerous studies have confirmed that gangliosides and their expression levels are controlled during development [6] and are cell type-specific [7], supporting the idea that these molecules are key players in cell commitment. While some biological roles of these lipids have been clearly recognized, as they have been shown to be involved in processes like cell proliferation [8], cell adhesion [9], apoptosis [10], and differentiation [11], less is known about their role in stem cell homeostasis and differentiation. Nonetheless, it has been shown that a reduction of ganglioside biosynthesis inhibits the neuronal differentiation of MSCs in the early stage of the process [12], and our group recently demonstrated that an increase of ganglioside GD1a is crucial for human bone marrow mesenchymal stem cell (MSC) differentiation [13]. Moreover, we demonstrated the pivotal role of sialidase NEU3 in regulating ganglioside GM3 content, which is a key in skeletal muscle cell differentiation and survival under hypoxia [14–17]. Clearly, as gangliosides are mainly distributed in the lipid rafts of cell plasma membranes, which are rich in key tyrosine kinase receptors, the present study further corroborates the notion that we are at the beginning of fully unveiling the role of these sphingolipids in stem cell biology.

2. Materials and Methods

2.1. Cell Isolation and Culture. Human tendon stem cells (hTSCs) were isolated from supraspinatus tendon specimens collected during arthroscopic rotator cuff repair, as previously reported [4]. The isolated hTSCs were cultured in minimal essential medium alpha modification (α-MEM) (Merck) supplemented with 2 mM L-glutamine (Euroclone), 1% antibiotic-antimycotic mixture (Euroclone), and 20% (v/v) fetal bovine serum (FBS) (HyClone, Thermo Fisher Scientific) at 37°C in a 5% CO_2 and 95% air-humidified atmosphere. The medium was changed every 2-3 days.

2.2. Osteogenic and Adipogenic Differentiation. hTSCs were seeded at a concentration of 3×10^4 cells/cm^2 in a growth medium, and after 24 hours, cells were switched to an osteogenic or adipogenic medium for 17 days or 21 days, respectively. Osteogenic differentiation was obtained by culturing cells in the presence of DMEM-low glucose (Merck) supplemented with 4 mM L-glutamine (Euroclone), 1% antibiotic-antimycotic mixture (Euroclone), 10% FBS (HyClone, Thermo Fisher Scientific), 10 nM cholecalciferol (Merck Millipore), and the mesenchymal stem cell osteogenesis kit (Merck Millipore) according to the manufacturer's instructions. Adipogenic differentiation was induced by culturing cells in the presence of DMEM-low glucose supplemented with 4 mM L-glutamine, 1% antibiotic-antimycotic mixture, 10% FBS, and the mesenchymal stem cell adipogenesis kit (Merck Millipore), according to the manufacturer's instructions. To evaluate the effects of ganglioside GM1 treatment (Santa Cruz Biotechnology) on differentiation, hTSCs were cultured for 17 days in an osteogenic medium or 21 days in adipogenic medium supplemented with 1, 10, 50, and 100 μM GM1. To evaluate the effects of the platelet-derived growth factor-BB (PDGF-BB, Thermo Fisher Scientific) on osteogenic differentiation, cells were cultured in an osteogenic medium containing PDGF-BB

at the final concentration of 10 ng/ml. The differentiation medium was changed every 2-3 days.

2.3. Metabolic Radiolabeling of Cell Sphingolipids. The metabolic radiolabeling of cell sphingolipids was performed as previously described by Riboni et al. [18]. Briefly, [3-^{3}H]-sphingosine (D-erythro > 97%, 50 μCi, 1.85 MBq, PerkinElmer) was dissolved in DMEM-low glucose with 10% FBS to a final concentration of 2.4 nM sphingosine, corresponding to 110.000 dpm/ml radioactivity. The medium was added to the cells and incubated for 2 hours (pulse) at 37°C, then it was replaced with DMEM-low glucose with 10% FBS without [^{3}H]-sphingosine for 48 hours (chase). After the incubation, cells were harvested by cell scraping in phosphate-buffered saline (PBS). Cell suspensions were frozen and lyophilized.

2.4. Extraction and Chromatographic Separation of Radiolabeled Sphingolipids. Total lipid extraction was performed as previously described by Bergante et al. [13]. Briefly, lipids were first extracted with 20 : 10 : 1 (v/v) chloroform/methanol/water, dried under a nitrogen stream, and then a two-phase partitioning was carried out in chloroform/methanol 2 : 1 (v/v) and 20% (v/v) water. After partitioning, gangliosides of the aqueous phase were separated and analyzed by high-performance thin-layer chromatography (HPTLC), using as running solvent chloroform/methanol/0.2% aqueous $CaCl_2$ 60 : 40 : 9 ($v/v/v$) [19, 20]. Radiolabeled sphingolipids were visualized with a Beta-Imager 2000 (Biospace). The radioactivity associated with individual lipids was determined with β-Vision software (Biospace).

2.5. RNA Extraction and Real-Time PCR. Total RNA was isolated using TRIzol Reagent (Ambion, Life Technologies), and 1 μg of extracted RNA was reverse transcribed to cDNA using the iScript cDNA synthesis kit (Bio-Rad) according to the manufacturer's instructions. Real-time PCR was performed in a 96-well plate with 10 ng of cDNA as a template, 0.2 μM primers, and 2x Power SYBR Green PCR Master Mix (Promega) in 20 μL final volume per well, using a StepOnePlus Real-Time PCR System (Applied Biosystems). The following primers were used to amplify the corresponding target genes: human alkaline phosphatase (ALP) forward 5'-CGCACGGAACTCCTGACC-3' and reverse 5'-GCCACCACCACCATCTCG-3', peroxisome proliferator-activated receptor-γ (PPAR-γ) forward 5'-TTCCTTCACTGATACACTGTCTGC-3' and reverse 5'-GGAGTGGGAGTGGTCTTCCATTAC-3', lipoprotein lipase (LPL) forward 5'-AGAGAGAACCAGACTCCAATG-3' and reverse 5'-GGCTCCAAGGCTGTATCC-3', beta 1,3-galactosyltransferase (GM1 synthase) forward 5'-CGCCTTCCAGGACTCCTACC-3' and reverse 5'-CCGTCTTGAGGACGTATCGG-3', osteocalcin forward 5'-GCAGCGAGGTAGTGAAGAG-3' and reverse 5'-GAAAGCCGATGTGGTCAGC-3', and S14 (used as endogenous control in all real-time PCR experiments) forward 5'-GTGTGACTGGTGGGATGAAGG-3' and reverse 5'-TTGATGTGTAGGGCGGTGATAC-3'.

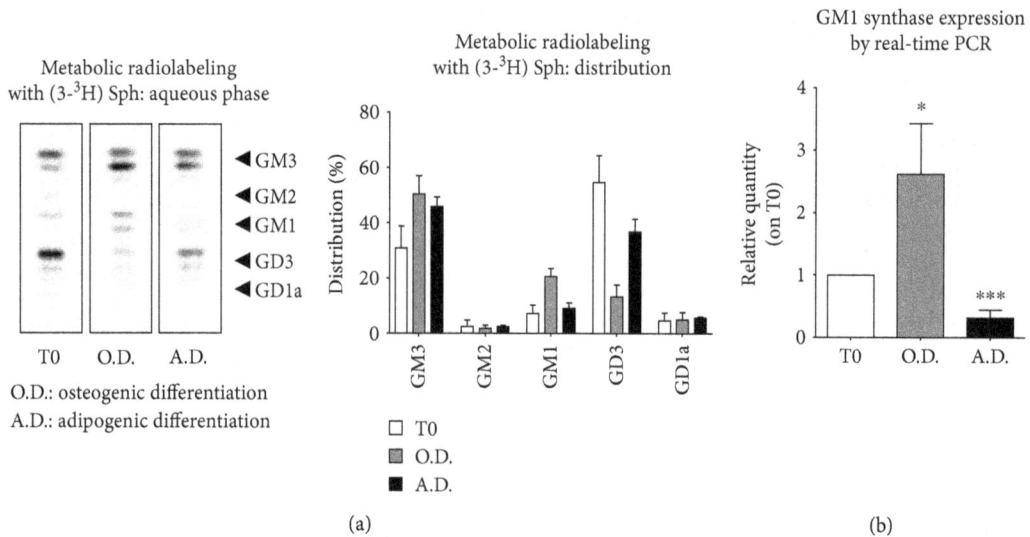

FIGURE 1: Ganglioside pattern upon differentiation of hTSCs to either osteoblasts or adipocytes. (a) Metabolic radiolabeled gangliosides separated by HPTLC and visualized with a Beta-Imager 2000 (Biospace). Doubled spots in cellular gangliosides correspond to the presence of species with different chain lengths of fatty acids. The graph on the right represents the percentage distribution of radiolabeled gangliosides. (b) Real-time PCR analysis of GM1 synthase gene expression in hTSCs differentiated toward osteoblasts (O.D.) or adipocytes (A.D.) as compared to that in undifferentiated cells (T0). Ribosomal protein S14 gene was used as housekeeper gene. All data are means ± SD of three different experiments. The statistical analysis was determined by Student's t-test. $^*p < 0.05$, $^{***}p < 0.001$.

2.6. Analysis of Mineralization.

Matrix mineralization of hTSCs was evaluated at the 17th day of osteogenic differentiation using the osteogenesis assay kit (Merck Millipore). Briefly, cells were fixed with 4% paraformaldehyde at room temperature for 15 minutes. In order to detect mineral deposition in the extracellular matrix, cells were washed twice with PBS and incubated with alizarin red stain solution for 20 minutes. The dye was then extracted from the stained monolayer according to the manufacturer's instructions and quantified using a Victor 3 instrument (Perkin Elmer).

2.7. Immunoblotting.

Cells were harvested in ice-cold PBS by cell scraping and centrifuged at 400 ×g for 10 minutes at 4°C. Cells were lysed in RIPA buffer (150 mM sodium chloride, 1% Triton X-100, 0.5% sodium deoxycholate, 0.1% sodium dodecyl sulphate, and 50 mM Tris pH 8) containing complete protease and phosphatase inhibitors (Merck). After cell lysis, the samples were centrifuged at 10,000 ×g for 15 minutes at 4°C. Protein amounts were measured using a Pierce BCA protein assay kit (Thermo Scientific). Proteins were loaded into a 10% SDS-PAGE gel, then transferred onto a nitrocellulose membrane (Trans-Blot, Bio-Rad Laboratories) by electroblotting. After blocking the membranes with 5% (w/v) of nonfat dry milk in Tris-buffered saline-Tween 0.1% (TBS-T) for 1 hour at room temperature, they were incubated overnight at 4°C with the following primary antibodies: rabbit phospho-PDGFR-β, 1 : 1000 dilution (Y751, Cell Signaling); rabbit PDGFR-β, 1 : 1000 dilution (Cell Signaling); and rabbit monoclonal early endosome antigen 1 (EEA1), 1 : 1000 dilution (Cell Signaling). The membranes were then washed in TBS-T three times and incubated for 1 hour at room temperature with specific secondary antibodies. In particular, phospho-PDGFR-β was incubated with the IRDye® 800CW goat anti-mouse IgG (LI-COR), the total PDGFR-β with the

IRDye 680RD goat anti-rabbit IgG (Li-COR), and EEA1 with the HRP-conjugated anti-rabbit IgG (Amersham), diluted 1 : 5000 in 5% (w/v) nonfat dry milk in TBS-T. The membranes were analyzed by the Odyssey® FC imaging system (LI-COR), and the densitometric analysis was performed with the specific Image Studio™ software (LI-COR).

3. Results

3.1. Ganglioside Changes in hTSC Differentiation toward Osteoblasts and Adipocytes.

To assess the ganglioside pattern distribution of hTSCs, cells were metabolically radiolabeled with the sphingolipid precursor [3-³H]-sphingosine and quantitatively analyzed by HTPLC coupled with a radiochromatoscanner, as described in "Materials and Methods." The ganglioside distribution in proliferating hTSCs was as follows: GM3 (30.79% ± 7.85), GM2 (2.53% ± 2.33), GM1 (7.28% ± 2.94), GD3 (43.83% ± 19.35), and GD1a (4.71% ± 2.80), with GM3 and GD3 being the main gangliosides (Figure 1(a) and 1(b), T0).

Next, changes in ganglioside pattern were evaluated upon differentiation of hTSCs to either osteoblasts or adipocytes, as previously reported [4], by metabolic radiolabeling after 17 and 21 days of cell culturing in either osteogenic (O.D.) or adipogenic (A.D.) medium (Figure 1(a)). When hTSCs were differentiated toward osteoblasts, a 1.6- and 2.8-fold increase of GM3 and GM1 gangliosides was observed, respectively, as well as a 3.7-fold decrease of GD3, as compared to proliferating undifferentiated cells. When hTSCs were differentiated toward adipocytes, a 1.7-fold increase in GM3 and 1.5-fold decrease in GD3 relative distribution were observed, as compared to undifferentiated cells, while no significant changes in the relative quantity of GM1 could be observed (Figure 1(a)). To test whether the observed increase of GM1 during osteogenesis was due to an upregulation of its biosynthesis, GM1 synthase expression was measured by real-time PCR, and a 2.6-fold increase could be observed at the end of the differentiation process, as compared to proliferating hTSCs. On the other hand, a 3.2-fold reduction of GM1 synthase expression was measured when hTSCs were induced to differentiate toward adipocytes (Figure 1(b)).

3.2. Effects of Exogenous GM1 on Osteogenic Differentiation of hTSCs. To test the role of GM1 increase during osteogenesis, exogenous 1, 10, 50, and 100 μM GM1 was supplemented in the osteogenic medium during the differentiation process. Osteogenic marker ALP gene expression was measured by real-time PCR after 17 days of differentiation and compared to undifferentiated cells (T0) and GM1-free osteogenic medium (O.D.). Results showed a significant 1.8- and 2.4-fold increase in ALP expression when cells were supplemented with 50 or 100 μM GM1 in addition to the osteogenic medium, respectively, as compared to O.D. (Figure 2(a)).

Afterward, cells were induced to differentiate to osteoblasts in the presence of 50 or 100 μM GM1 and were evaluated for their capacity to sustain the mineralization of the extracellular matrix using a standard alizarin red staining, as described in "Materials and Methods." Dye relative quantification showed an increase of red staining in hTSCs differentiated in the presence of GM1, which was significantly higher (1.7-fold) in 100 μM GM1-treated cells (Figure 2(b)). On the contrary, exogenous GM1 strongly inhibited the gene expression of the adipogenic markers LPL and PPAR-γ (Figures 2(c) and 2(d)).

3.3. Mechanism of GM1-Activated Osteogenesis. To test whether osteogenesis was activated by GM1 through the inhibition of PDGFR-β, hTSCs were induced to differentiate in the presence of the ganglioside and then subjected to PDGFR-β analysis by Western blot. Results revealed that GM1-treated cells showed a 40% decrease in PDGFR-β phosphorylation, measured as the pPDGFR/PDGFR ratio, as compared to untreated cells, supporting the hypothesis of a GM1-induced inhibition of PDGFR-β (Figure 3(a)). Furthermore, it was assessed whether exogenous GM1 was able to counteract PDGF-induced activation of PDGFR-β, which is known to inhibit osteogenesis [21]. To this purpose, hTSCs were induced to differentiate for 17 days in normal osteogenic medium in the presence of 10 ng/ml PDGF-BB, which caused a 43% decrease in ALP expression (Figure 3(b)) and a 40% decrease in osteocalcin expression by real-time PCR (Figure 3(c)). On the other hand, addition of 100 μM GM1 to the osteogenic medium containing 10 ng/ml PDGF-BB completely restored the differentiation capability of hTSCs, as ALP and osteocalcin expression levels were comparable to differentiated untreated controls (Figure 3(b) and 3(c)).

4. Discussion

In this work, we investigated the role of gangliosides in the osteogenic differentiation of adult human tendon stem cells that we isolated and characterized for the first time from human supraspinatus tendons [4]. The method used for

ganglioside pattern analysis required an initial metabolic radiolabeling of cell sphingolipids by adding [3-^{3}H]-sphingosine in the culture medium that has been effectively used in our laboratories for many years [13–15]. As a result, cells synthesize radiolabeled sphingolipids that can be separated by HPTLC chromatography and accurately measured with a radiochromatoscanner. The use of metabolic radiolabeling significantly improves the sensitivity of the method, reducing the number of stem cells required for each analysis. Results demonstrated that the two main gangliosides of hTSCs, GM3 and GD3, increased and decreased, respectively, when cells were differentiated toward osteoblasts or adipocytes, suggesting that the modulation of these gangliosides is possibly linked to a general change of the biological status of the cell and not to the commitment toward a specific cell lineage. On the other hand, a marked increase of ganglioside GM1 was observed only during osteogenesis, supporting the possible role of this ganglioside in driving the process (Figure 1). The increase in GM1 content was accompanied by an increase of its synthase, which was instead reduced during adipogenesis (Figure 1). Interestingly, the addition of exogenous GM1 to the differentiation medium improved osteogenesis, as confirmed by a significant increase of ALP gene expression, which is a specific osteoblast marker, as well as by an increase of the extracellular matrix mineralization, as assessed by alizarin red staining (Figure 2). On the contrary, gene expression of the adipogenic markers PPAR-γ and LPL decreased upon GM1 supplementation to the adipogenic differentiation medium, supporting the idea that the ganglioside could inhibit the process (Figure 2). We then investigated the mechanism of GM1-induced increase of osteogenesis in hTSCs. Along this line, it has been reported that gangliosides can regulate the activity of the epidermal growth factor receptor [22], the fibroblast growth factor receptor [23], the nerve growth factor receptor (NGF) [24], the platelet-derived growth factor receptor (PDGFR) [25], and the insulin receptor (IR) [26]. In particular, it has been shown that GM1 is crucial in PDGFR regulation through different mechanisms of action that appear to be cell type-dependent. In this context, it has been demonstrated that, in fibroblasts, GM1 is able to inhibit the ligand-mediated phosphorylation of tyrosine residues of the cytoplasmic tail of the receptor [27], as well as the ligand-induced intracellular association of SH2-containing proteins with PDGFR in human glioma cells [28]. On the contrary, in Swiss-3T3 cells, it has been demonstrated that GM1-mediated inhibition of PDGFR requires the extracellular and/or the transmembrane domains of the receptor [29]. Moreover, in the same cell line, it has been shown that GM1 regulates PDGFR signaling by controlling the distribution of the receptor in- and outside of lipid rafts and that PAG regulates the membrane partitioning and the mitogenic signaling of PDGFR through an increase in GM1 levels in caveolae [30, 31]. PDGF/PDGFR signaling is reported to be involved in the regulation of various cell functions, including osteogenesis and adult stem cell differentiation toward osteoblasts. In particular, it has been observed that the downregulation of PDGRα promotes osteogenic differentiation of MSCs through the BMP/smad signaling pathway [32], and the blocking of the PDGFR-β

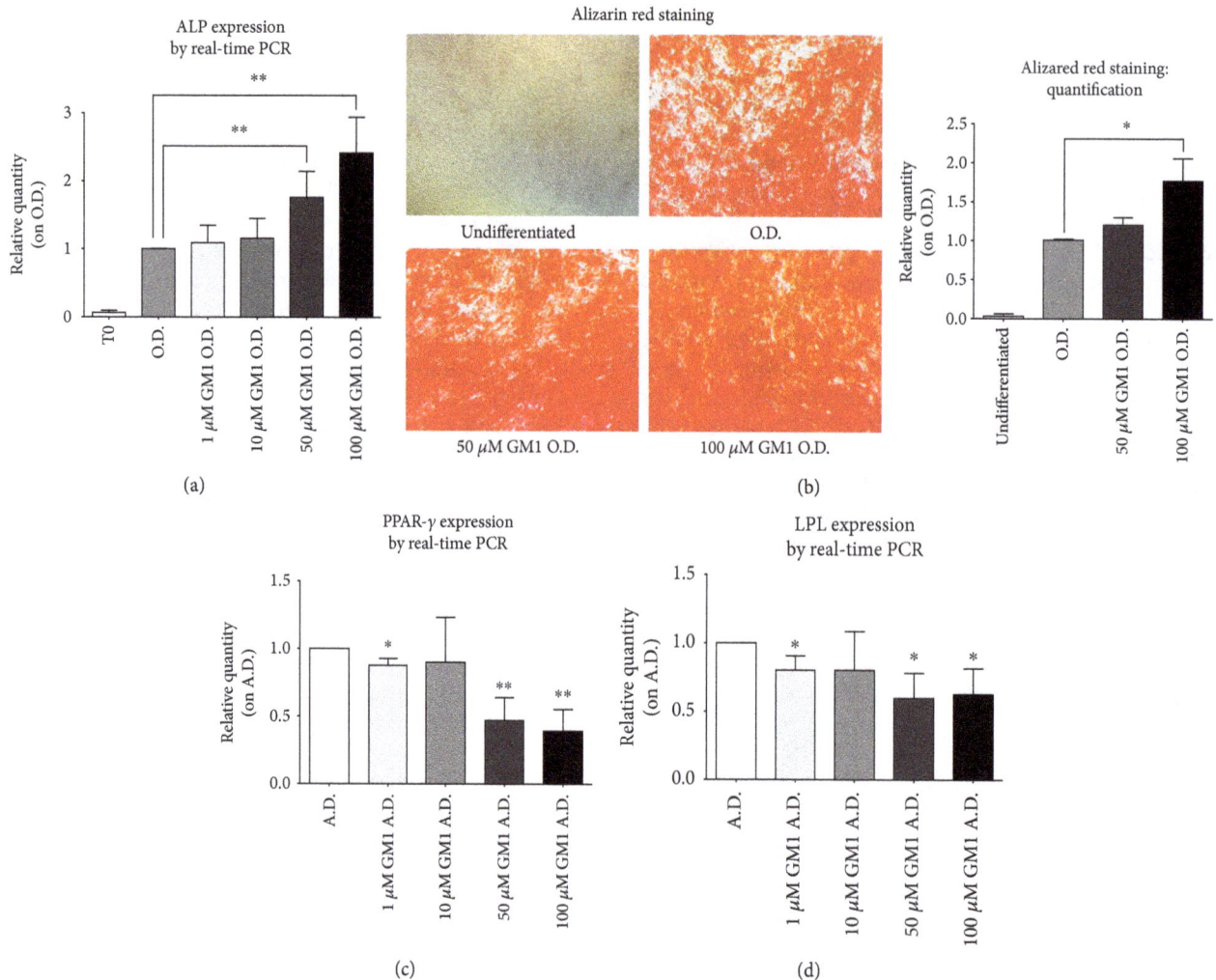

FIGURE 2: Evaluation of hTSC differentiation either to osteoblasts and adipocytes upon GM1 treatment. (a) Gene expression of the osteogenic marker ALP by real-time PCR. hTSCs were differentiated toward osteoblasts for 17 days in osteogenic medium supplemented with exogenous 1, 10, 50, and 100 μM GM1. The results were compared to hTSCs differentiated in GM1-free osteogenic medium (O.D.). Ribosomal protein S14 gene was used as endogenous control. (b) Analysis and quantification of calcium deposits in hTSCs after osteogenic differentiation by alizarin red staining. Undifferentiated hTSCs and hTSCs differentiated in the presence of 50 μM and 100 μM GM1 were compared to hTSCs differentiated in GM1-free osteogenic medium (O.D.) and considered as controls. (c, d) Gene expression analysis of adipogenic markers, PPAR-γ and LPL, by real-time PCR. hTSCs were differentiated toward adipocytes for 21 days in adipogenic medium supplemented with exogenous 1, 10, 50, and 100 μM GM1. The results were compared to hTSCs differentiated in GM1-free adipogenic medium (A.D.). Ribosomal protein S14 gene was used as endogenous control. All data are means ± SD of four different experiments. The statistical analysis was determined by Student's t-test. $^{*}p < 0.05$, $^{**}p < 0.01$.

pathway markedly promotes osteoblast differentiation and matrix mineralization in mouse osteoblastic MC3T3-E1 cells [33]. Moreover, PDGFR-β inhibition increases the osteogenic differentiation of primary rat osteoblastic cells [34] and human MSCs [21]. Altogether, these results support the hypothesis that GM1 could exert its effects on osteogenesis through the inhibition of the PDGF receptor also in hTSCs. To test this hypothesis, we assessed the activation levels of the PDGFR-β receptor during osteogenesis in the presence of exogenous GM1 in the culture medium. Indeed, we observed a significant decrease in the activation of the receptor when GM1 was added to the differentiation medium (Figure 3). To further confirm our hypothesis, we assessed whether GM1 was able to counteract the inhibition of osteogenesis caused by the activation of PDGFR-β upon addition

of its ligand (PDGF-BB) in the differentiation medium. Results showed that PDGF-BB stimulation inhibited osteogenesis, as confirmed by a significant decrease of ALP and osteocalcin gene expression. As anticipated, the addition of GM1 to the osteogenic medium containing PDGF-BB completely restored the differentiation capabilities of hTSCs, as we could observe ALP and osteocalcin expression levels similar to untreated control cells (Figure 3).

5. Conclusions

In conclusion, our results show that ganglioside GM1 significantly increases during osteogenic differentiation of hTSCs. Most importantly, the ganglioside increase is instrumental for driving the process through the inhibition of PDGFR-β.

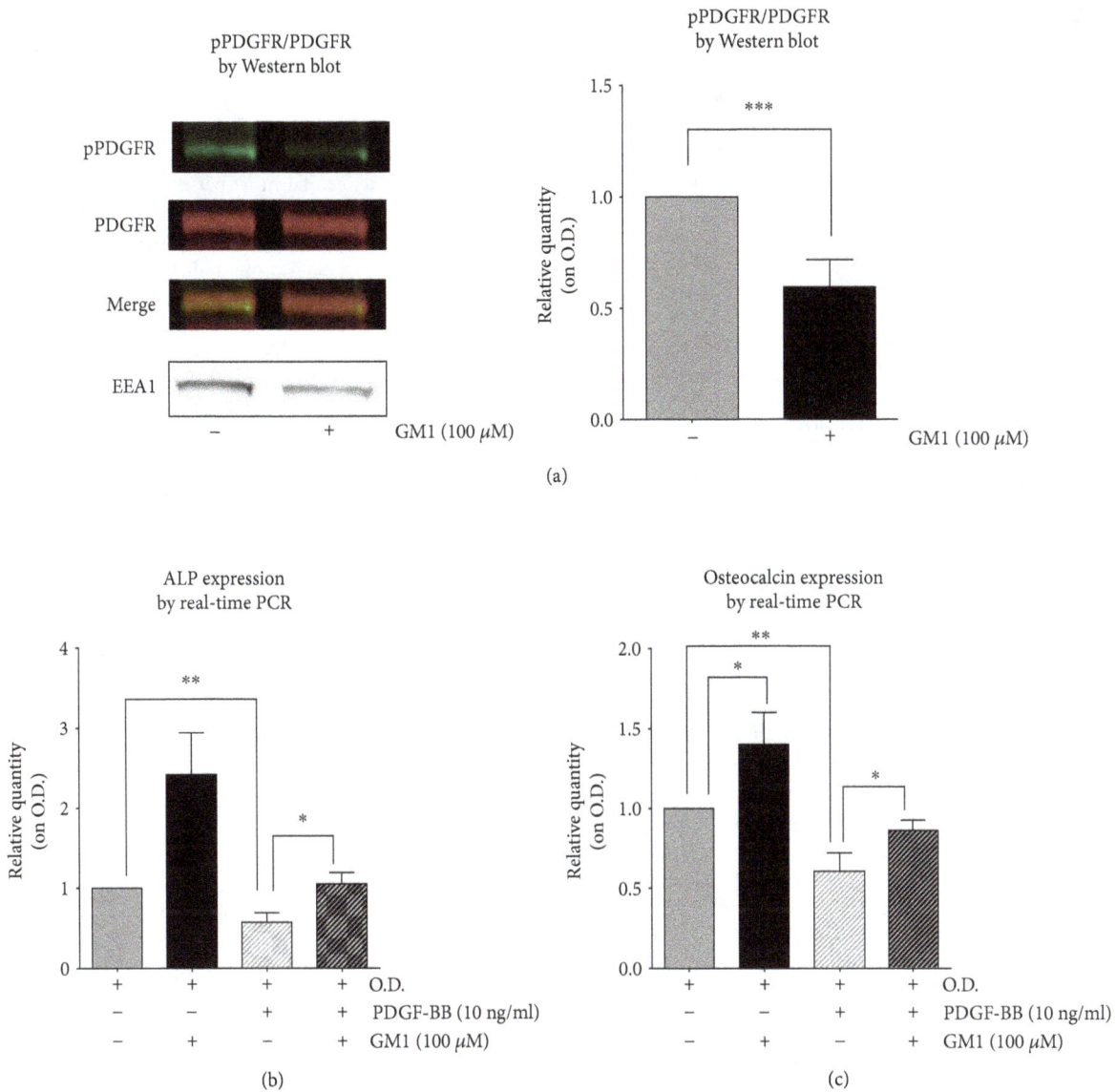

FIGURE 3: Effects of GM1 treatment on PDGFR activation. (a) Western blot analysis and quantification of PDGFR-β activation. hTSCs were differentiated toward osteoblasts in osteogenic medium supplemented with 100 μM GM1, as compared to hTSCs differentiated in GM1-free osteogenic medium (O.D.). Total proteins were extracted and analyzed with anti-phosphorylated-PDGFR-β (Tyr 751) antibody (green) and anti-PDGFR-β (28E1) antibody (red). EEA1 expression was used as internal control. Data are means ± SD of four different experiments. (b, c) Gene expression analysis of the osteogenic markers ALP and osteocalcin by real-time PCR. hTSCs were differentiated toward osteoblasts in osteogenic medium supplemented with 100 μM GM1 or 10 ng/ml PDGF-BB or with both 100 μM GM1 and 10 ng/ml PDGF-BB. The results were compared to hTSCs differentiated in free osteogenic medium (O.D.). Ribosomal protein S14 gene was used as housekeeper. All data are means ± SD of three different experiments. The statistical analysis was determined by Student's t-test. $^*p < 0.05$, $^{**}p < 0.01$, $^{***}p < 0.001$.

Indeed, the addition of exogenous GM1 to the differentiation medium greatly increased the osteogenic capabilities of hTSCs, supporting its possible use as a new factor to be added in the differentiation medium to improve this process. Further studies are ongoing in our laboratories to fully elucidate the mechanism of GM1 regulation of PDGFR-β activation and the possible therapeutic application of GM1 in regenerative medicine.

Acknowledgments

This work was partially supported by the "Line 2 Grants, Type B" from the Department of Biomedical Sciences for Health, University of Milan (Italy) and by the local research funds of the IRCCS Policlinico San Donato, a clinical research hospital partially funded by the Italian Ministry of Health.

References

[1] J. Apostolakos, T. J. Durant, C. R. Dwyer et al., "The enthesis: a review of the tendon-to-bone insertion," *Muscles, Ligaments and Tendons Journal*, vol. 4, no. 3, pp. 333–342, 2014.

[2] P. Randelli, F. Randelli, V. Ragone et al., "Regenerative medicine in rotator cuff injuries," *BioMed Research International*, vol. 2014, Article ID 129515, 9 pages, 2014.

[3] J. A. Cadby, E. Buehler, C. Godbout, P. R. van Weeren, and J. G. Snedeker, "Differences between the cell populations from the peritenon and the tendon core with regard to their potential implication in tendon repair," *PLoS One*, vol. 9, no. 3, article e92474, 2014.

[4] P. Randelli, E. Conforti, M. Piccoli et al., "Isolation and characterization of 2 new human rotator cuff and long head of biceps tendon cells possessing stem cell-like self-renewal and multipotential differentiation capacity," *The American Journal of Sports Medicine*, vol. 41, no. 7, pp. 1653–1664, 2013.

[5] P. H. Lopez and R. L. Schnaar, "Gangliosides in cell recognition and membrane protein regulation," *Current Opinion in Structural Biology*, vol. 19, no. 5, pp. 549–557, 2009.

[6] R. K. Yu, "Chapter 3 development regulation of ganglioside metabolism," *Progress in Brain Research*, vol. 101, pp. 31–44, 1994.

[7] J. Inokuchi, M. Nagafuku, I. Ohno, and A. Suzuki, "Heterogeneity of gangliosides among T cell subsets," *Cellular and Molecular Life Sciences*, vol. 70, no. 17, pp. 3067–3075, 2013.

[8] D. H. Kwak, S. Lee, S. J. Kim et al., "Ganglioside GM3 inhibits the high glucose- and TGF-β1-induced proliferation of rat glomerular mesangial cells," *Life Sciences*, vol. 77, no. 20, pp. 2540–2551, 2005.

[9] T. Kazarian, A. A. Jabbar, F. Q. Wen, D. A. Patel, and L. A. Valentino, "Gangliosides regulate tumor cell adhesion to collagen," *Clinical & Experimental Metastasis*, vol. 20, no. 4, pp. 311–319, 2003.

[10] F. Malisan and R. Testi, "GD3 in cellular ageing and apoptosis," *Experimental Gerontology*, vol. 37, no. 10-11, pp. 1273–1282, 2002.

[11] S. M. Kim, J. U. Jung, J. S. Ryu et al., "Effects of gangliosides on the differentiation of human mesenchymal stem cells into osteoblasts by modulating epidermal growth factor receptors," *Biochemical and Biophysical Research Communications*, vol. 371, no. 4, pp. 866–871, 2008.

[12] G. Moussavou, D. H. Kwak, M. U. Lim et al., "Role of gangliosides in the differentiation of human mesenchymal-derived stem cells into osteoblasts and neuronal cells," *BMB Reports*, vol. 46, no. 11, pp. 527–532, 2013.

[13] S. Bergante, E. Torretta, P. Creo et al., "Gangliosides as a potential new class of stem cell markers: the case of GD1a in human bone marrow mesenchymal stem cells," *Journal of Lipid Research*, vol. 55, no. 3, pp. 549–560, 2014.

[14] L. Anastasia, N. Papini, F. Colazzo et al., "NEU3 sialidase strictly modulates GM3 levels in skeletal myoblasts C2C12 thus favoring their differentiation and protecting them from apoptosis," *The Journal of Biological Chemistry*, vol. 283, no. 52, pp. 36265–36271, 2008.

[15] R. Scaringi, M. Piccoli, N. Papini et al., "NEU3 sialidase is activated under hypoxia and protects skeletal muscle cells from apoptosis through the activation of the epidermal growth factor receptor signaling pathway and the hypoxia-inducible factor (HIF)-1α," *The Journal of Biological Chemistry*, vol. 288, no. 5, pp. 3153–3162, 2013.

[16] N. Papini, L. Anastasia, C. Tringali et al., "MmNEU3 sialidase over-expression in C2C12 myoblasts delays differentiation and induces hypertrophic myotube formation," *Journal of Cellular Biochemistry*, vol. 113, no. 9, pp. 2967–2978, 2012.

[17] M. Piccoli, E. Conforti, A. Varrica et al., "NEU3 sialidase role in activating HIF-1α in response to chronic hypoxia in cyanotic congenital heart patients," *International Journal of Cardiology*, vol. 230, pp. 6–13, 2017.

[18] L. Riboni, P. Viani, and G. Tettamanti, "[51] Estimating sphingolipid metabolism and trafficking in cultured cells using radiolabeled compounds," *Methods in Enzymology*, vol. 311, pp. 656–682, 2000.

[19] N. Papini, L. Anastasia, C. Tringali et al., "The plasma membrane-associated sialidase MmNEU3 modifies the ganglioside pattern of adjacent cells supporting its involvement in cell-to-cell interactions," *The Journal of Biological Chemistry*, vol. 279, no. 17, pp. 16989–16995, 2004.

[20] R. K. Yu and T. Ariga, "Ganglioside analysis by high-performance thin-layer chromatography," *Methods in Enzymology*, vol. 312, pp. 115–134, 2000.

[21] F. Fierro, T. Illmer, D. Jing et al., "Inhibition of platelet-derived growth factor receptorβ by imatinib mesylate suppresses proliferation and alters differentiation of human mesenchymal stem cells *in vitro*," *Cell Proliferation*, vol. 40, no. 3, pp. 355–366, 2007.

[22] E. G. Bremer, J. Schlessinger, and S. Hakomori, "Ganglioside-mediated modulation of cell growth. Specific effects of GM3 on tyrosine phosphorylation of the epidermal growth factor receptor," *The Journal of Biological Chemistry*, vol. 261, no. 5, pp. 2434–2440, 1986.

[23] E. Meuillet, G. Cremel, D. Hicks, and H. Dreyfus, "Ganglioside effects on basic fibroblast and epidermal growth factor receptors in retinal glial cells," *Journal of Lipid Mediators and Cell Signalling*, vol. 14, no. 1-3, pp. 277–288, 1996.

[24] G. Ferrari, B. L. Anderson, R. M. Stephens, D. R. Kaplan, and L. A. Greene, "Prevention of apoptotic neuronal death by G_{M1} ganglioside. Involvement of Trk neurotrophin receptors," *The Journal of Biological Chemistry*, vol. 270, no. 7, pp. 3074–3080, 1995.

[25] J. Brooklyn, E. G. Bremer, and A. J. Yates, "Gangliosides inhibit platelet-derived growth factor-stimulated receptor dimerization in human glioma U-1242MG and Swiss 3T3 cells," *Journal of Neurochemistry*, vol. 61, no. 1, pp. 371–374, 1993.

[26] X. Q. Wang, S. Lee, H. Wilson et al., "Ganglioside GM3 depletion reverses impaired wound healing in diabetic mice by activating IGF-1 and insulin receptors," *The Journal of Investigative Dermatology*, vol. 134, no. 5, pp. 1446–1455, 2014.

[27] A. J. Yates, H. E. Saqr, and J. Van Brocklyn, "Ganglioside modulation of the PDGF receptor. A model for ganglioside functions," *Journal of Neuro-Oncology*, vol. 24, no. 1, pp. 65–73, 1995.

[28] T. Farooqui, T. Kelley, K. M. Coggeshall, A. A. Rampersaud, and A. J. Yates, "GM1 inhibits early signaling events mediated by PDGF receptor in cultured human glioma cells," *Anticancer Research*, vol. 19, no. 6B, pp. 5007–5013, 1999.

[29] J. L. Oblinger, C. L. Boardman, A. J. Yates, and R. W. Burry, "Domain-dependent modulation of PDGFRβ by ganglioside GM1," *Journal of Molecular Neuroscience*, vol. 20, no. 2, pp. 103–114, 2003.

[30] T. Mitsuda, K. Furukawa, S. Fukumoto, H. Miyazaki, T. Urano, and K. Furukawa, "Overexpression of ganglioside GM1 results in the dispersion of platelet-derived growth factor receptor from glycolipid-enriched microdomains and in the suppression of cell growth signals," *The Journal of Biological Chemistry*, vol. 277, no. 13, pp. 11239–11246, 2002.

[31] L. Veracini, V. Simon, V. Richard et al., "The Csk-binding protein PAG regulates PDGF-induced Src mitogenic signaling via GM1," *The Journal of Cell Biology*, vol. 182, no. 3, pp. 603–614, 2008.

[32] A. Li, X. Xia, J. Yeh et al., "PDGF-AA promotes osteogenic differentiation and migration of mesenchymal stem cell by down-regulating PDGFRα and derepressing BMP-Smad1/5/8 signaling," *PLoS One*, vol. 9, no. 12, article e113785, 2014.

[33] Y. Y. Zhang, Y. Z. Cui, J. Luan, X. Y. Zhou, G. L. Zhang, and J. X. Han, "Platelet-derived growth factor receptor kinase inhibitor AG-1295 promotes osteoblast differentiation in MC3T3-E1 cells via the Erk pathway," *Bioscience Trends*, vol. 6, no. 3, pp. 130–135, 2012.

[34] S. O'Sullivan, D. Naot, K. Callon et al., "Imatinib promotes osteoblast differentiation by inhibiting PDGFR signaling and inhibits osteoclastogenesis by both direct and stromal cell-dependent mechanisms," *Journal of Bone and Mineral Research*, vol. 22, no. 11, pp. 1679–1689, 2007.

Focal Adhesion Kinase and ROCK Signaling are Switch-Like Regulators of Human Adipose Stem Cell Differentiation towards Osteogenic and Adipogenic Lineages

Laura Hyväri [ID],[1,2] Miina Ojansivu [ID],[1,2] Miia Juntunen [ID],[1,2] Kimmo Kartasalo [ID],[3,4] Susanna Miettinen [ID],[1,2] and Sari Vanhatupa [ID][1,2]

[1]Adult Stem Cell Research Group, BioMediTech Institute and Faculty of Medicine and Life Sciences, University of Tampere, Tampere, Finland
[2]Science Center, Tampere University Hospital, Tampere, Finland
[3]Computational Biology Group, BioMediTech Institute and Faculty of Medicine and Life Sciences, University of Tampere, Tampere, Finland
[4]BioMediTech Institute and Faculty of Biomedical Sciences and Engineering, Tampere University of Technology, Tampere, Finland

Correspondence should be addressed to Susanna Miettinen; susanna.miettinen@uta.fi

Academic Editor: Kenichi Tamama

Adipose tissue is an attractive stem cell source for soft and bone tissue engineering applications and stem cell therapies. The adipose-derived stromal/stem cells (ASCs) have a multilineage differentiation capacity that is regulated through extracellular signals. The cellular events related to cell adhesion and cytoskeleton have been suggested as central regulators of differentiation fate decision. However, the detailed knowledge of these molecular mechanisms in human ASCs remains limited. This study examined the significance of focal adhesion kinase (FAK), Rho-Rho-associated protein kinase (Rho-ROCK), and their downstream target extracellular signal-regulated kinase 1/2 (ERK1/2) on hASCs differentiation towards osteoblasts and adipocytes. Analyses of osteogenic markers *RUNX2A*, alkaline phosphatase, and matrix mineralization revealed an essential role of active FAK, ROCK, and ERK1/2 signaling for the osteogenesis of hASCs. Inhibition of these kinases with specific small molecule inhibitors diminished osteogenesis, while inhibition of FAK and ROCK activity led to elevation of adipogenic marker genes *AP2* and *LEP* and lipid accumulation implicating adipogenesis. This denotes to a switch-like function of FAK and ROCK signaling in the osteogenic and adipogenic fates of hASCs. On the contrary, inhibition of ERK1/2 kinase activity deceased adipogenic differentiation, indicating that activation of ERK signaling is required for both adipogenic and osteogenic potential. Our findings highlight the reciprocal role of cell adhesion mechanisms and actin dynamics in regulation of hASC lineage commitment. This study enhances the knowledge of molecular mechanisms dictating hASC differentiation and thus opens possibilities for more efficient control of hASC differentiation.

1. Introduction

Mesenchymal stem cells (MSCs) are multipotent adult stem cells that give rise to osteoblasts, adipocytes, and chondrocytes *in vitro*. MSCs can be harvested from multiple adult tissues, for example, bone marrow, adipose tissue, dental tissues, and umbilical cord [1]. MSCs derived from fat tissue, adipose-derived stromal/stem cells (ASCs), are increasingly used in regenerative medicine due to their desirable immunomodulatory properties and ease of harvest [1]. Regulation of MSC differentiation has been extensively studied, but the research has been mainly conducted with the bone marrow mesenchymal stem cells (BMSC) of human or rodent origin. Although the central transcription factors and signaling pathways are conserved between cell types and species, the extrapolation of these previous results to human ASCs cannot be made without reservation. It has been discovered that MSCs of different species are not fully comparable regarding their differentiation potential [2, 3] or immunosuppressive capacity [4]. Additionally, the differentiation potential of MSCs has been shown to vary even within species depending on the harvest site [5]. Thus, there is a need for in vitro studies elucidating the molecular mechanisms regulating differentiation potential specifically in human ASCs.

Self-renewal and differentiation of mesenchymal stem cells are tightly regulated by signals from the surrounding environment. Especially signals that regulate cell adhesion and cytoskeletal arrangements have been suggested to be important regulators of MSC differentiation [6]. Cells grow and function in association with extracellular matrix (ECM) components and respond to a wide range of external signals by converting their morphology, behavior, and fate decision accordingly [7–9]. One of the most important response mechanisms is based on the function of transmembrane adhesion receptors of the integrin family and integrin-based focal adhesion (FA) complexes. FAs work in the regulation of cytoskeletal networking and cellular signaling through a central mediator, focal adhesion kinase (FAK) [10]. FAK signaling functions through autophosphorylation of tyrosine 397 that induces interaction of FAK with Src, a nonreceptor tyrosine kinase that stabilizes as a response of this interaction and further phosphorylates other tyrosines of FAK. This leads to full activity of both kinases and subsequent activation of numerous intracellular pathways [11]. In mesenchymal stem cells (MSCs), FAK signaling is interconnected with various pathways including mitogen-activated kinases (MAPKs) and Rho-family GTPases RhoA, Rac, and Cdc42 [12].

The regulation of the cell cytoskeleton and morphology is primarily controlled by the RhoA-ROCK pathway [13], which sustains the integrity of the cytoskeleton by stimulating actomyosin contractility [14, 15]. ROCK isoforms are protein serine/threonine kinases that phosphorylate substrates such as myosin light chain (MLC) phosphatase to drive the assembly of the actin cytoskeleton [13]. The RhoA-ROCK signaling is also an important regulator of stem cell commitment [7, 16–18], and the cell shape determined by RhoA function has been proposed to be a major switch between adipogenic and osteogenic differentiation of human MSCs (hMSCs) [7]. In addition, ROCK signaling is related to the substrate stiffness-driven lineage commitment of MSCs through mechanosensing of the microenvironment via interplay with integrin-FAK signaling [19].

MAPK pathway component extracellular signal-regulated kinase 1/2 (ERK1/2) is linked to vital cellular functions such as proliferation, survival, apoptosis, motility, transcription, metabolism, and differentiation [20]. ERK1/2 has been shown to be a downstream effector of FAK-mediated signaling in MSCs [18, 21]. It has also been suggested as a mechanosensing protein, regulated by the RhoA-ROCK-mediated actin dynamics in hMSCs [22–24]. ERK1/2 activity is linked to the expression of osteogenic markers in hASCs [25]. However, the role of ERK signaling in the adipogenic differentiation fate differs

depending on the experimental design and the cell type studied [25–28].

In previous studies, the cellular mechanisms of adhesion and cytoskeletal arrangements have been studied in multiple cell types and varying experimental conditions and configurations. In this study, our objective was to clarify the role of these mechanisms in the differentiation fate decision of adipose tissue-derived stem cells. The current study carefully analyzed the significance of FAK, ROCK, and ERK1/2 proteins in the adipogenic and osteogenic differentiation of hASCs. The key results demonstrated the reciprocal regulation of FAK and ROCK signaling in the interface of hASC osteogenesis and adipogenesis. Our results also consistently indicated that in hASCs, ERK1/2 activity is required for the full osteogenic and adipogenic potential. As a conclusion, our results suggested that ERK1/2 activation together with cell adhesion and actin regulation by FAK-RhoA-ROCK signaling are fine tuning regulators of hASC fate decision. This investigation enhanced the understanding of the signaling mechanisms governing stem cell commitment and gave insight for future development of in vitro models, tissue engineering constructs, and stem cell therapies.

2. Materials and Methods

2.1. Cell Isolation and Culture. The study was carried out in accordance with the Ethics Committee of the Pirkanmaa Hospital District, Tampere, Finland (ethical approval R15161). The hASCs were isolated from adipose tissue samples of six female donors (age, 44 ± 11 years, donor information in Table S1) with a written informed consent of the donors. Isolation of the stem cells was performed as described previously [29]. The isolated hASCs were maintained and expanded in human serum containing basic culture medium (BM) (composition in Table 1) and passaged after reaching 70–80% confluence.

2.2. Flow Cytometric Analysis of Surface Marker Expression. The cells were identified as MSCs by flow cytometry (FACSAria; BD Biosciences, Erembodegem, Belgium) at passage 1 to confirm the MSC immunophenotype of the cells. Cells were single stained using monoclonal antibodies against CD3-PE, CD14-PE-Cy7, CD19-PE-Cy7, CD45R0-APC, CD54-FITC, CD73-PE, CD90-APC (BD Biosciences, Franklin Lakes, NJ, USA), CD11a-APC, CD80-PE, CD86-PE, CD105-PE (R&D Systems, Minneapolis, MN, USA), CD34-APC, and HLA-DR-PE (ImmunoTools, Friesoythe, Germany). The FACS analysis was performed on 10,000 cells per sample and positive expression was defined as fluorescence level greater than 99% of the comparable unstained cell sample.

2.3. Osteogenic and Adipogenic Differentiation Cultures. Human ASCs were seeded into CellBIND polystyrene plates (Corning Inc., Corning, NY, USA) in BM prior to the experiments. Osteogenic and adipogenic inductions were initiated on the following day by introducing the osteogenic medium (OM) and adipogenic medium (AM) to the cells (compositions in Table 1). 0.25 mM IBMX (3-isobutyl-1-

TABLE 1: Culture media compositions.

Component	BM	OM	AM	Manufacturer
Dulbecco's Modified Eagle Medium/Ham's Nutrient Mixture F-12 (DMEM/F-12)				Thermo Fisher Scientific, Waltham, MA, USA
GlutaMAX	1%	1%	1%	
Insulin	—	—	100 nM	
Human serum (HS)	5%	5%	5%	PAA Laboratories GmbH, Pasching, Austria
Penicillin/streptomycin	1%	1%	1%	Lonza, Basel, Switzerland
L-Ascorbic acid 2-phosphate	—	200 μM	—	
β-Glycerophosphate	—	10 mM	—	
Dexamethasone (DEX)	—	5 nM	1 μM	Sigma-Aldrich, Saint Louis, MO, USA
Pantothenate	—	—	17 μM	
Biotin	—	—	33 μM	
3-Isobutyl-1-methylxanthine (IBMX)	—	—	0.25 M	

methylxanthine; Sigma-Aldrich, Saint Louis, MO, USA) was added to the adipogenic differentiation cultures upon first change of culture media. 5 nM Dexamethasone (DEX; Sigma-Aldrich) was applied to OM when used. Fresh differentiation media were applied to the cells twice a week during the experiments. As a control, the hASCs were cultured in BM condition. The experiments were conducted at passages 3–5.

2.4. Small Molecule Inhibitors.

BM, OM, and AM were supplemented with small molecule inhibitors targeted to FAK, ROCK, and ERK1/2 proteins and added to the cell cultures. FAK and ROCK signaling were inhibited using PF-562271 (Selleck Chemicals, Houston, Texas, USA) and Y-27632 (Selleck Chemicals), respectively. Inhibition of ERK1/2 activation was conducted with PD98059 (Calbiochem/EMD Millipore, Billerica, Massachusetts, USA) which is a specific inhibitor of ERK1/2 upstream kinase mitogen-activated protein kinase 1 (MEK1). BM, OM, and AM conditions without the inhibitors were used as controls. Fresh media supplemented with the inhibitors were applied to the cells twice a week during the experiments.

2.5. Live/Dead Staining.

The viability of the hASCs seeded 260 cells/cm^2 in 24-well plate and cultured 7 days in BM, OM, or AM and left untreated (control) or treated with FAK inhibitor PF-562271, ROCK inhibitor Y-27632, or MEK/ERK inhibitor PD98059 was studied with LIVE/DEAD Viability/Cytotoxicity Kit (Molecular Probes; Thermo Fisher Scientific). The viable cells (green fluorescence) and dead cells (red fluorescence) were imaged using an Olympus microscope (IX51, Olympus) equipped with a fluorescence unit and camera (DP30BW, Olympus) with 4x magnification.

2.6. Fluorescence Staining of the Actin Cytoskeleton.

The hASCs were cultured 7 days in BM, OM, or AM and left untreated (control) or treated with 2 μM FAK inhibitor PF-562271, 15 μM ROCK inhibitor Y-27632, and 30 μM MEK/ERK inhibitor PD98059. The cells were fixed and permeabilized with 4% PFA (Sigma-Aldrich) supplemented with 0.1% Triton X-100 for 15 min at RT. Blocking was done with 1% bovine serum albumin (BSA; Sigma-Aldrich) for 1 h at +4°C. For actin staining, the cells were incubated in tetramethyl-rhodamine B isothiocyanate- (TRITC-) conjugated phalloidin (P1951; Sigma-Aldrich) for 45 min at RT followed by 4′,6-diamidino-2-phenylindole (DAPI, Sigma-Aldrich) staining to visualize the nuclei.

2.7. Cell Proliferation and Quantitative Analysis of Alkaline Phosphatase Activity.

Cell proliferation of control and inhibitor-treated hASCs (seeded 260 cells/cm^2 in 24-well plate) was assessed with CyQUANT cell proliferation assay (Molecular Probes; Thermo Fisher Scientific, Waltham, MA, USA) after 7 and 14 days of culture as described previously [29, 30]. The activity of alkaline phosphatase (ALP) was analyzed from the same cell lysates as cell proliferation as described previously [29].

2.8. Alizarin Red Staining and Quantification of Mineralization.

The cells (seeded 260 cells/cm^2 and cultured with control and inhibitor conditions) were stained with Alizarin Red (AR) after 14 and 21 days of culture for the analysis of mineralization. The staining was done as described previously [31]. Briefly, the cells were fixed with 70% ethanol, stained with 2% Alizarin Red S (pH 4.1–4.3; Sigma-Aldrich), and photographed after three washes with water and one with ethanol. Quantitative results were obtained by extracting the dye with 100 mM cetylpyridinium chloride (Sigma-Aldrich) for 3 hours and measuring the absorbances of the samples at 544 nm.

2.9. Oil Red O Staining.

hASCs (seeded 260 cells/cm^2 in 24-well plate) were cultured in BM, OM, and AM supplemented with inhibitor molecules for 21 days and stained with Oil Red O (ORO) staining, which indicates lipid droplet formation, as described previously [29]. Following ORO stain, the hASCs were counterstained with DAPI (Sigma-Aldrich; dilution 1 : 2000) for 5 minutes before the last washing steps. Fluorescence microscope images were taken with an

TABLE 2: The primer sequences and accession numbers for qRT-PCR.

Gene	5'-Sequence-3'	Product size (bp)	Accession number
AP2	Forward GGTGGTGGAATGCGTCATG	71	NM_001442
	Reverse CAACGTCCCTTGGCTTATGC		
LEP	Forward ACAATTGTCACCAGGATCAATGAC	73	NM_000230
	Reverse TCCAAACCGGTGACTTTCTGT		
RPLP0	Forward AATCTCCAGGGGCACCATT	70	NM_001002
	Reverse CGCTGGCTCCCACTTTGT		
RUNX2A	Forward CTTCATTCGCCTCACAAACAAC	62	NM_001024630.3
	Reverse TCCTCCTGGAGAAAGTTTGCA		

bp: base pair.

Olympus microscope (IX51, Olympus, Tokyo, Japan) equipped with a fluorescence unit and a camera (DP30BW, Olympus).

2.10. Quantification of Lipid Formation. Lipid formation was quantified based on image analysis of samples stained with ORO and DAPI. Image quantification was performed with a custom analysis pipeline designed for CellProfiler (version 2.1.1, 64-bit Windows; http://www.cellprofiler.org [32]). Lipid maturation was assessed by applying a $10\,\mu m$ diameter threshold for lipid droplet clusters. See Supplemental Materials for a detailed description of the analysis pipeline.

2.11. qRT-PCR. The quantitative real-time reverse transcriptase polymerase chain reaction (qRT-PCR) analysis was performed after 7 and 14 days of culture (hASCs seeded $3160\,cells/cm^2$ in 6-well plate) as described previously [33]. The expressions of *human runt-related transcription factor 2a (RUNX2A), human adipocyte fatty acid-binding protein (FABP4 or AP2)*, and *human leptin (LEP)* were normalized with the expression of *human acidic ribosomal phosphoprotein P0 (RPLP0)*. Gene sequences and accession numbers are presented in Table 2.

2.12. Western Blotting and Immunodetection. Human ASCs (seeded $3160\,cells/cm^2$ in 6-well plate) were starved for 24 hours in BM, OM, or AM containing 1% human serum before the 7d inhibitor-supplemented culture, which was also conducted in starvation media. Samples lysed with 2X LAEMMLI sample buffer were analyzed with Western blotting (WB) as described earlier [34]. Briefly, samples were separated with SDS electrophoresis and transferred into polyvinylidene fluoride membrane ($0.2\,\mu m$ PVDF Single application; Bio-Rad, Hercules, CA, USA). Membrane was blocked with 5% milk in Tris-buffered saline supplemented with 0.05% Tween 20 (Sigma-Aldrich). Membranes were incubated with primary antibodies followed by secondary antibody incubation and chemiluminescence detection (ECL Prime Western Blotting Detection Reagent; GE Healthcare, Little Chalfont, UK) and visualized with Chemi Doc MP System (Bio-Rad). Antibodies and dilutions are presented in Table 3.

2.13. Statistical Analysis. All results are represented as mean and standard deviation (SD). Statistical analyses were

TABLE 3: Primary and secondary antibodies used in Western blot analysis.

Antibody type	Antibody	Host species	Dilution	Incubation
Primary	Anti-β-actin[1]	Mouse	1:2000	RT, 2 h
Primary	Anti-FAK[2]	Rabbit	1:1000	+4°C, overnight
Primary	Anti-p-FAK[2]	Rabbit	1:1000	+4°C, overnight
Primary	Anti-ERK2[1]	Rabbit	1:1000	RT, 2 h
Primary	Anti-p-ERK1/2[2]	Rabbit	1:2000	+4°C, overnight
Primary	Anti-MLC2	Rabbit	1:800	+4°C, overnight
Primary	Anti-p-MLC2	Rabbit	1:800	+4°C, overnight
Secondary	Anti-rabbit IgG[2]	Goat	1:2000	RT, 1 h
Secondary	Anti-mouse IgG[1]	Goat	1:2000	RT, 1 h

[1] Santa Cruz Biotechnology, Dallas, Texas, USA. [2] Cell Signaling Technology, Danvers, Massachusetts, USA.

conducted using GraphPad Prism 5 (La Jolla, CA, USA). Statistical differences between the inhibitor-treated samples and the respective controls were tested using the nonparametric Mann–Whitney test followed by Bonferroni post hoc test. Statistical differences with $p < 0.05$ were considered significant. Detailed information of the biological and technical replicates used in statistical analysis is given in Table S2.

3. Results

3.1. Characterization of hASCs. Surface marker expression of hASCs was analyzed by flow cytometry. The hASCs were characterized as MSCs due to positive expression of CD73, CD90, and CD105; lack of CD3, CD11, CD14, CD19, CD45, CD80, CD86, and HLA-DR expression; and moderate expression of CD34 and CD54 (Table S3).

3.2. Inhibition of FAK, ROCK, and ERK1/2 Activity Reduces Proliferation of hASCs. Cell proliferation capacity was evaluated in BM, OM, and AM with gradient concentrations of FAK, ROCK, and ERK inhibitors PF-562271, Y-27632, and PD98059, respectively. CyQUANT assay indicated that

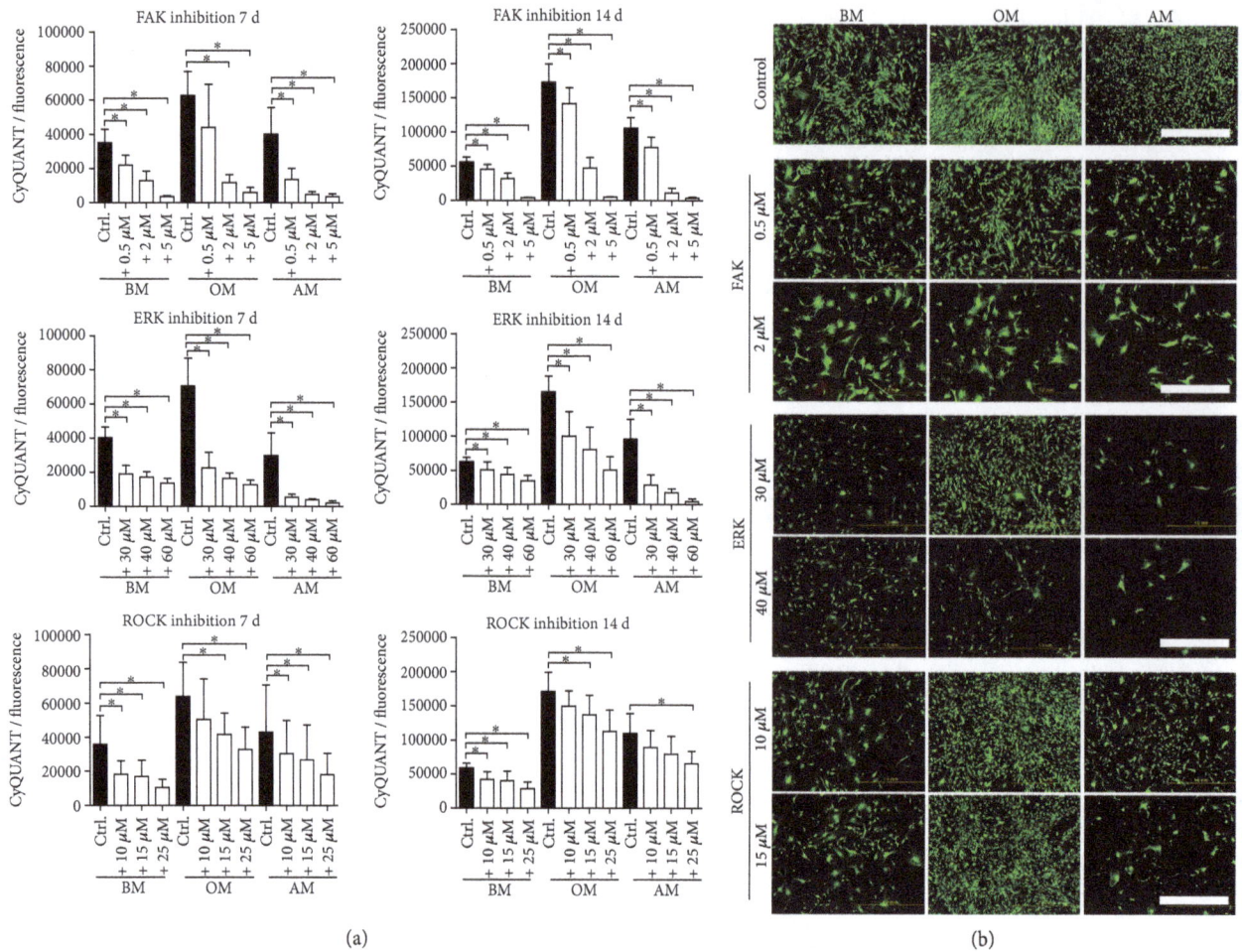

FIGURE 1: Cell viability and proliferation after 7 and 14 days of culture in response to inhibition of FAK, ERK1/2, and ROCK signaling. (a) hASCs were cultured 7 or 14 d in BM, OM, and AM supplemented with FAK, ERK1/2, and ROCK inhibitors. The inhibitor effect on proliferation was studied in each culture condition separately by comparing the different inhibitor concentrations with the untreated medium control. Significance level 5%, designated with an asterisk (*). FAK, ERK, and ROCK inhibitors: $N = 12$ (independent biological replicates from 4 donors). (b) Representative fluorescence images of LIVE/DEAD-stained hASCs. hASCs were cultured in BM, OM, or AM supplemented with the abovementioned inhibitors. Cell viability was analyzed with LIVE/DEAD assay at 7 d. Green dye represents living cells, red dye dead cells. Scale bar 1.0 mm. BM: basic medium; OM: osteogenic medium; AM: adipogenic medium.

the inhibitors have a regulatory function on cell proliferation (Figure 1(a)). The cell numbers were reduced dose dependently in the inhibitor-treated conditions compared to the control conditions. Despite a decrease in the cell number as a response to increased inhibitor concentrations, adherent cells remained viable with a negligible amount of dead cells (Figure 1(b)), as assessed with the LIVE/DEAD method. In addition to the inhibitor function on cell number, the inhibitor treatment also affected the typical fibroblast-like morphology of hASCs. Based on the immunofluorescence staining of actin cytoskeleton (Figure 2), ROCK inhibition caused the most prominent changes to the morphology of the hASCs. Y-27632 treated cells appeared spindle-like in OM and AM media, and the cells in OM had formed a network of star-shaped cells with long extensions.

3.3. FAK, ROCK, and ERK1/2 Functions Are Essential to hASC Osteogenesis.
The early osteogenic differentiation potential of hASCs cultured in BM, OM, and AM in the

presence or absence of the FAK, ROCK, and ERK inhibitors was assessed by quantitative real-time reverse transcriptase polymerase chain reaction analysis of the bone associated marker gene RUNX2A (Figure 3(a)) and by quantitative activity assay of ALP (Figure 3(b)) which is an early marker of osteogenesis [35]. At 7 days of culture, RUNX2A expression was markedly upregulated in the OM condition but downregulated by the addition of all studied inhibitors. However, statistical analyses were not done due to the low sample number. The enzymatic activity of ALP was the most prominent in the OM control medium after two weeks of culture, and addition of the inhibitors reduced the enzymatic activity dose dependently. ALP activation was markedly lower in BM and AM conditions, yet a similar trend in the inhibitor effect was seen.

Deposition of calcium phosphate mineral is characteristic to the maturation of osteoblasts and hence, late osteogenic differentiation capacity was studied by Alizarin Red staining protocol after 14 and 21 days of culture. Strong staining for

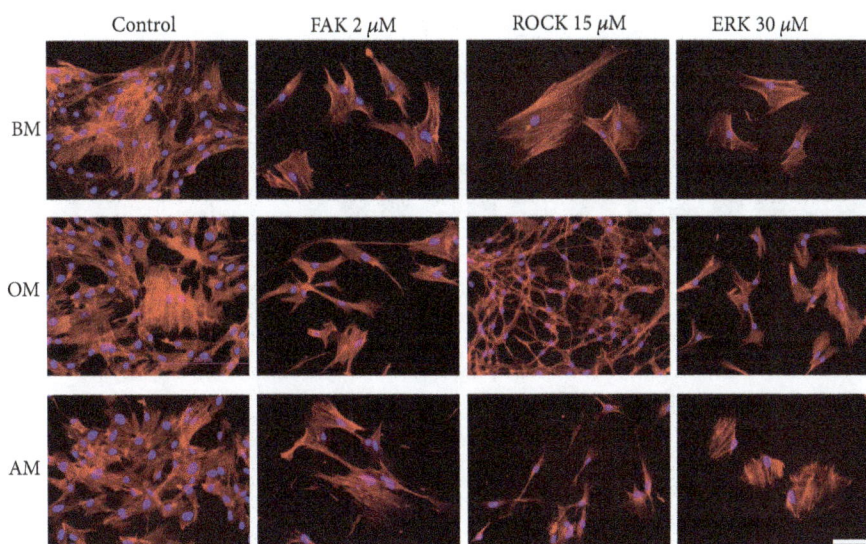

FIGURE 2: Immunofluorescence staining of actin cytoskeleton and nuclei. hASCs were treated with 2 μM FAK, 15 μM ROCK, or 30 μM ERK inhibitors, and the cytoskeleton was stained with phalloidin (red) and nuclei with DAPI (blue) at day 7. Scale bar 100 μm. BM: basic medium; OM: osteogenic medium; AM: adipogenic medium.

mineralization of the ECM occurred in the OM control medium at 21 d, as indicated by the quantitative analysis and the corresponding red-stained samples (Figure 3(c)). Mineral accumulation was significantly weakened in the inhibitor-supplemented OM conditions. BM and AM, lacking the osteogenic agents, were not able to support matrix mineralization. Although the inhibitors caused statistically significant reduction of mineralization in BM and AM conditions, the absolute values in the control conditions were too low to have any relevance for the mineralization. 2-week culture period was too short for mineral formation in the studied conditions.

3.4. Inhibition of FAK and ROCK Enhance Adipogenic Outcome of the hASCs. Adipogenic differentiation was analyzed in terms of the expression profiles of adipogenic marker genes *AP2* [36] and *LEP* [37] (Figure 4). As expected, the expression of adipogenic marker genes was most elevated in the hASCs cultured in AM. Based on our results, FAK inhibition increased the expression of *AP2* at both time points in all culture conditions. FAK inhibition also upregulated *LEP* in OM condition at both time points, but in AM, *LEP* expression was only induced at day 14. Inhibition of the Rho-ROCK signaling using Y-27632 led to enhanced *AP2* expression but had an opposite downregulating effect on *LEP* in AM condition. ERK inhibition, on the other hand, augmented *AP2* expression at 7 d but downregulated *AP2* on 14 d. Moreover, ERK inhibition also repressed *LEP* expression at both time points in AM condition suggesting that inhibition of ERK predominantly had a repressing effect on these adipogenic marker genes. Statistical analyses were not done due to the low sample number.

To further study adipogenic differentiation of the hASCs, accumulation of lipid droplets was analyzed after three weeks of culture with a fat-soluble diazol dye Oil Red O (ORO), Figure 5(a) [38]. We also quantified the lipid accumulation

by creating and optimizing a CellProfiler pipeline to analyze ORO-stained fluorescence images. We analyzed both total lipid droplet area in the cultures (Figure 5(b)) and the area of lipid droplet clusters exceeding 10 μm diameter limit (Figure S1) to visualize the ongoing adipogenic differentiation and maturation of adipocytes which is distinguished by the increasing number of lipid droplets as well as the enlargement of the individual fat vacuoles [39]. Lipid droplet cluster areas over 10 μm in diameter were further normalized with cell nuclei number to obtain results representative of the single-cell level (Figure 5(b)).

Interestingly, FAK inhibitor treatment significantly increased the proportion of large LDs in OM condition. In AM conditions 0.5 μM FAK inhibitor treatment also elevated lipid formation. However, the quantitative results showed that 2 μM FAK inhibitor led to a reduced area of LDs in AM condition. ROCK inhibition resulted in increased adipogenesis on both culture and single-cell level in OM and AM conditions. ERK inhibition reduced the area of ORO-stained LDs in the culture, also when normalized with the cell number.

3.5. Western Blot Analysis of the Inhibitor Functionality and Cross Talk between Signal Pathways. The functionality of small molecule inhibitors was confirmed by WB analysis of hASCs cultured in starvation media (Figure 6 and Figure S2). The ratio of phosphorylated and unphosphorylated forms of these proteins was analyzed with semiquantification of the band intensities using ImageJ software [40] (Figure 6(b)). Based on the visual inspection and the semiquantified results, the level of the target protein phosphorylation was clearly decreased by the specific inhibitory molecules confirming the inhibitor functionality.

Furthermore, our results pointed out that FAK, ROCK, and ERK inhibitors affected also other studied phosphoproteins and basal protein levels indicating a prospective cross

(a) *RUNX2A* expression

(b) ALP activity

(c) Mineralization

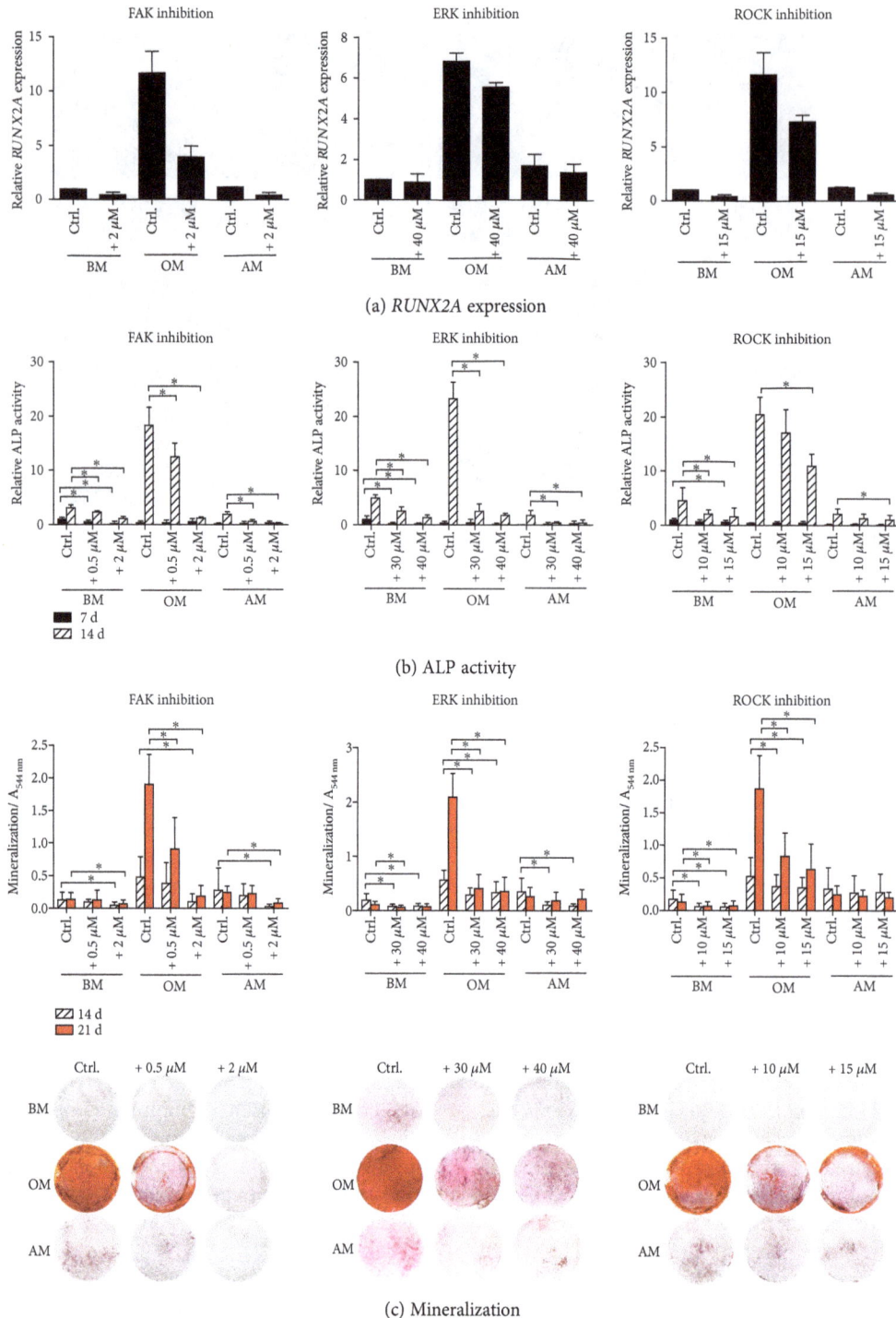

FIGURE 3: Osteogenic differentiation of hASCs in BM, OM, and AM culture conditions supplemented with FAK, ERK, and ROCK inhibitors. (a) The cells were cultured in BM, OM, or AM supplemented with $2\,\mu$M FAK, $40\,\mu$M ERK, or $15\,\mu$M ROCK inhibitors in addition to medium controls. *RUNX2A* expression was analyzed with qRT-PCR at 7 d. FAK and ROCK: $N = 5$ (independent experiments, 5 donors), ERK: $N = 3$ (independent experiments, 3 donors). (b) ALP activity was analyzed with ALP assay at 7 d and 14 d. The ALP absorbance values were normalized with corresponding CyQUANT results, and the results are presented relative to the 7 d BM sample. Significance level 5%, designated with an asterisk (*). FAK, ERK, ROCK: $N = 9$ (independent biological replicates from 3 donors). (c) Matrix mineralization was analyzed with AR staining after 14 d and 21 d of culture. Quantitative results of AR staining are presented as graphs and corresponding representative images of the stained wells (21 d, area $1.9\,\text{cm}^2$) are presented below; bright red dye represents mineral. Significance level 5%. FAK, ROCK: $N = 18$ (independent biological replicates from 6 donors, control condition values of the graphs are the same since the experiments were conducted at the same time), ERK: $N = 15$ (independent biological replicates from 5 donors). BM: basic medium; OM: osteogenic medium; AM: adipogenic medium; ALP: alkaline phosphatase; AR: Alizarin Red.

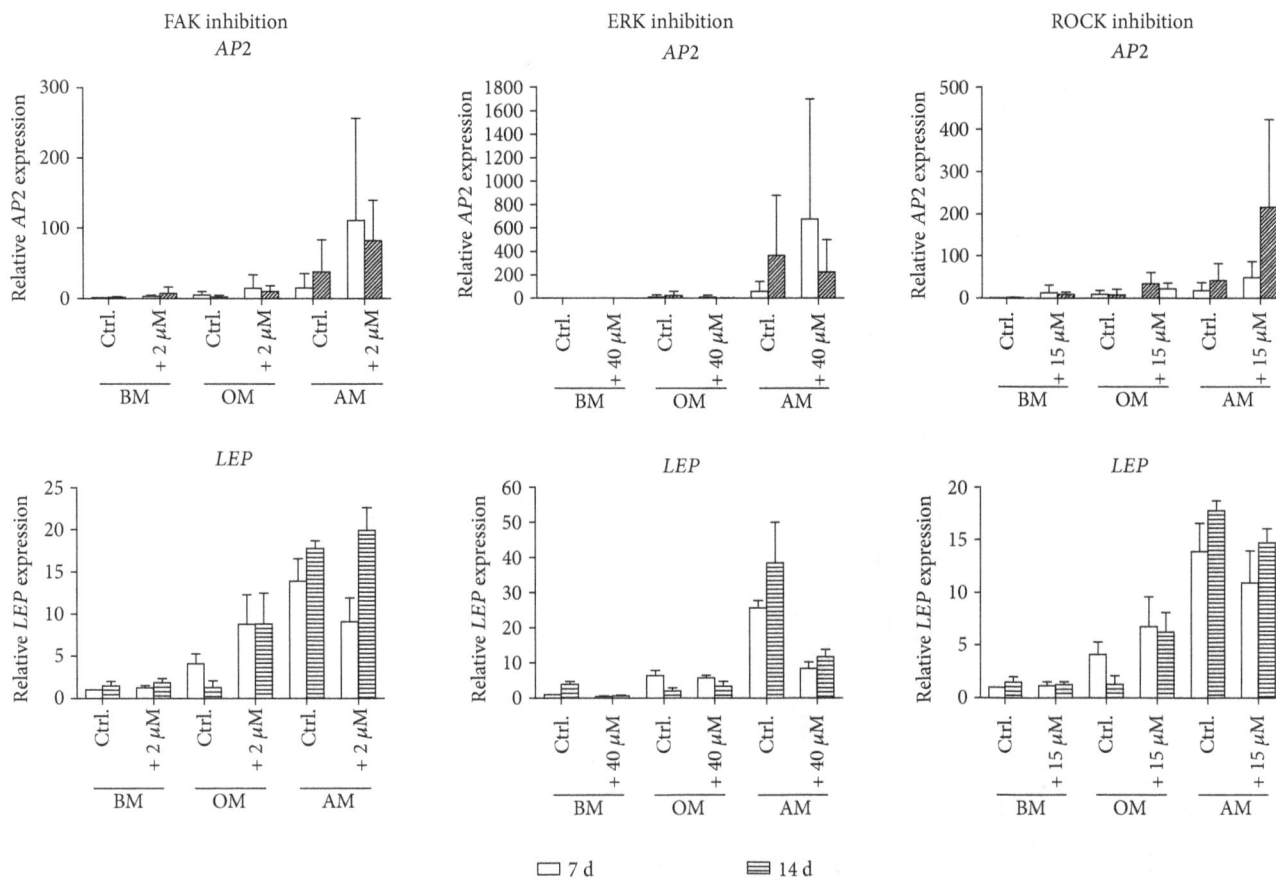

FIGURE 4: Expression of adipogenic marker genes *AP2* and *LEP* in hASCs treated with FAK, ERK, and ROCK inhibitors. The hASCs were cultured in BM, OM, or AM supplemented with 2 μM FAK, 40 μM ERK, or 15 μM ROCK inhibitors in addition to medium controls. *AP2* and *LEP* expressions were analyzed with qRT-PCR. The expression of *AP2* and *LEP* are normalized with the expression of the housekeeping gene *RPLP0*, and the results are presented relative to the 7 d BM sample. FAK and ROCK: $N = 5$ (independent experiments, 5 donors), ERK: $N = 3$ (independent experiments, 3 donors). BM: basic medium; OM: osteogenic medium; AM: adipogenic medium.

talk between signaling pathways. For instance, FAK inhibition had a modest decreasing effect on p-ERK1/2 in OM condition and FAK inhibitor also reduced ROCK downstream target p-MLC2 in BM and AM conditions. ROCK inhibition had a complementary decreasing effect on FAK phosphorylation in OM conditions, and also ERK inhibition decreased p-FAK levels in OM and AM conditions.

4. Discussion

Despite the fact that hASCs are already used in clinical treatments, the knowledge of the regulatory mechanisms of hASC differentiation originates from research done with varying cell types of human and nonhuman origin. Our aim was to carefully analyze the significance of cell adhesion and cytoskeleton in hASC osteogenic and adipogenic differentiation by using small molecular inhibitors for central proteins in cell adhesion and cytoskeletal dynamics.

Previous studies have noted the importance of FAK signaling in the osteogenic potential of hMSCs [18, 21, 41]. Our results support these findings by showing that the expression of the osteogenic marker gene *RUNX2A*, the enzymatic activity of ALP, and eventually mineralization

were distinctly decreased as a result of FAK inhibition in OM condition. In the presence of higher amounts of inhibitor, the cells failed to deposit virtually any mineral, presumably because of the decreased cell number. Role of FAK in the adipogenic differentiation has been investigated mainly with rodent cells and with diverging experimental setups [42–44]. Li and Xie [42] reported that firm adhesion is required for osteogenesis whereas morphological change accompanied with calpain-mediated cleavage of FAK is essential for preadipocytic differentiation and final maturation of adipocytes. On the contrary, a more recent *in vivo* study by Luk and coworkers [44] showed that the adipocyte survival was decreased by FAK knockout. We discovered that in human ASCs, inhibition of FAK activity induced expressions of adipogenic marker genes *AP2* and *LEP* in OM and AM conditions. Moreover, the CellProfiler analysis and normalized lipid droplet values revealed that FAK inhibition significantly induced lipid droplet maturation in OM condition, and 0.5 μM concentration had moderately inducing effect in AM as well. However, the total lipid droplet area in the culture was reduced with FAK inhibition, likely due to the decreased number of adherent cells, since the inhibition also affects the cell adhesion sites. These results together with

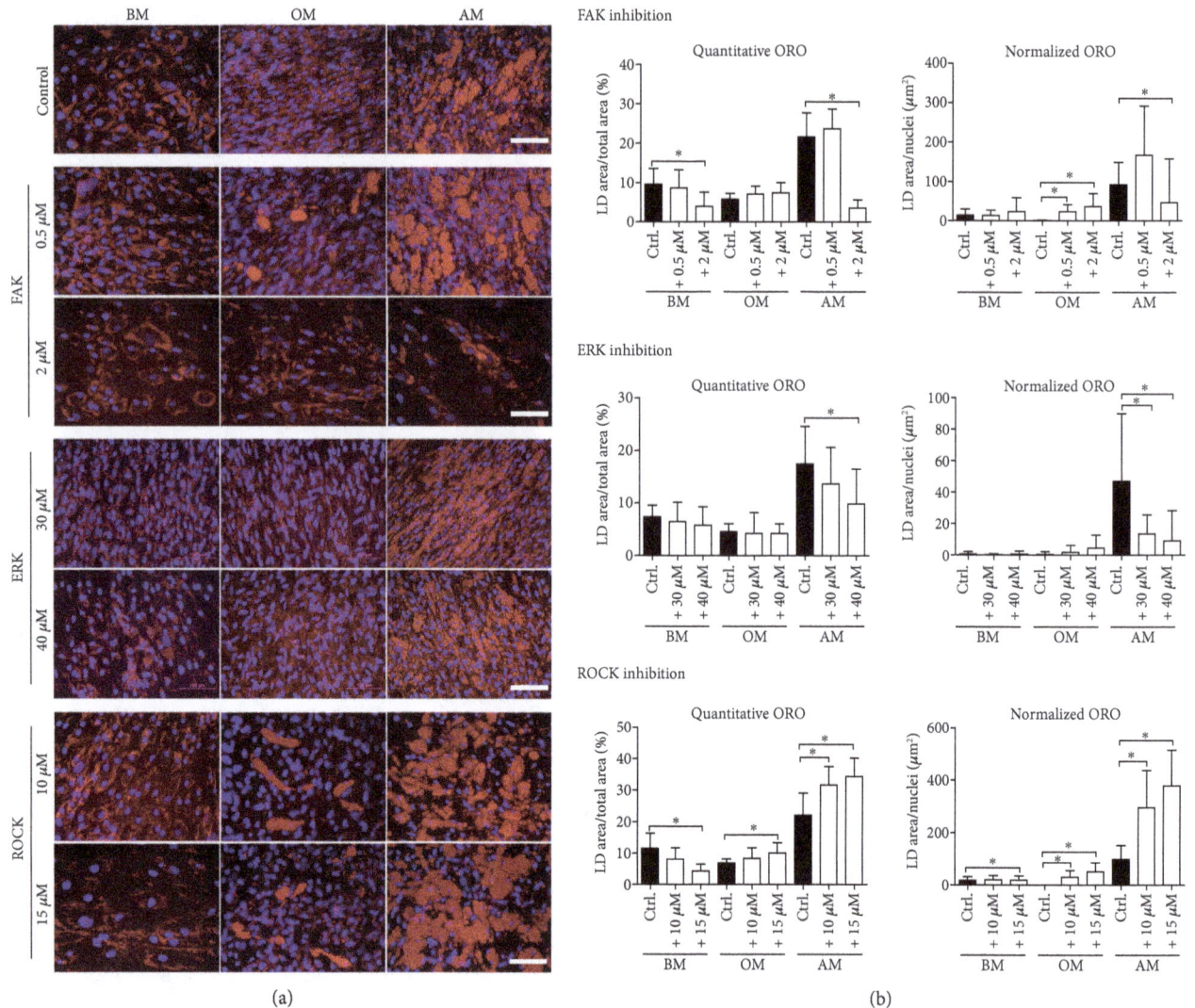

(a)   (b)

FIGURE 5: ORO staining of hASCs and quantification of lipid accumulation from ORO-stained fluorescence images. (a) Representative ORO- and DAPI-stained fluorescence images of FAK, ERK, and ROCK inhibitor-treated hASCs at 21 d. Human ASCs were stained with ORO for intracellular lipid accumulation followed by nuclei staining with DAPI. Fluorescence images were taken with Alexa546 for ORO (red) and DAPI (blue) filters. Scale bars 100 μm. (b) ORO-stained samples of FAK, ERK, and ROCK inhibitor-treated hASCs were imaged with fluorescence microscope using Alexa546 and DAPI filters and analyzed with a custom analysis pipeline designed for CellProfiler. Quantitative ORO graph presents the area of all stained LDs as percentages of the total image area. Normalized ORO graph describes LD formation on the single cell level: the area of LD clusters over 10 μm in diameter is normalized with the corresponding nuclei count. Significance level 5%, designated with an asterisk (*). FAK, ROCK: $N = 13 - 16$ (images from 2 donors), ERK: $N = 19 - 21$ (images from 3 donors). BM: basic medium; OM: osteogenic medium; AM: adipogenic medium; ORO: Oil Red O; LD: lipid droplet.

previous findings suggest that weakening of the adhesion is needed to guide the differentiation towards adipogenic lineage, whereas too robust disruption in the adhesion affects the survival of the cells. Our results support the role of FAK signaling as a central regulator of the differentiation fate of hASCs.

FAK signaling works in cooperation with Rho-ROCK signaling to regulate cytoskeletal dynamics and cell morphology [18, 19]. We found out that both ROCK and FAK inhibition suppresses phospho-MLC2 suggesting that the actin tension is regulated by FAK-ROCK-MLC signaling cascade. Additionally, ROCK inhibition was shown to reduce phospho-FAK levels. Presumably diminished actin tension

by ROCK inhibition affects upstream FA assembly and thus levels of FAK protein activation. These findings indicate a bidirectional regulation between actin assembly and cell adhesion mechanisms in hASCs. In addition to the cooperation of FAK and ROCK signaling, Rho-ROCK pathway itself has been shown to be an important regulator of the balance between osteogenesis and adipogenesis in MSCs [7, 13–15]. In the present study, we found out that the functionality of the ROCK signaling cascade was required in the commitment of hASCs to the osteoblastic lineage since inhibition of ROCK signaling caused a dose-dependent decrease of RUNX2A expression, reduced ALP activity, and hindered the mineral formation. Our results showed that ROCK

(a)

(b)

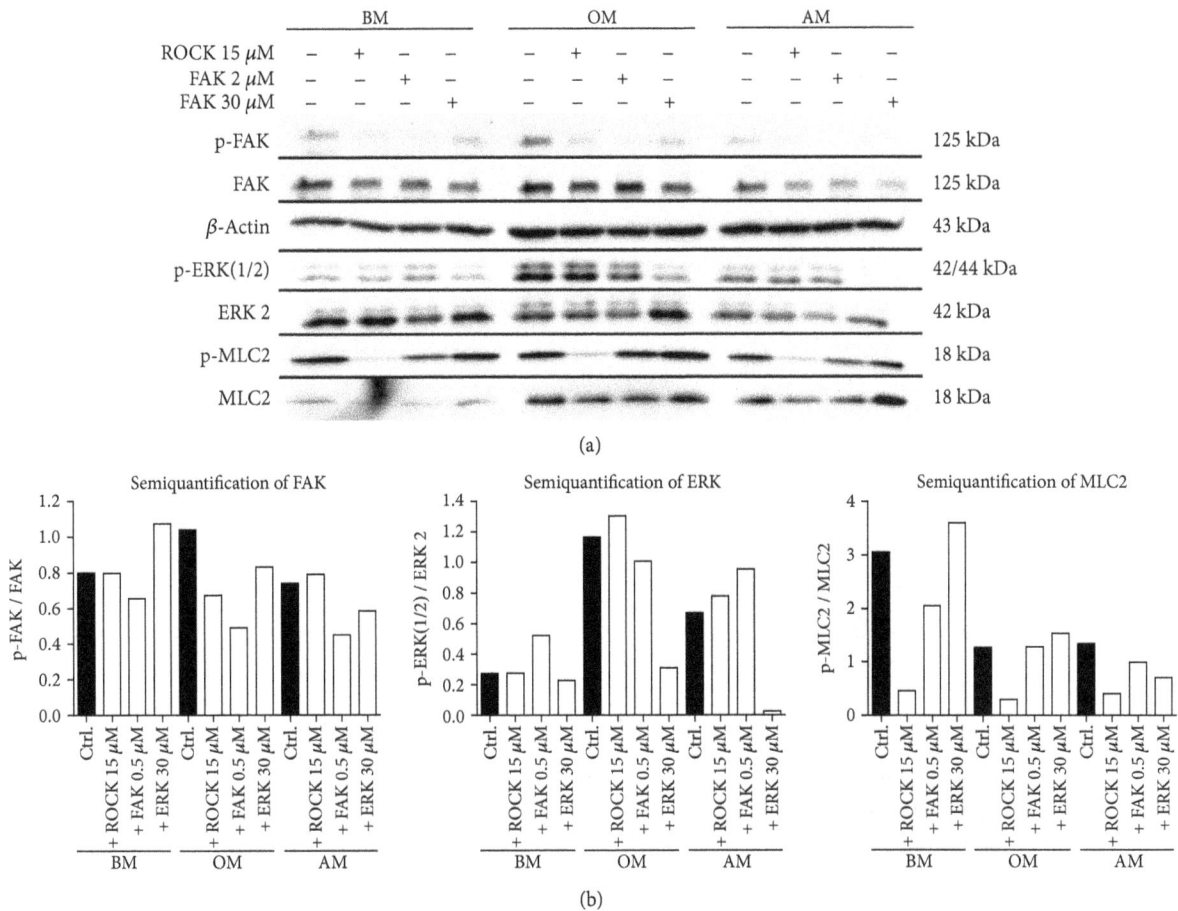

FIGURE 6: Intracellular protein activation at day 7 as a response to FAK, ROCK, and ERK inhibition. hASCs were cultured 7 days in BM, OM, and AM media containing 1% human serum supplemented with 15 μM ROCK inhibitor, 2 μM FAK inhibitor, or 30 μM ERK inhibitor. (a) Representative WB results of immunoblotted p-FAK, FAK, β-actin, p-ERK(1/2), ERK 2, p-MLC2, and MLC2. (b) Semiquantified WB results representing the ratio of phosphorylated and basal form of FAK, ERK, and MLC2 proteins. BM: basic medium; OM: osteogenic medium; AM: adipogenic medium.

inhibition efficiently suppressed the phosphorylation of MLC2, which is involved in actin filament bundling [13]. Thus, hindered actin filament bundling and the disruption of the actomyosin contractility might have led to the observed inhibition of the osteogenesis in our study. Osteogenic differentiation of hMSCs has been demonstrated even without soluble differentiation factors with patterning of the culture platform [7, 45, 46] denoting the importance of the cell shape in the differentiation process. We discovered that the morphology of hASCs was clearly affected by the ROCK inhibitor. Y-27632-treated hASCs appeared spindle-like stellar cells in OM and AM conditions when observed during the culture. These cytoskeletal modifications corresponded to the hindered osteogenic course and likely turned the regulatory switch towards adipogenesis. Indeed, the analysis of the adipogenic gene expression and lipid formation revealed that inhibition of ROCK reciprocally induced substantial adipogenic differentiation in AM but also in the OM condition. These results strongly demonstrate that actin cytoskeleton is an important regulator driving the switch between the osteogenic and adipogenic course of hASC differentiation.

ERK has been suggested to be a mechanosensing protein downstream FAK-Rho-ROCK signaling axis guiding the differentiation fate of hMSCs [23, 24]. In this study, we saw that the inhibition of FAK and ROCK phosphorylation affected phospho-ERK levels suggesting that ERK is regulated in cooperation by the cell adhesion mechanisms and the contractility of the actin cytoskeleton. Interestingly, ERK inhibition also slightly reduced phospho-FAK levels in OM and AM conditions with a currently unknown mechanism. ERK1/2 activity has been linked to the expression of osteogenic markers in hASCs [25] and previous studies have noted that ERK inhibition obstructs osteogenesis in hMSCs [25, 28, 47]. The present study also showed that inhibition of ERK1/2 activation efficiently and dose dependently inhibited the ALP activity and mineral deposition and downregulated RUNX2A expression in OM condition. Additionally, ERK1/2 has been suggested to have a regulatory role on MSC adipogenesis, though it has remained contradictory whether the role is activatory or inhibitory [25–28]. ERK1/2 pathway has been suggested to work as a molecular switch between adipogenic and osteogenic lineage commitment of BMSCs when cultured with osteogenic supplements [28].

On the other hand, a more recent study of Xu and coworkers [23] suggested that ERK1/2 is a positive regulator of the hBMSC adipogenesis. Our results consistently indicated that ERK1/2 activity is required for the full osteogenic but also adipogenic potential of hASCs. Inhibition of ERK activity reduced the expression of adipogenic marker genes and lipid accumulation. To our knowledge, this is the first study where ERK inhibition is shown to diminish hASC adipogenesis in both osteogenic and adipogenic culture conditions. Although the proteins investigated in this study are interconnected, the role of ERK in the hASC differentiation was not parallel with the switch-like regulation of FAK and ROCK pathways. However, the mechanism of ERK signaling in adipogenesis needs to be further studied.

5. Conclusions

This study set out to determine the significance of cell adhesion and cytoskeletal modifications regulated by FAK and ROCK signaling and their downstream target EKR1/2 for adipogenic and osteogenic differentiation potential of hASCs. The results show that ERK1/2 pathway plays a crucial positive role in both osteogenic and adipogenic courses of hASC differentiation, whereas FAK and ROCK work as molecular switches since they function as positive regulators of osteogenesis but negative regulators of adipogenesis. The investigation of these signaling proteins at the molecular level also highlights the interesting interconnection of FAK, ROCK, and ERK1/2 signaling in hASCs and implicates the complex interplay between these crucial regulators of differentiation fate. This study confirms the molecular mechanisms of cell adhesion and actin tension in human ASCs and gives us tools to modify and guide the cell proliferation and differentiation in stem cell-based applications and therapies.

Acknowledgments

The authors thank Ms. Anna-Maija Honkala, Ms. Sari Kalliokoski, and Tampere Imaging Facility, BioMediTech and Faculty of Medicine and Life Sciences, University of Tampere for technical assistance. This study was financially supported by the Competitive State Research Financing of the Expert Responsibility area of Tampere University Hospital, Tekes (The Finnish Funding Agency for Innovation), Academy of Finland, and Jane and Aatos Erkko Foundation. Research funding of Doctoral Programme in Biomedicine and Biotechnology, University of Tampere, and Doctoral Programme of Computing and Electrical Engineering, Tampere University of Technology, are gratefully acknowledged.

Supplementary Materials

Figure S1: quantification of lipid droplets over $10\,\mu m$ in diameter from the ORO-stained fluorescence images. Related to Figure 5(b). Figure S2: intracellular protein activation at day 7 as a response to FAK, ROCK, and ERK inhibition. Related to Figure 6. Table S1: donor information. Information of donor gender, age, and adipose tissue harvest site. Related to Materials and Methods section. Table S2: statistical analysis. Information of donor number, biological replicates, and technical replicates of statistical analyses. Related to Section 2.13. Table S3: surface marker expression. Related to Section 3.1. (*Supplementary Materials*)

References

[1] I. Ullah, R. B. Subbarao, and G. J. Rho, "Human mesenchymal stem cells - current trends and future prospective," *Bioscience Reports*, vol. 35, no. 2, pp. 1–18, 2015.

[2] M. J. Martínez-Lorenzo, M. Royo-Cañas, E. Alegre-Aguarón et al., "Phenotype and chondrogenic differentiation of mesenchymal cells from adipose tissue of different species," *Journal of Orthopaedic Research*, vol. 27, no. 11, pp. 1499–1507, 2009.

[3] A. Scuteri, E. Donzelli, D. Foudah et al., "Mesengenic differentiation: comparison of human and rat bone marrow mesenchymal stem cells," *International Journal of Stem Cells*, vol. 7, no. 2, pp. 127–134, 2014.

[4] G. Ren, J. Su, L. Zhang et al., "Species variation in the mechanisms of mesenchymal stem cell-mediated immunosuppression," *Stem Cells*, vol. 27, no. 8, pp. 1954–1962, 2009.

[5] R. Vishnubalaji, M. al-Nbaheen, B. Kadalmani, A. Aldahmash, and T. Ramesh, "Comparative investigation of the differentiation capability of bone-marrow- and adipose-derived mesenchymal stem cells by qualitative and quantitative analysis," *Cell and Tissue Research*, vol. 347, no. 2, pp. 419–427, 2012.

[6] N. J. Walters and E. Gentleman, "Evolving insights in cell-matrix interactions: elucidating how non-soluble properties of the extracellular niche direct stem cell fate," *Acta Biomaterialia*, vol. 11, pp. 3–16, 2015.

[7] R. McBeath, D. M. Pirone, C. M. Nelson, K. Bhadriraju, and C. S. Chen, "Cell shape, cytoskeletal tension, and RhoA regulate stem cell lineage commitment," *Developmental Cell*, vol. 6, no. 4, pp. 483–495, 2004.

[8] P. S. Mathieu and E. G. Loboa, "Cytoskeletal and focal adhesion influences on mesenchymal stem cell shape, mechanical properties, and differentiation down osteogenic, adipogenic, and chondrogenic pathways," *Tissue Engineering. Part B, Reviews*, vol. 18, no. 6, pp. 436–444, 2012.

[9] E. K. F. Yim and M. P. Sheetz, "Force-dependent cell signaling in stem cell differentiation," *Stem Cell Research & Therapy*, vol. 3, no. 5, p. 41, 2012.

[10] B. Geiger, J. P. Spatz, and A. D. Bershadsky, "Environmental sensing through focal adhesions," *Nature Reviews. Molecular Cell Biology*, vol. 10, no. 1, pp. 21–33, 2009.

[11] K. R. Legate, S. A. Wickstrom, and R. Fassler, "Genetic and cell biological analysis of integrin outside-in signaling," *Genes & Development*, vol. 23, no. 4, pp. 397–418, 2009.

[12] P. Tomakidi, S. Schulz, S. Proksch, W. Weber, and T. Steinberg, "Focal adhesion kinase (FAK) perspectives in mechanobiology: implications for cell behaviour," *Cell and Tissue Research*, vol. 357, no. 3, pp. 515–526, 2014.

[13] K. Riento and A. J. Ridley, "Rocks: multifunctional kinases in cell behaviour," *Nature Reviews Molecular Cell Biology*, vol. 4, no. 6, pp. 446–456, 2003.

[14] R. W. Tilghman and J. T. Parsons, "Focal adhesion kinase as a regulator of cell tension in the progression of cancer," *Seminars in Cancer Biology*, vol. 18, no. 1, pp. 45–52, 2008.

[15] A. V. Schofield, R. Steel, and O. Bernard, "Rho-associated coiled-coil kinase (ROCK) protein controls microtubule dynamics in a novel signaling pathway that regulates cell migration," *The Journal of Biological Chemistry*, vol. 287, no. 52, pp. 43620–43629, 2012.

[16] E. J. Arnsdorf, P. Tummala, R. Y. Kwon, and C. R. Jacobs, "Mechanically induced osteogenic differentiation - the role of RhoA, ROCKII and cytoskeletal dynamics," *Journal of Cell Science*, vol. 122, no. 4, pp. 546–553, 2009.

[17] A. Santos, A. D. Bakker, J. M. A. de Blieck-Hogervorst, and J. Klein-Nulend, "WNT5A induces osteogenic differentiation of human adipose stem cells via rho-associated kinase ROCK," *Cytotherapy*, vol. 12, no. 7, pp. 924–932, 2010.

[18] Y.-R. V. Shih, K. F. Tseng, H. Y. Lai, C. H. Lin, and O. K. Lee, "Matrix stiffness regulation of integrin-mediated mechanotransduction during osteogenic differentiation of human mesenchymal stem cells," *Journal of Bone and Mineral Research*, vol. 26, no. 4, pp. 730–738, 2011.

[19] H. Lv, L. Li, M. Sun et al., "Mechanism of regulation of stem cell differentiation by matrix stiffness," *Stem Cell Research & Therapy*, vol. 6, no. 1, p. 103, 2015.

[20] J. W. Ramos, "The regulation of extracellular signal-regulated kinase (ERK) in mammalian cells," *The International Journal of Biochemistry & Cell Biology*, vol. 40, no. 12, pp. 2707–2719, 2008.

[21] R. M. Salasznyk, R. F. Klees, W. A. Williams, A. Boskey, and G. E. Plopper, "Focal adhesion kinase signaling pathways regulate the osteogenic differentiation of human mesenchymal stem cells," *Experimental Cell Research*, vol. 313, no. 1, pp. 22–37, 2007.

[22] P. Müller, A. Langenbach, A. Kaminski, and J. Rychly, "Modulating the actin cytoskeleton affects mechanically induced signal transduction and differentiation in mesenchymal stem cells," *PLoS One*, vol. 8, no. 7, article e71283, 2013.

[23] B. Xu, Y. Ju, and G. Song, "Role of p38, ERK1/2, focal adhesion kinase, RhoA/ROCK and cytoskeleton in the adipogenesis of human mesenchymal stem cells," *Journal of Bioscience and Bioengineering*, vol. 117, no. 5, pp. 624–631, 2014.

[24] R. Panayiotou, F. Miralles, R. Pawlowski et al., "Phosphorylation acts positively and negatively to regulate MRTF-A subcellular localisation and activity," *eLife*, vol. 5, 2016.

[25] Q. Liu, L. Cen, H. Zhou et al., "The role of the extracellular signal-related kinase signaling pathway in osteogenic differentiation of human adipose-derived stem cells and in adipogenic transition initiated by dexamethasone," *Tissue Engineering. Part A*, vol. 15, no. 11, pp. 3487–3497, 2009.

[26] F. Bost, M. Aouadi, L. Caron et al., "The extracellular signal-regulated kinase isoform ERK1 is specifically required for in vitro and in vivo adipogenesis," *Diabetes*, vol. 54, no. 2, pp. 402–411, 2005.

[27] R. L. Kortum, D. L. Costanzo, J. Haferbier et al., "The molecular scaffold kinase suppressor of Ras 1 (KSR1) regulates adipogenesis," *Molecular and Cellular Biology*, vol. 25, no. 17, pp. 7592–7604, 2005.

[28] R. K. Jaiswal, N. Jaiswal, S. P. Bruder, G. Mbalaviele, D. R. Marshak, and M. F. Pittenger, "Adult human mesenchymal stem cell differentiation to the osteogenic or adipogenic lineage is regulated by mitogen-activated protein kinase," *The Journal of Biological Chemistry*, vol. 275, no. 13, pp. 9645–9652, 2000.

[29] B. Lindroos, S. Boucher, L. Chase et al., "Serum-free, xeno-free culture media maintain the proliferation rate and multipotentiality of adipose stem cells in vitro," *Cytotherapy*, vol. 11, no. 7, pp. 958–972, 2009.

[30] L. Tirkkonen, S. Haimi, S. Huttunen et al., "Osteogenic medium is superior to growth factors in differentiation of human adipose stem cells towards bone-forming cells in 3D culture," *European Cells and Materials*, vol. 25, pp. 144–158, 2013.

[31] M. Ojansivu, S. Vanhatupa, L. Björkvik et al., "Bioactive glass ions as strong enhancers of osteogenic differentiation in human adipose stem cells," *Acta Biomaterialia*, vol. 21, pp. 190–203, 2015.

[32] L. Kamentsky, T. R. Jones, A. Fraser et al., "Improved structure, function and compatibility for CellProfiler: modular high-throughput image analysis software," *Bioinformatics*, vol. 27, no. 8, pp. 1179-1180, 2011.

[33] L. Kyllönen, S. Haimi, B. Mannerström et al., "Effects of different serum conditions on osteogenic differentiation of human adipose stem cells in vitro," *Stem Cell Research & Therapy*, vol. 4, no. 1, p. 17, 2013.

[34] S. Vanhatupa, M. Ojansivu, R. Autio, M. Juntunen, and S. Miettinen, "Bone morphogenetic protein-2 induces donor-dependent osteogenic and adipogenic differentiation in human adipose stem cells," *Stem Cells Translational Medicine*, vol. 4, no. 12, pp. 1391–1402, 2015.

[35] U. Stucki, J. Schmid, C. F. Hammerle, and N. P. Lang, "Temporal and local appearance of alkaline phosphatase activity in early stages of guided bone regeneration. A descriptive histochemical study in humans," *Clinical Oral Implants Research*, vol. 12, no. 2, pp. 121–127, 2001.

[36] B. Galateanu, S. Dinescu, A. Cimpean, A. Dinischiotu, and M. Costache, "Modulation of adipogenic conditions for prospective use of hADSCs in adipose tissue engineering," *International Journal of Molecular Sciences*, vol. 13, no. 12, pp. 15881–15900, 2012.

[37] P. J. Simons, P. S. van den Pangaart, C. P. A. A. van Roomen, J. M. F. G. Aerts, and L. Boon, "Cytokine-mediated modulation of leptin and adiponectin secretion during in vitro adipogenesis: evidence that tumor necrosis factor-α- and interleukin-1β-treated human preadipocytes are potent leptin producers," *Cytokine*, vol. 32, no. 2, pp. 94–103, 2005.

[38] A. Mehlem, C. E. Hagberg, L. Muhl, U. Eriksson, and A. Falkevall, "Imaging of neutral lipids by oil red O for analyzing the metabolic status in health and disease," *Nature Protocols*, vol. 8, no. 6, pp. 1149–1154, 2013.

[39] H. Varinli, M. J. Osmond-McLeod, P. L. Molloy, and P. Vallotton, "LipiD-QuanT: a novel method to quantify lipid accumulation in live cells," *Journal of Lipid Research*, vol. 56, no. 11, pp. 2206–2216, 2015.

[40] C. A. Schneider, W. S. Rasband, and K. W. Eliceiri, "NIH image to ImageJ: 25 years of image analysis," *Nature Methods*, vol. 9, no. 7, pp. 671–675, 2012.

[41] S. Viale-Bouroncle, M. Gosau, and C. Morsczeck, "Laminin regulates the osteogenic differentiation of dental follicle cells via integrin-α2/-β1 and the activation of the FAK/ERK signaling pathway," *Cell and Tissue Research*, vol. 357, no. 1, pp. 345–354, 2014.

[42] J. J. Li and D. Xie, "Cleavage of focal adhesion kinase (FAK) is essential in adipocyte differentiation," *Biochemical and Biophysical Research Communications*, vol. 357, no. 3, pp. 648–654, 2007.

[43] W. Luo, H. Shitaye, M. Friedman et al., "Disruption of cell-matrix interactions by heparin enhances mesenchymal progenitor adipocyte differentiation," *Experimental Cell Research*, vol. 314, no. 18, pp. 3382–3391, 2008.

[44] C. T. Luk, S. Y. Shi, E. P. Cai et al., "FAK signalling controls insulin sensitivity through regulation of adipocyte survival," *Nature Communications*, vol. 8, article 14360, 2017.

[45] M. J. Dalby, N. Gadegaard, R. Tare et al., "The control of human mesenchymal cell differentiation using nanoscale symmetry and disorder," *Nature Materials*, vol. 6, no. 12, pp. 997–1003, 2007.

[46] K. A. Kilian, B. Bugarija, B. T. Lahn, and M. Mrksich, "Geometric cues for directing the differentiation of mesenchymal stem cells," *Proceedings of the National Academy of Sciences of the United States of America*, vol. 107, no. 11, pp. 4872–4877, 2010.

[47] H. Gu, F. Guo, X. Zhou et al., "The stimulation of osteogenic differentiation of human adipose-derived stem cells by ionic products from akermanite dissolution via activation of the ERK pathway," *Biomaterials*, vol. 32, no. 29, pp. 7023–7033, 2011.

Zebularine Promotes Hepatic Differentiation of Rabbit Bone Marrow Mesenchymal Stem Cells by Interfering with p38 MAPK Signaling

Yong-Heng Luo(iD),[1] **Juan Chen**(iD),[1] **En-Hua Xiao**(iD),[1] **Qiu-Yun Li**,[1] and **Yong-Mei Luo**(iD)[2]

[1]*Department of Radiology, Second Xiangya Hospital of Central South University, Changsha, Hunan 410011, China*
[2]*Department of safety & environmental protection, Shenzhen Zhongjin Lingnan Nonfemet Company Ltd, Shenzhen, Guangdong 518040, China*

Correspondence should be addressed to En-Hua Xiao; xiaoenhua64@csu.edu.cn

Academic Editor: Mustapha Najimi

Demethylating agent zebularine is reported to be capable of inducing differentiation of stem cells by activation of methylated genes, though its function in hepatocyte differentiation is unclear. p38 signal pathway is involved in differentiation of hepatocytes and regulating of DNA methyltransferases 1 (DNMT1) expression. However, little is known about the impact of zebularine on bone marrow mesenchymal stem cells (BMMSCs) and p38 signaling during hepatic differentiation. The present study investigated the effects of zebularine on hepatic differentiation of rabbit BMMSCs, as well as the role of p38 on DNMT1 and hepatic differentiation, with the aim of developing a novel strategy for improving derivation of hepatocytes. BMMSCs were treated with zebularine at concentrations of 10, 20, 50, and 100 μM in the presence of hepatocyte growth factor; changes in the levels of hepatic-specific alpha-fetoprotein and albumin were detected and determined by RT-PCR, WB, and immunofluorescence staining. Expression of DNMT1 and phosphorylated p38 as well as urea production and ICG metabolism was also analyzed. Zebularine at concentrations of 10, 20, and 50 μM could not affect cell viability after 48 h. Zebularine treatment leads to an inhibition of DNMT activity and increase of hepatic-specific proteins alpha-fetoprotein and albumin in BMMSCs in vitro; zebularine addition also induced expression of urea production of and ICG metabolism. p38 signal was activated in BMMSCs simulated with HGF; inhibition of p38 facilitated the synthesis of DNMT1 and albumin in cells. Zebularine restrained DNMT1 and phosphorylated p38 which were induced by HGF. Therefore, this study demonstrated that treatment with zebularine exhibited terminal hepatic differentiation of BMMSCs in vitro in association with hepatocyte growth factor; p38 pathway at least partially participates in zebularine-induced hepatic differentiation of rabbit BMMSCs.

1. Introduction

Liver regeneration is critical for graft survival and competent organ function. Bone marrow mesenchymal stem cells (BMMSCs) have immense potential in the field of regenerative medicine for its multilineage potential. BMMSCs, therefore, are increasingly being considered in cell-based therapeutic strategies for liver regeneration. However, their low hepatic differentiation efficiency in vitro is a significant obstacle to hepatocyte transplantation. Current evidence suggests that epigenetic programming plays an important role in stem cell biology by maintaining pluripotency and

promoting stem cell differentiation into more mature cell progenies [1, 2]. A key epigenetic reprogramming mechanism is DNA methylation. DNA methyltransferase inhibitors (DNMTi) initiate differentiation by decreasing the global methylation status of the cells, and therefore, genes are more prone to transcription. Recently, it was shown that DNMTi, such as 5-azacytidine and zebularine, are capable of inducing the differentiation of stem cells [3–6]. Though previous studies have demonstrated that treatment of BMMSCs isolated from different sources with 5-azacytidine resulted in the expression of hepatic-specific proteins in these cells in vitro [6, 7], its use can be limited by its instabilities and toxicities.

Zebularine (1-(β-d-ribofuranosyl)-1, 2-dihydropyrimidin-2-one) is a second-generation hydrophilic inhibitor of DNA methylation [8]. In contrast to 5-azacytidine and other DNMTi, zebularine is quite stable [9] and has low toxicity [10], making it an attractive candidate for liver regeneration. However, to date, no data have been published regarding the course of action of zebularine in liver regeneration. It would be worthwhile to investigate whether treatment of BMMSCs with zebularine can direct them toward specific hepatic lineage.

Hepatocyte growth factor (HGF) played a critical role in the development and regeneration of the liver and induced expression of the hepatic phenotype in mesenchymal stem cells in vitro [11, 12]. Mitogen-activated protein kinases (MAPKs) play important roles in the cellular response to growth factors, cytokines and chemicals, or environmental stress. p38 signal pathway is one of the major MAPK pathways. In addition to inflammation and stress responses, p38 is involved in the control of cell cycle and proliferation [13]. Previous studies have indicated the reciprocal regulation of HGF and activated p38 in cell proliferation [14–16]. Transforming growth factor-β (TGF-β) downregulated activation of HGF precursors and influenced hepatocyte plasticity via p38 signal pathway [15, 17, 18]. Besides that, HGF phosphorylated p38, but p-p38 suppressed the activation of DNA synthesis by HGF, while the p38 inhibitor SB203580 increased HGF-induced DNA synthesis [19]. Taken together, the data presented here highlight the important role that p38 signal pathway plays in the differentiation and proliferation of hepatocytes. However, little is known about the impact of zebularine on HGF-induced hepatic differentiation and p38 activation.

In this study, we investigated the effects of zebularine on DNA methyltransferases 1 (DNMT1) and hepatic differentiation of BMMSCs. Activation of p38 and its role on DNMT1 and hepatic differentiation were also analyzed. The objective is to come up with a novel strategy that would be highly potent in terms of differentiating the BMMSCs into hepatocytes while being least toxic to biological systems.

2. Materials and Methods

2.1. Reagents. We purchased sheep anti-rabbit antibodies of CD29, CD34, CD44, CD45, and fluorescein isothiocyanate-(FITC-) labeled IgG secondary antibody from eBioscience (San Diego, CA). Sheep polyclonal anti-human antibodies to alpha-fetoprotein (AFP), albumin (ALB) and β-actin, and FITC-labeled IgG secondary antibody were obtained from Sigma (St. Louis, MO). Antibodies to DNMT1 and phosphorylated p38 were obtained from Cell Signaling Technology (Beverly, MA). HGF was purchased from Proteintech (Rocky Hill, NJ). Zebularine was purchased from Berry and Associates (Dexter, MI).

The p38 inhibitor SB203580 was obtained from Merck (Germany). A stock solution of SB203580 was prepared in dimethyl sulfoxide (DMSO). SB203580 was diluted in Dulbecco modified Eagle medium (DMEM; Gibco, Rockville, MD) and was added to cell culture 1 h before stimulation with HGF and kept further during the exposure to this compound. A stock solution of zebularine for cellular assays was prepared in DMSO and then diluted in the optimal medium to the final concentrations. Indocyanine green (ICG) was obtained from Aladdin (Shanghai, China).

2.2. Cell Culture. The biological study was approved by the Medicine Human Ethics Committee of the Second Xiangya Hospital of the Central South University. Rabbit bone marrow was obtained from three New Zealand rabbits (male, two-month-old, less than 1 kg in weight) obtained from the Laboratory Animal Unit of the Second Xiangya Hospital of the Central South University. BMMSCs were harvested from expansion culture of cell suspension and were propagated in DMEM supplemented with 10% fetal bovine serum (FBS; Gibco, Rockville, MD), 100 U/ml penicillin, and 100 mg/ml streptomycin. The third to fifth generation of cells were collected for study. BMMSCs were identified by the flow cytometric analysis of CD29, CD34, CD44, and CD45. The experiments were performed at least three times in cell strains from the three rabbits and obtained similar results.

Primary rabbit hepatocytes were isolated from anesthetised rabbits by in situ perfusion of the liver with 0.05% collagenase as previously described [20]. Cell suspensions were seeded in collagen-coated (100 mg) petri dishes at a concentration of 9×10^6 viable cell in a 1:1 (v/v) Ham's F12 and William's E medium. Plates were thereby incubated at 37°C under 5% CO_2 and 95% air. The culture medium was replenished every other day.

2.3. Flow Cytometry. Approximately 1×10^6 cells of the third generation cells were harvested and resuspended in 1 ml phosphate-buffered saline (PBS). Cells were incubated with primary antibodies of CD29 (1:100), CD34 (1:100), CD44 (1:100), CD45 (1:100), and ALB (1:200) for 1 h at 4°C. Subsequently, the cells were washed with PBS for 3 times and incubated with FITC-conjugated secondary sheep antibody (1:200) for 40 min at 4°C.

2.4. Treatment of BMMSCs with Zebularine. Cytotoxicity of zebularine was evaluated by trypan blue exclusion test prior to the experiment. Six concentrations (0, 10, 20, 50, 100, and 200 μM) of zebularine were used for assessment. Zebularine was supplemented to cells to final concentrations and incubated in CO_2 incubator at 37°C. Cell viability was measured after treatment for 48 h. A hemocytometer was used to count the unstained (viable) and the stained (dead) cells. The percentage of cell viability was calculated according to the formula cell viability (%) = (the number of the viable cells/total cells) × 100%.

HGF (60 μg/l) was utilized as the hepatocyte-inducing protocol. BMMSCs were seeded in cell culture flasks and grown to subconfluence. The cells were incubated with zebularine (0, 10, 20, 50, and 100 μM) in the presence of HGF for 24 h at 37°C in a humidified atmosphere containing 5% CO_2. After incubation, the medium was aspirated, and the cells were then washed twice and cultured in medium with HGF. The noninduced BMMSCs and primary rabbit hepatocytes were used as negative or positive controls. The experiments were terminated after 21 days.

2.5. Quantitative Real-Time Polymerase Chain Reaction (RT-PCR). Cells in each group were collected on days 7, 14, and 21. The total RNA was harvested using Trizol according to instructions of the manufacturer (Invitrogen, Carlsbad, CA). After RNA gel electrophoresis, the qualified RNA was subjected to reverse transcription using the PrimeScript RT reagent kit (Takara, Shiga, Japan). Polymerase chain reaction conditions were initial denaturation at 95°C for 10 min, followed by 40 cycles at 95°C for 5 s and 60°C for 30 s. Amplification of the housekeeping gene β-actin mRNA was carried out with forward (CATCCTGCGTCTGGACCTGG) and reverse (TAATGTCACGCACGATTTCC) primers. The forward and reverse primer sequences were CCCTCATCCTC CTGCTACATT and CGGAACAAACTGGGTAAAGGT for AFP, AAGACGTGTGTTGCCGATGA and GCCTTT CAAATGGCAGG for ALB. The comparative threshold cycle (Ct) method was used to determine the relative ratio of expression for each gene.

2.6. Western Blot. Cell proteins were extracted using lysis buffer (20 mM Tris, 150 mM NaCl, 1 mM EDTA, 1% Triton X-100) supplemented with phosphatase inhibitors (1 mM sodium vanadate, 50 mM NaF) and protease inhibitors (0.1% phenylmethylsulfonyl fluoride; Complete protease inhibitor, Roche). After being boiled in Laemmli sample buffer, 10 mg of protein extracts was subjected to SDS-PAGE gel. Next, proteins were transferred to a polyvinylidene difluoride membrane by a Bio-Rad gel-blotting apparatus (Bio-Rad, Hercules, CA, USA). The blots were blocked with 5% nonfat dry milk at room temperature for 1 h and then incubated overnight with the desired primary antibodies at 4°C. After being washed thrice for 10 min each with TBST, peroxidase was detected by chemiluminescence and visualized by exposure to X-ray films (Kodak, USA). Quantification of Western blot products was performed by a laser densitometry (Bio-Rad, USA) and presented as a ratio between optical density of target protein band and β-actin band.

2.7. Immunofluorescence Staining. After being rinsed in PBS, cells cultured on coverslips in each group were fixed in 40 g/l paraformaldehyde, permeabilized by triton X-100, and blocked in phosphate-buffered saline buffer supplemented with 5% bovine serum albumin. Cells were labeled with primary sheep anti-rabbit antibodies against ALB (1 : 100) for 1 h at 4°C. After washing, cells were incubated with FITC-conjugated secondary antibodies for ALB. DAPI was used as a nuclear counterstain. Cells were visualized using a fluorescence microscope (Axio Vert 200, Zeiss, Germany).

2.8. ICG Uptake. ICG was dissolved in 0.01 M PBS to produce a 5 mg/ml stock solution and was diluted in optimal medium to a final concentration of 1 mg/ml. The seeded scaffolds were immersed in the ICG solution and incubated for 30 min at 37°C. After being washed using PBS, the cells were finally examined and imaged microscopically.

2.9. Urea Production. The differentiated BMMSCs were incubated with 1 ml medium containing 5 mM NH4Cl (Sigma) for 24 h at 37°C on days 0, 7, 14, and 21. After incubation, the supernatants were collected and the urea concentrations

were analyzed using a colorimetric assay kit (GBD Corporation, San Diego, CA). The content of urea was presented in terms of pg protein/cell/day.

2.10. Statistical Analysis. All data are presented as means ± SD. Statistical analyses were performed with SPSS 19.0 (Chicago, IL, USA). Comparisons between results from multiple treatment groups were performed using one-way analysis of variance (ANOVA), and LSD test was performed as a post hoc test to show individual differences. Statistical significance was defined as $p < 0.05$.

3. Results

3.1. BMMSC Phenotyping. The BMMSCs are characterized by expression of CD29 but negative for CD45. To address the cell phenotyping, flow cytometry analysis of CD29 and CD45 was performed. The cells showed high expression of CD29 (93.99% ± 3.21%) and CD44 (90.57% ± 3.03%) while there was no obvious expression of CD34 (3.08% ± 1.66%) and CD45 (3.81% ± 1.95%, Figure 1(a)).

3.2. Toxicity of Zebularine on BMMSCs. Cell viability in 200 μM group is lower than that in 0, 10, 20, 50, and 100 μM groups (all $p < 0.05$, Figure 1(b)), which means concentration of 200 μM is toxic to cells. Cell viability in 100 μM group is lower than that in 0 μM group ($p < 0.05$); however, the difference is not significant when compared with control, 10, 20, and 50 μM groups (all $p > 0.05$). There is no significant difference in the cell viability among 0, 10, 20, and 50 μM groups (all $p > 0.05$) and for that reason were not considered as cytotoxic. Therefore, zebularine with concentrations of 0, 10, 20, 50, and 100 μM was used in the subsequent studies.

3.3. Zebularine Induced the Differentiation of BMMSCs into Hepatocytes. AFP, a characteristic marker of hepatocyte during embryonic development and fetal stages, was recruited when hepatic transdifferentiation was studied. Noninduced BMMSCs expressed little AFP mRNA. Treatment with HGF in the absence of zebularine (0 μM) increased the mRNA expression of AFP and reached a peak on day 14 ($p < 0.05$, Figure 2(a)). Pretreatment of zebularine at concentrations of 10 and 20 μM also improved AFP expression on day 7 ($p < 0.05$, respectively), but there is no significant difference between the two concentrations ($p < 0.05$). On day 14, zebularine exhibited significant effect on AFP expression, with the highest expression level in 10 and 20 μM groups, but there is no significant difference between 10 and 20 μM groups ($p > 0.05$). Zebularine did not change the peak time. On day 21, mRNA expression of AFP decreased in all induced groups but still higher than that of noninduced group ($p < 0.05$, respectively), which indicated that induction of AFP persists long after the drug removal.

Differentiation of BMMSCs was also traced up by determining expression for ALB, a typical marker for mature hepatocytes. The mRNA expression of ALB increased on day 14 and reached a peak on day 21 in the 0 μM group ($p < 0.05$, Figure 2(b)). Zebularine induced upregulation of ALB mRNA in a dose-dependent manner. Pretreatment with

(a)

(b)

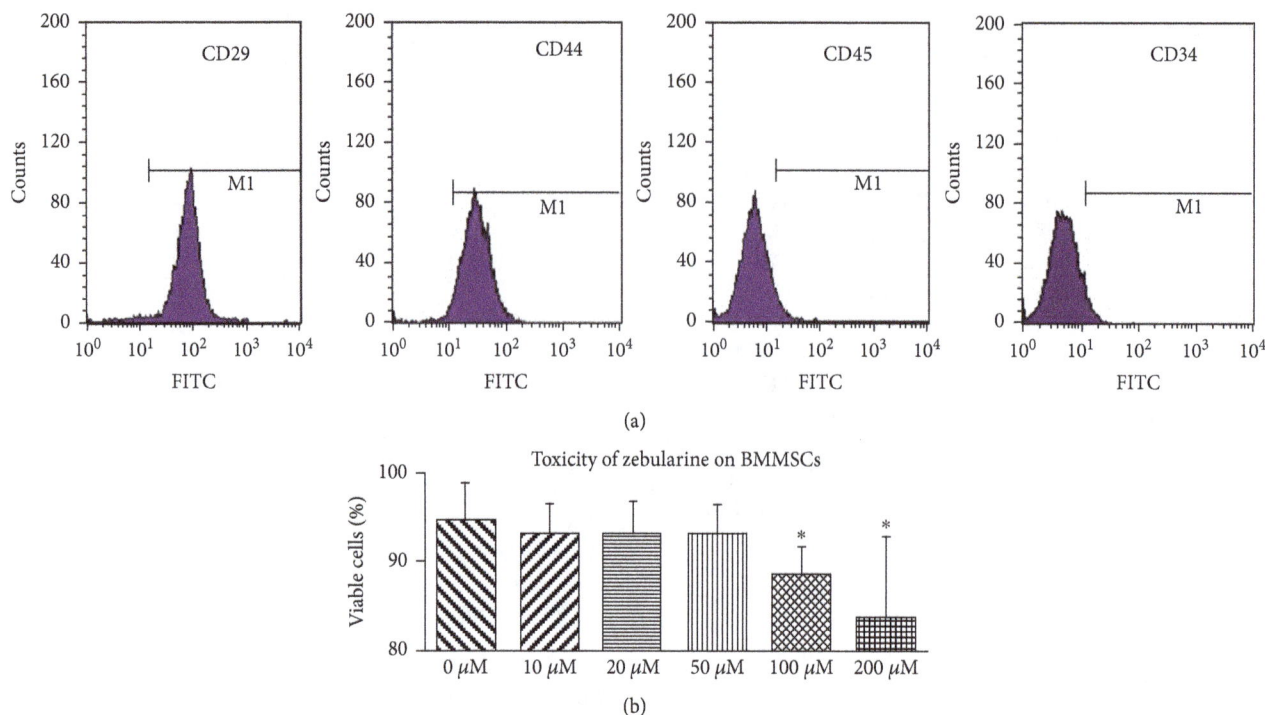

FIGURE 1: Positive expression rates of BMMSC surface marker antigens CD29, CD44, CD45, and CD34 and toxicity of zebularine on BMMSCs. Asterisk indicates $p < 0.05$ compared with the $0\,\mu$M group.

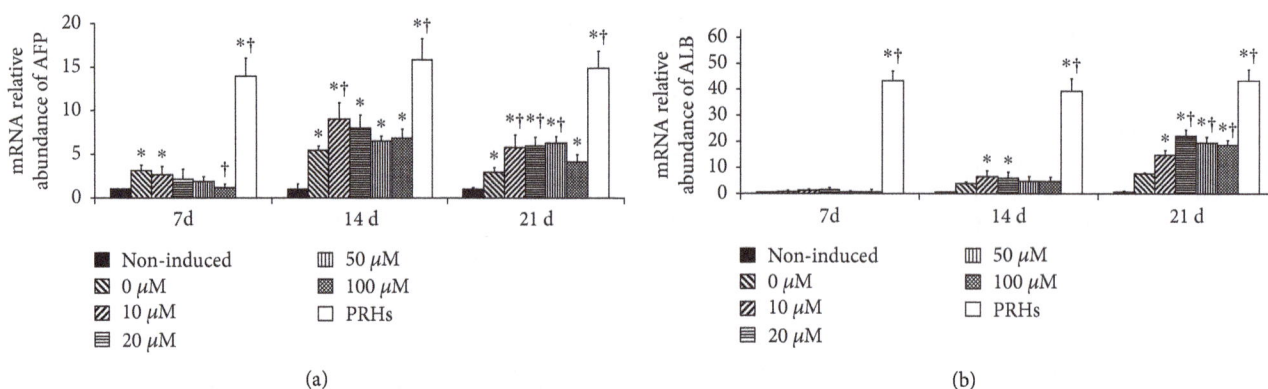

(a)

(b)

FIGURE 2: Zebularine promoted the mRNA expression of AFP and ALB. Noninduced BMMSCs and primary rabbit hepatocytes (PRHs) were used as negative or positive controls. (a) On day 7, noninduced BMMSCs expressed little AFP; increased AFP mRNA expression was observed in 0 and 10 μM groups. On day 14, zebularine exhibited significant effect on AFP expression, with the highest expression level in 10 and 20 μM groups. (b) Noninduced BMMSCs expressed little ALB. The mRNA levels of ALB started to increase at 14 days after pretreatment of zebularine at concentrations of 10 and 20 μM. Exposure to zebularine exhibited significant effect on ALB expression after 21 days, with the highest expression level in the 20 μM group. Asterisk indicates $p < 0.05$ compared with the control group; dagger indicates $p < 0.05$ compared with the $0\,\mu$M (HGF) group.

different doses of zebularine did not improve ALB expression on day 7 ($p > 0.05$, respectively). The mRNA levels of ALB started to increase at 14 days after stimulation of zebularine at concentrations of 10 and 20 μM ($p < 0.05$, respectively). Exposure to zebularine exhibited significant effect on ALB expression after 21 days. With a decreased AFP expression and an increased ALB expression, BMMSCs were inclined to differentiate into mature hepatocyte-like cells. There were higher levels of AFP in 20, 50, and 100 μM groups compared with that in the $0\,\mu$M (HGF only) group (all $p < 0.05$), with the

highest level in the 20 μM group. Therefore, zebularine at a concentration of 20 μM was used in subsequent experiments.

To further quantify the effects of zebularine on ALB expression, Western blot assays were performed. Noninduced BMMSCs expressed little ALB. The protein expression of ALB increased on day 14 and reached a peak on day 21 in the $0\,\mu$M (HGF only) group ($p < 0.05$, Figure 3(a)). Zebularine at 20 μM clearly reinforced the HGF-induced upregulation of ALB protein expression ($p < 0.05$). Furthermore, the peak of expression of ALB

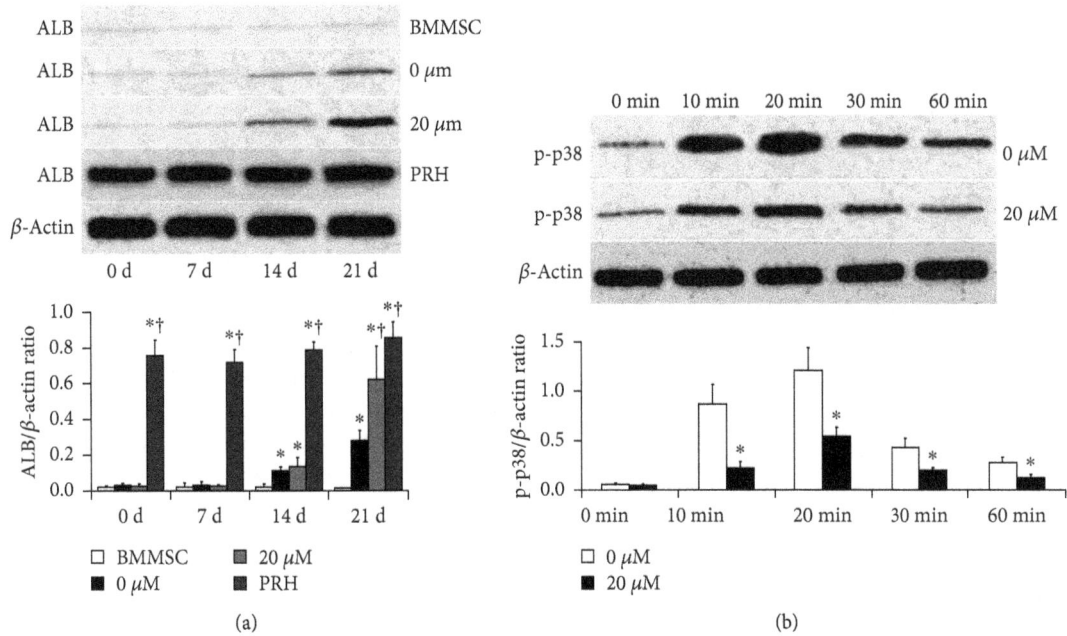

FIGURE 3: Zebularine promoted protein expression of ALB in BMMSCs and attenuated activation of the p38 signal pathway induced by HGF. (a) The protein expression of ALB increased on day 14 and reached a peak on day 21 in the $0\,\mu$M (HGF only) group. Zebularine at $20\,\mu$M clearly reinforced the HGF-induced upregulation of ALB protein expression. However, the peak of expression of ALB in both 0 and $20\,\mu$M groups was lower than that in primary rabbit hepatocytes. (b) HGF ($0\,\mu$M group) increased the expression of phosphorylated p38 in cultured BMMSCs. However, addition of zebularine ($20\,\mu$M group) significantly suppressed p38 pathway activation in the cells stimulated with HGF. Asterisk indicates $p < 0.05$ compared with min 0; dagger indicates $p < 0.05$ compared with HGF ($0\,\mu$M group).

in the $20\,\mu$M group (zebularine + HGF) was higher than that in the $0\,\mu$M (HGF only) group ($p < 0.05$) on day 21, which followed the same trend with mRNA expression. However, the peak of expression of ALB in both 0 and $20\,\mu$M groups was lower than that in primary rabbit hepatocytes (both $p < 0.05$).

3.4. Zebularine Inhibited Activation of the p38 Pathway in BMMSCs.
To address the involvement of p38 in hepatic differentiation, phospho-specific antibody for the activated form of p38 was used in Western blot analyses of cell lysates. BMMSCs were stimulated with zebularine and/or HGF; the p-p38 level was measured at various time points from 0 to 60 min. HGF increased the expression of phosphorylated p38 in cultured BMMSCs. However, addition of zebularine significantly suppressed p38 pathway activation in the cells stimulated with HGF ($p < 0.05$, Figure 3(b)).

3.5. Zebularine and p38 Specific Inhibitor SB203580 Inhibited Expression of DNMT1.
Cells were treated with zebularine, SB203580, and zebularine + SB203580 in the presence of HGF. Expression level of DNMT1 protein was also measured via Western blot (Figure 4). HGF increased the expression of DNMT1 ($p < 0.05$). HGF-induced upregulation of DNMT1 was inhibited by zebularine and SB203580 (both $p < 0.05$). Zebularine had a stronger effect on DNMT1 than SB203580 did ($p < 0.05$), though the difference between zebularine and zebularine + SB203580 groups was not significant ($p > 0.05$). DNMT1 level was similar in noninduced BMMSCs and primary rabbit hepatocytes ($p > 0.05$).

We also found that ALB protein expression was upregulated by SB203580 ($p < 0.05$, Figure 4), while the strengthening effect of SB203580 on cell differentiation was weaker than that of zebularine ($p < 0.05$). However, the difference between zebularine and zebularine + SB203580 groups was not significant ($p < 0.05$). Furthermore, the peak of expression of ALB in the induced groups was lower than that in primary rabbit hepatocytes (all $p < 0.05$). Similar results were found on immunofluorescence microscopic evaluation of ALB expression (Figure 5).

3.6. ICG Metabolism and Urea Production.
Cellular uptake and releasing of ICG, which determines the liver-specific metabolic function, were used to identify differentiated hepatocytes in vitro. Induced cells were positive for ICG after incubation in ICG solution for 30 min (Figure 6(a)). ICG in the differentiated cells was released after 6 h (Figure 6(b)). In addition, urea production was investigated. Zebularine treatment induced urea production in the cells on days 14 and 21 (Figure 6(c), both $p < 0.05$). However, urea production in cells in induced groups was lower than that in primary rabbit hepatocytes (all $p > 0.05$).

4. Discussion

Though hepatocyte transplantation is considered to be an alternative to orthotopic liver transplantation, the shortage of donor cells for hepatocyte transplantation has not been resolved. Therefore, the derivation of hepatocytes from stem cells is of value in the creation of an unlimited source of

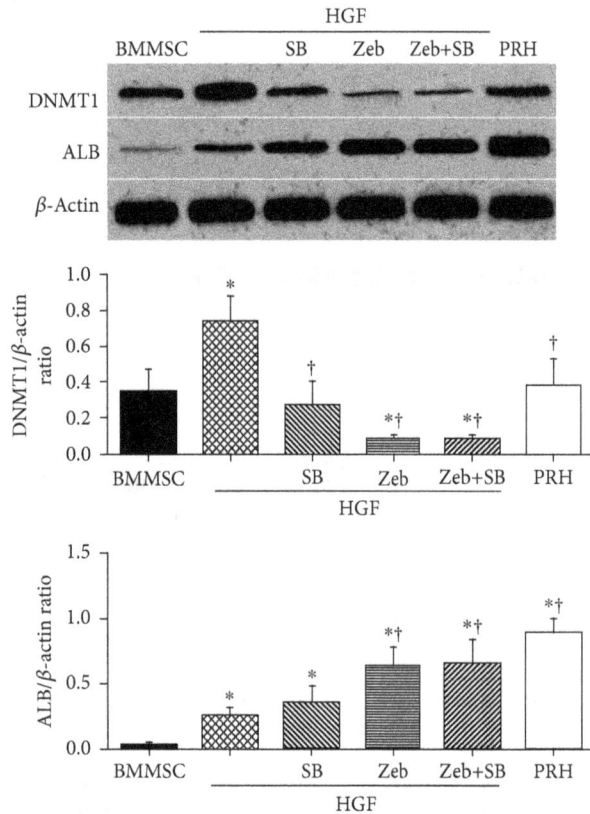

FIGURE 4: Zebularine and SB203580 inhibited expression of DNMT1 and upregulated expression of ALB in BMMSCs. Noninduced BMMSCs and primary rabbit hepatocytes (PRH) were used as negative or positive controls. HGF increased the expression of DNMT1. HGF-induced expression of DNMT1 was inhibited by zebularine and SB203580. ALB protein expression was regulated by SB203580 and zebularine. The peak of expression of ALB in the induced groups was lower than that in primary rabbit hepatocytes. Asterisk indicates $p < 0.05$ compared with the control group; dagger indicates $p < 0.05$ compared with the HGF group.

donor cells for hepatocyte transplantation therapy. Nowadays, autologous BMMSCs have been widely applied in the liver repair, but its efficacy is often limited by the low transdifferentiation rate [21–23]. Cytokines, including HGF, epidermal growth factor (EGF), and vascular endothelial growth factor (VEGF) 165 [11], have been shown to induce hepatic differentiation of BMMSCs, though their application is limited by short half-life in vivo and hemodynamic abnormalities and potentially severe side effects when used in large doses.

By activation of methylated genes in stem cells, DNMTi serve as prime candidates for cellular differentiation agents. The effect of zebularine on inhibiting DNA methylation was demonstrated in mammalian stem cell lines [24, 25]. However, a number of studies have investigated the effect of zebularine on hepatic tumors and cardiomyocyte differentiation. It has been reported that zebularine inhibits liver tumor cell proliferation, induces apoptosis, and promotes their maturation and differentiation in a concentration-, time-, and dose-dependent manner [26, 27]. In another study, it has been demonstrated that different doses of

zebularine have opposite roles in immunogenicity [28]. In the present study, low concentrations of zebularine could not affect cell viability. When concentration of zebularine increased, the cell viability decreased. This phenomenon may be due to higher doses of zebularine mediating cell cytotoxicity by embedding into DNA and RNA and directly inhibiting cell proliferation. Meanwhile, lower doses of zebularine primarily inhibit DNA methylation, resulting in the recovery of gene normal expression. We could detect a decrease of DNMT1 in BMMSCs by using zebularine. More interestingly, inhibition of DNMT activity by zebularine treatment leads to an increase of AFP and ALB in rabbit cells and therefore support the hepatic differentiation. These data were supported by immunostaining. To the best of our knowledge, this is the first report to show that zebularine leads to remarkable increment in hepatic differentiation of BMMSCs. Also, we observed that zebularine addition induced expression of urea production of and ICG metabolism in our cells, suggesting that zebularine-treated cells possess hepatic-like functionality.

Previous studies have demonstrated that treatment of BMMSCs by zebularine resulted in the expression of cardiac-specific proteins in vitro [29], suggesting that DNA methylation is not the only factor that determines gene expression during cell differentiation process; appropriate microenvironment and the induced culture conditions also have effects on the cell differentiation process. Anyway, combination of zebularine and cell factors is a better method than that of only growth factor supplement for higher transdifferentiation rate, and zebularine could be used as a new method or it can be used in combination with other systems to enhance hepatic differentiation.

The balance between proliferation and differentiation as well as between apoptosis and cell survival is required for DNMTi to promote liver regeneration. Indeed, inhibited HGF signaling, disrupted hepatocyte proliferation, and hepatocyte apoptosis increased the susceptibility of the liver to failure [30]. In hepatic failure and acute liver injury, increased blood HGF level plays an important functional role in liver regeneration but also induces expression of TGF-β family [30], which induces apoptosis during fibrogenesis and provides growth control in regeneration processes. Expression of p38 signal was required for TGF-β-induced hepatocyte apoptosis. Previous studies have indicated the reciprocal regulation of HGF and p38 MAPK [16, 19, 31]. In this study, the p38 signal was activated in BMMSCs simulated with HGF; the time to peak is 20 min, which is similar to the finding in human BMMSCs [32]. These results suggest that p38 could be involved in the transformation of BMMSCs from different species.

p38 is also involved in regulating of DNMT expression, though its role is often controversial in different cell types and in different laboratories. For example, reports revealed that phosphorylated p38 induces toxic injuries through mediating DNMT1, DNMT3a, and DNMT3b expressions [33, 34], while others documented that activated p38 represses the induction of DNMT1 [35, 36]. In our study, inhibition of p38 by SB203580 significantly decreased the expression of DNMT1. Here, we used SB203580 to determine

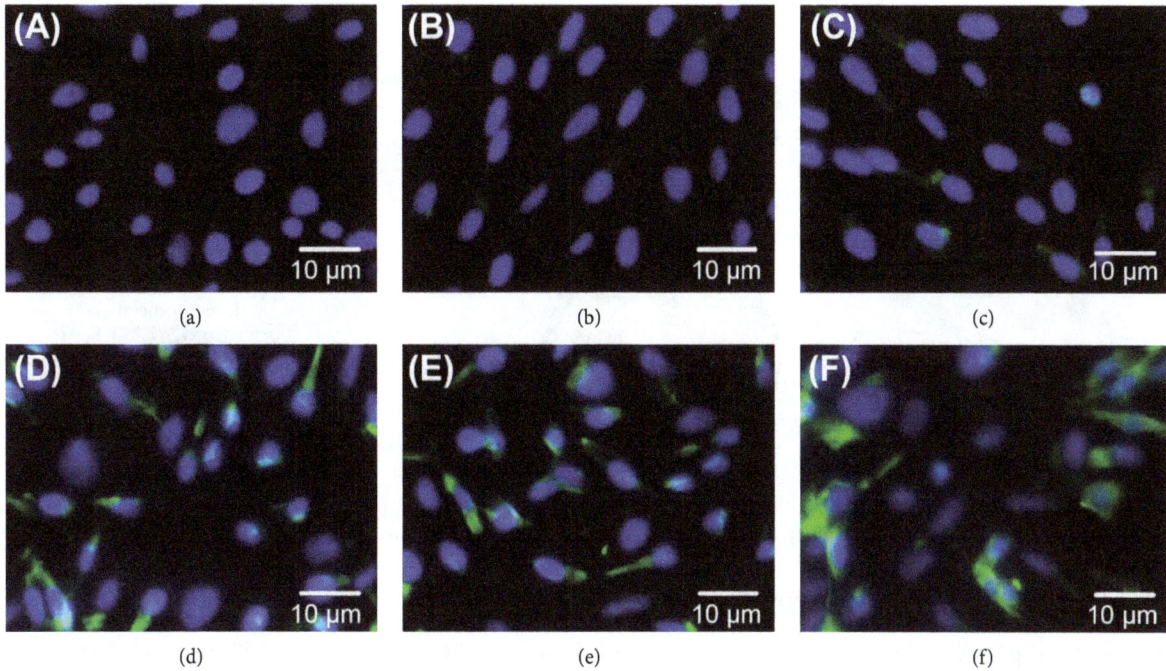

(a) (b) (c)

(d) (e) (f)

FIGURE 5: Recruitment of ALB in the cytoplasm of BMMSCs on the 21st day. (a) Noninduced BMMSCs, (b) HGF, (c) HGF + SB203580, (d) HGF + zebularine, (e) HGF + zebularine + SB203580, and (f) primary rabbit hepatocytes. Cells analyzed by immunofluorescence with ALB (green) as a hepatocyte marker and DAPI to stain nuclear (blue). There were (18.67 ± 6.19)%, (26.71 ± 7.31)%, (70.04 ± 6.09)%, (71.82 ± 5.67)%, and (89.36 ± 5.38)% positive cells in HGF, HGF + SB203580, HGF + zebularine, HGF + zebularine + SB203580, and primary rabbit hepatocyte groups, respectively.

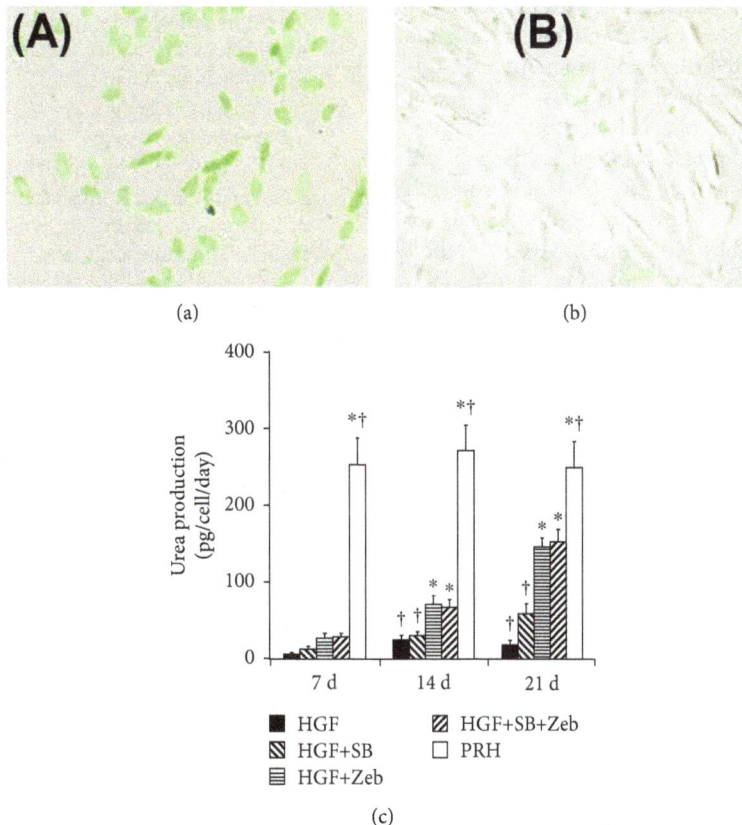

(a) (b)

(c)

FIGURE 6: ICG metabolism and urea production. BMMSC-derived cells were positive for ICG after incubation in ICG solution for 30 min (a). ICG in the differentiated cells was released after 6 h (b). Zebularine treatment induced urea production in the cells (c). Asterisk indicates $p < 0.05$ compared with the HGF group; dagger indicates $p < 0.05$ compared with the zebularine group.

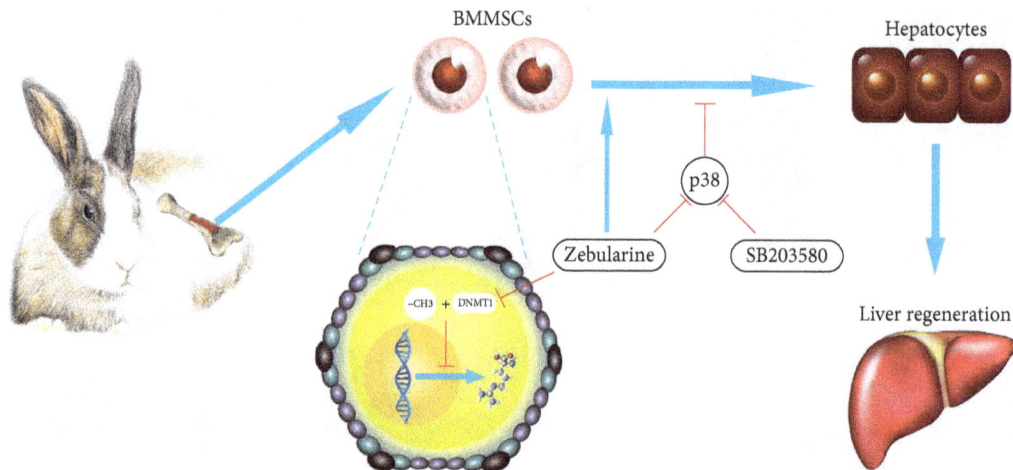

FIGURE 7: Graphical abstract. The increase in the level of DNMT1 and phosphorylated p38 in BMMSCs was restrained by zebularine. Zebularine leads to remarkable increment in hepatic differentiation of BMMSCs, partly through regulation of HGF-induced p38 activation.

the specificity of the p38 signaling pathway in mediating hepatic differentiation of BMMSCs. We found that SB203580 inhibited p38 phosphorylation and expression of hepatic-specific proteins induced by HGF, with a weaker force than zebularine. These data demonstrated that the p38 pathway at least partially participates in zebularine-induced hepatic differentiation of rabbit BMMSCs (Figure 7).

There are several questions that remain unanswered. For instance, the maturation degree and substitution function of hepatocyte-like cells from BMMSCs still fell short of primary rabbit hepatocytes. The concentration and induction time needs further improvement in order to obtain better transdifferentiation rate. Besides, we used BMMSCs from rabbit in vitro to explore the potential of zebularine as the differentiation inducer; potential response between zebularine and cells in vivo has not been investigated. Our next research interests may involve the therapeutic potential of hepatocyte-like cells induced by zebularine in vivo in a rabbit model of liver injury, as well as induction of BMMSCs derived from human. Further studies are needed to investigate how zebularine restrains p38 and the detailed interactions between its downstream targets.

In conclusion, we demonstrated that zebularine significantly increases the expression of hepatic-associated marker proteins in BMMSCs and enhances the urea production and ICG metabolic function of these cells. Zebularine exerts its demethylating effect through inhibition of DNNT1, partially by interfering with p38 MAPK signaling. The results obtained from this study would serve as an attempt in the therapeutic march to enhance regeneration of injured liver.

Acknowledgments

This study was supported by the National Nature Science Foundation of China (nos. 81571784, 30870695), the Foundation of Hunan Province and Technology Department, China (no. 2015SF2020-4), and the Foundation of Hunan Provincial Development and Reform Commission, China (no. 201583).

References

[1] M. S. Roost, R. C. Slieker, M. Bialecka et al., "DNA methylation and transcriptional trajectories during human development and reprogramming of isogenic pluripotent stem cells," *Nature Communications*, vol. 8, no. 1, p. 908, 2017.

[2] I. Mortada and R. Mortada, "Epigenetic changes in mesenchymal stem cells differentiation," *European Journal of Medical Genetics*, vol. 61, no. 2, pp. 114–118, 2018.

[3] J. K. Christman, "5-Azacytidine and 5-aza-2′-deoxycytidine as inhibitors of DNA methylation: mechanistic studies and their implications for cancer therapy," *Oncogene*, vol. 21, no. 35, pp. 5483–5495, 2002.

[4] C. B. Yoo, J. C. Cheng, and P. A. Jones, "Zebularine: a new drug for epigenetic therapy," *Biochemical Society Transactions*, vol. 32, no. 6, pp. 910–912, 2004.

[5] S. Ehnert, C. Eipel, K. Abshagen et al., "Hepatic differentiation of adipose-derived mesenchymal stem cells reduces recruitment of immune cells after transplantation into livers of CCl4 treated mice," *Zeitschrift für Gastroenterologie*, vol. 49, no. 1, 2011.

[6] Y. He, J. Cui, T. He, and Y. Bi, "5-Azacytidine promotes terminal differentiation of hepatic progenitor cells," *Molecular Medicine Reports*, vol. 12, no. 2, pp. 2872–2878, 2015.

[7] C. Seeliger, M. Culmes, L. Schyschka et al., "Decrease of global methylation improves significantly hepatic differentiation of Ad-MSCs: possible future application for urea detoxification," *Cell Transplantation*, vol. 22, no. 1, pp. 119–131, 2013.

[8] J. B. Andersen, V. M. Factor, J. U. Marquardt et al., "An integrated genomic and epigenomic approach predicts therapeutic response to zebularine in human liver cancer," *Science Translational Medicine*, vol. 2, no. 54, article 54ra77, 2010.

[9] H. Dock, A. Theodorsson, and E. Theodorsson, "DNA methylation inhibitor zebularine confers stroke protection in ischemic rats," *Translational Stroke Research*, vol. 6, no. 4, pp. 296–300, 2015.

[10] D. Neureiter, S. Zopf, T. Leu et al., "Apoptosis, proliferation and differentiation patterns are influenced by zebularine and SAHA in pancreatic cancer models," *Scandinavian Journal of Gastroenterology*, vol. 42, no. 1, pp. 103–116, 2007.

[11] Y. Tan, E.-h. Xiao, L.-z. Xiao et al., "VEGF165 expressing bone marrow mesenchymal stem cells differentiate into hepatocytes

under HGF and EGF induction in vitro," *Cytotechnology*, vol. 64, no. 6, pp. 635–647, 2012.

[12] J. S. Ye, X. S. Su, J. F. Stoltz, N. de Isla, and L. Zhang, "Signalling pathways involved in the process of mesenchymal stem cells differentiating into hepatocytes," *Cell Proliferation*, vol. 48, no. 2, pp. 157–165, 2015.

[13] Y.-H. Luo, P.-B. Ouyang, J. Tian, X.-J. Guo, and X.-C. Duan, "Rosiglitazone inhibits TGF-β 1 induced activation of human Tenon fibroblasts via p38 signal pathway," *PLoS One*, vol. 9, no. 8, article e105796, 2014.

[14] K.-W. Goh and Y.-H. Say, "γ-Synuclein confers both pro-invasive and doxorubicin-mediated pro-apoptotic properties to the colon adenocarcinoma LS 174T cell line," *Tumor Biology*, vol. 36, no. 10, pp. 7947–7960, 2015.

[15] Y. Yu, J. Duan, Y. Li et al., "Silica nanoparticles induce liver fibrosis via TGF-β_1/Smad3 pathway in ICR mice," *International Journal of Nanomedicine*, vol. 12, pp. 6045–6057, 2017.

[16] W. Kuang, Q. Deng, C. Deng, W. Li, S. Shu, and M. Zhou, "Hepatocyte growth factor induces breast cancer cell invasion via the PI3K/Akt and p 38 MAPK signaling pathways to up-regulate the expression of COX2," *American Journal of Translational Research*, vol. 9, no. 8, pp. 3816–3826, 2017.

[17] A. Kaimori, J. Potter, J. Y. Kaimori, C. Wang, E. Mezey, and A. Koteish, "Transforming growth factor-β1 induces an epithelial-to-mesenchymal transition state in mouse hepatocytes in vitro," *Journal of Biological Chemistry*, vol. 282, no. 30, pp. 22089–22101, 2007.

[18] D. Black, S. Lyman, T. Qian et al., "Transforming growth factor beta mediates hepatocyte apoptosis through Smad 3 generation of reactive oxygen species," *Biochimie*, vol. 89, no. 12, pp. 1464–1473, 2007.

[19] M. Aasrum, I. J. Brusevold, T. Christoffersen, and G. H. Thoresen, "HGF-induced DNA synthesis in hepatocytes is suppressed by p 38," *Growth Factors*, vol. 34, no. 5-6, pp. 217–223, 2016.

[20] M. Daujat, L. Pichard, C. Dalet et al., "Expression of five forms of microsomal cytochrome P^{-450} in primary cultures of rabbit hepatocytes treated with various classes of inducers," *Biochemical Pharmacology*, vol. 36, no. 21, pp. 3597–3606, 1987.

[21] P. C. Lin, T. W. Chiou, Z. S. Lin et al., "A proposed novel stem cell therapy protocol for liver cirrhosis," *Cell Transplantation*, vol. 24, no. 3, pp. 533–540, 2015.

[22] G. Kim, Y. W. Eom, S. K. Baik et al., "Therapeutic effects of mesenchymal stem cells for patients with chronic liver diseases: systematic review and meta-analysis," *Journal of Korean Medical Science*, vol. 30, no. 10, pp. 1405–1415, 2015.

[23] Z. Shan, Y. Hirai, M. Nakayama et al., "Therapeutic effect of autologous compact bone-derived mesenchymal stem cell transplantation on prion disease," *Journal of General Virology*, vol. 98, no. 10, pp. 2615–2627, 2017.

[24] H. Ruan, S. Qiu, B. C. Beard, and M. E. Black, "Creation of zebularine-resistant human cytidine deaminase mutants to enhance the chemoprotection of hematopoietic stem cells," *Protein Engineering Design and Selection*, vol. 29, no. 12, pp. 573–582, 2016.

[25] L. Zhou, X. Dong, L. Wang et al., "Casticin attenuates liver fibrosis and hepatic stellate cell activation by blocking TGF-β/Smad signaling pathway," *Oncotarget*, vol. 8, no. 34, pp. 56267–56280, 2017.

[26] K. Nakamura, K. Aizawa, K. H. Aung, J. Yamauchi, and A. Tanoue, "Zebularine upregulates expression of CYP genes through inhibition of DNMT1 and PKR in HepG2 cells," *Scientific Reports*, vol. 7, no. 1, article 41093, 2017.

[27] G. Mohan, A. A. Shamsuddin, D. Hasan Adli et al., "Promoting effect of small molecules in cardiomyogenic and neurogenic differentiation of rat bone marrow-derived mesenchymal stem cells," *Drug Design Development and Therapy*, vol. 10, no. 1, pp. 81–91, 2015.

[28] M. Fardi, S. Solali, and M. Farshdousti Hagh, "Epigenetic mechanisms as a new approach in cancer treatment: an updated review," *Genes & Diseases*, 2018.

[29] R. Khanabdali, A. Saadat, M. Fazilah et al., "Promoting effect of small molecules in cardiomyogenic and neurogenic differentiation of rat bone marrow-derived mesenchymal stem cells," *Drug Design, Development and Therapy*, vol. 10, pp. 81–91, 2016.

[30] W. M. Lee, R. H. Squires Jr, S. L. Nyberg, E. Doo, and J. H. Hoofnagle, "Acute liver failure: summary of a workshop," *Hepatology*, vol. 47, no. 4, pp. 1401–1415, 2008.

[31] S. S. Dykes, J. J. Steffan, and J. A. Cardelli, "Lysosome trafficking is necessary for EGF-driven invasion and is regulated by p38 MAPK and Na+/H+ exchangers," *BMC Cancer*, vol. 17, no. 1, p. 672, 2017.

[32] K. K. Aenlle, K. M. Curtis, B. A. Roos, and G. A. Howard, "Hepatocyte growth factor and p38 promote osteogenic differentiation of human mesenchymal stem cells," *Molecular Endocrinology*, vol. 28, no. 5, pp. 722–730, 2014.

[33] M. Arechederra, N. Priego, A. Vázquez-Carballo et al., "p38 MAPK down-regulates fibulin 3 expression through methylation of gene regulatory sequences: role in migration and invasion," *The Journal of Biological Chemistry*, vol. 290, no. 7, pp. 4383–4397, 2015.

[34] C. M. Liu, J. Q. Ma, W. R. Xie et al., "Quercetin protects mouse liver against nickel-induced DNA methylation and inflammation associated with the Nrf 2/HO-1 and p 38/STAT1/NF-κB pathway," *Food and Chemical Toxicology*, vol. 82, pp. 19–26, 2015.

[35] C. Li, P. J. R. Ebert, and Q. J. Li, "T cell receptor (TCR) and transforming growth factor β (TGF-β) signaling converge on DNA (cytosine-5)-methyltransferase to control forkhead box protein 3 (foxp 3) locus methylation and inducible regulatory T cell differentiation," *Journal of Biological Chemistry*, vol. 288, no. 26, pp. 19127–19139, 2013.

[36] Q. Xi, N. Gao, Y. Yang et al., "Anticancer drugs induce hypomethylation of the acetylcholinesterase promoter via a phosphorylated-p 38-DNMT1-AChE pathway in apoptotic hepatocellular carcinoma cells," *The International Journal of Biochemistry & Cell Biology*, vol. 68, pp. 21–32, 2015.

Intraparenchymal Neural Stem/Progenitor Cell Transplantation for Ischemic Stroke Animals

Hailong Huang ⓘ,[1] Kun Qian,[2] Xiaohua Han ⓘ,[1] Xin Li,[1] Yifeng Zheng,[3] Zhishui Chen,[4,5,6] Xiaolin Huang ⓘ,[1] and Hong Chen ⓘ[1]

[1]*Department of Rehabilitation Medicine, Tongji Hospital, Tongji Medical College, Huazhong University of Science and Technology, Wuhan 430030, China*
[2]*Department of Reproductive Medicine, Tongji Hospital, Tongji Medical College, Huazhong University of Science and Technology, Wuhan 430030, China*
[3]*Department of Neurosurgery, Tongji Hospital, Tongji Medical College, Huazhong University of Science and Technology, Wuhan 430030, China*
[4]*Institute of Organ Transplantation, Key Laboratory of the Ministry of Health and the Ministry of Education, Tongji Hospital, Tongji Medical College, Huazhong University of Science and Technology, Wuhan 430030, China*
[5]*Key Laboratory of Organ Transplantation, Ministry of Education, Wuhan 430030, China*
[6]*Key Laboratory of Organ Transplantation, Ministry of Health, Wuhan 430030, China*

Correspondence should be addressed to Xiaolin Huang; xiaolinh2006@126.com and Hong Chen; chenhong1129@hotmail.com

Academic Editor: Heinrich Sauer

Intraparenchymal transplantation of neural stem/progenitor cells (NSPCs) has been extensively investigated in animal models of ischemic stroke. However, the reported therapeutic efficacy was inconsistent among studies. To evaluate this situation, PubMed, Embase, and Web of Science databases were searched for preclinical studies using NSPC intraparenchymal transplantation in ischemic stroke animals. Data of study quality score, neurobehavioral (mNSS, rotarod test, and cylinder test) and histological (infarct volume) outcomes, cell therapy-related serious adverse events, and related cellular mechanisms were extracted for meta-analysis and systematic review. A total of 62 studies containing 73 treatment arms were included according to our criterion, with a mean quality score of 5.10 in 10. Among these studies, almost half of the studies claimed no adverse events of tumorigenesis. The finally pooled effect sizes for neurobehavioral and histological assessments were large (1.27 for mNSS, 1.63 for the rotarod test, 0.71 for the cylinder test, and 1.11 for infarct volume reduction). With further analysis, it was found that the administration time poststroke, NSPC donor species, and transplantation immunogenicity had close correlations with the degree of infarct volume reduction. The NSPC dosage delivered into the brain parenchyma was also negatively correlated with the effect of the cylinder test. Intriguingly, endogenous apoptosis inhibition and axonal regeneration played the most critical role in intraparenchymal NSPC transplantation among the cellular mechanisms. These results indicate that intraparenchymal NSPC transplantation is beneficial for neurobehavioral and histological improvement and is relatively safe for ischemic stroke animals. Therefore, intraparenchymal NSPC transplantation is a promising treatment for stroke patients.

1. Introduction

Ischemic stroke is one of the leading causes of death and disability around the world [1, 2]. After stroke, approximately 90% of survivors experience motor dysfunction [3], which lasts for the rest of their life and affects their daily life quality severely. However, there are few effective treatments for the ischemic stroke. Stem cell transplantation to rescue the motor function deficits poststroke has attracted a growing interest [4–6].

Among the various cell populations used for stroke cell therapy, neural stem/progenitor cells (NSPCs) and mesenchymal stem cells (MSCs) are both investigated extensively. Meta-analysis indicates that MSC therapy lies mainly in the time-dependent bystander mediators poststroke [7–9] as MSCs possess the poor potential of neural lineage differentiation. In contrast, NSPCs were regarded as a more appropriate source because of their capabilities of differentiation to neural cell phenotypes *in vitro* and *in vivo* [10, 11]. Transplanted NSPCs can migrate to peri-ischemic areas and ameliorate functional deficits [11–13]. Multiple but inconsistent mechanisms by which NSPCs enhance functional recovery were proposed, from neuroprotection [14] to neuroregeneration [15]. Similarly, the curative benefit is conflicting among studies when the following factors are involved, including donor cell states, dosage, immunogenicity, administration time after stroke onset, and immunosuppressive medicine usage. Therefore, there is a need for systematic analysis of the studies on intraparenchymal NSPC transplantation.

We conducted a meta-analysis to determine whether intraparenchymal NSPC transplantation is beneficial in preclinical studies based on neurobehavioral tests (mNSS, rotarod test, and cylinder test) and histological outcome (infarct volume). In addition, we pooled results about the cellular mechanisms and serious adverse events (SAEs). We hope that this analysis provides information for potential future clinical trials involving stem cell transplantation in stroke.

2. Methods

This meta-analysis was carried out following the guidelines of Preferred Reporting Items for Systematic Reviews and Meta-Analyses (PRISMA, http://www.prisma-statement.org/, Table S1 in Supplementary Materials available online) [16].

2.1. Search Strategy. We searched for correlative studies about neural stem/progenitor cell (NSPC) transplantation in animal models of ischemic stroke in three databases (PubMed, Embase, and Institute for Scientific Information Web of Science databases, up until July 11, 2018) by independent investigators. The search strategy was as follows: ((neural stem cells) OR (stem cell, neural) OR (neural progenitor cell) OR (neural precursor cell) OR NSPC) AND (stroke OR ischemic stroke OR brain ischemia OR brain infarction OR cerebral ischemia OR intracranial ischemia OR cerebrovascular OR middle cerebral artery OR anterior cerebral artery). The default language for all included studies was English. After studies were extracted, the titles, abstracts, and the secondary references were reviewed carefully. If controversy existed in whether the study is eligible, the study would be examined again and all investigators would discuss to reach a consensus.

2.2. Inclusion and Exclusion Criteria. This meta-analysis included controlled studies claiming that NSPCs and other vehicles (culture medium, PBS, or saline) were delivered intraparenchymally in ischemic stroke animals (nonhuman). For all included studies, neurobehavioral function

assessments must be served as one kind of outcome indicators. We excluded studies with brain lesions other than cerebral ischemia or with cell therapy paradigm using mature cells or genetically modified cells other than those for labeling or tracing in vivo or preconditioned cell transplantation. We also excluded studies without precise animal numbers or outcome values for individual comparison.

2.3. Study Quality Assessment. To estimate methodological quality for all included studies, the CAMARADES (Collaborative Approach to Meta-Analysis and Review of Animal Data from Experimental Studies) checklist was applied as follows: (1) publication on a peer-reviewed journal, (2) control of temperature, (3) randomization to treatment groups, (4) allocation concealment, (5) blinded assessment of outcomes, (6) avoidance of neuroprotective anesthetics (mostly known as ketamine), (7) use of animals with relevant comorbidities, (8) sample size calculation, (9) compliance with animal welfare regulations, and (10) statement of conflict of interest. We endowed each item one point and got the total score of every study after retrieving the full text, as well as the supplementary data and secondary references.

2.4. Data Extraction. Besides the study quality score, we extracted the following data from each study: first author, published year, recipient species, animal models, donor species, cell characteristics (intervention time relative to stroke onset, graft sites, and cell dose), administration of immunosuppressive drugs, and sensorimotor or histological outcomes at the final time point recorded (showing the four most used data of mNSS, rotarod test, cylinder test, and infarct volume). For the safety of intraparenchymal NSPC transplantation, data of treatment-related serious adverse events (tumor/teratoma formation, seizure, infection, or death) were considered. In addition, the data of cellular treatment effects [17] (Table S2 in Supplementary Materials available online) were extracted for further analysis. The outcome values of the rotarod test were multiplied by −1 given its positive relationship with the behavioral outcome in contrast to the other three measures [7]. GetData Graph Digitizer (version 2.24) was used to quantify the mean value and standard deviation (SD) or standard error (SE) from figures, if no detailed data was referred to in the text. When all data were shown in SE, SD could be recalculated with the following formula [18]:

$$SD = \sqrt{N} \times SE, \tag{1}$$

where N means the group size.

2.5. Statistical Analysis. All statistical analyses were performed using Stata (ver. 12.0, StataCorp). We evaluated the standard mean difference (SMD), 95% confidence interval (CI), and significance in a DerSimonian and Laird random-effects model by the statistics of Hedges' g across all studies. The therapeutic effects of intraparenchymally transplanted NSPCs in ischemic stroke were determined by obtaining mean effect sizes, with a value of <0.2 defined as a small effect, 0.2–0.8 as a medium effect, and

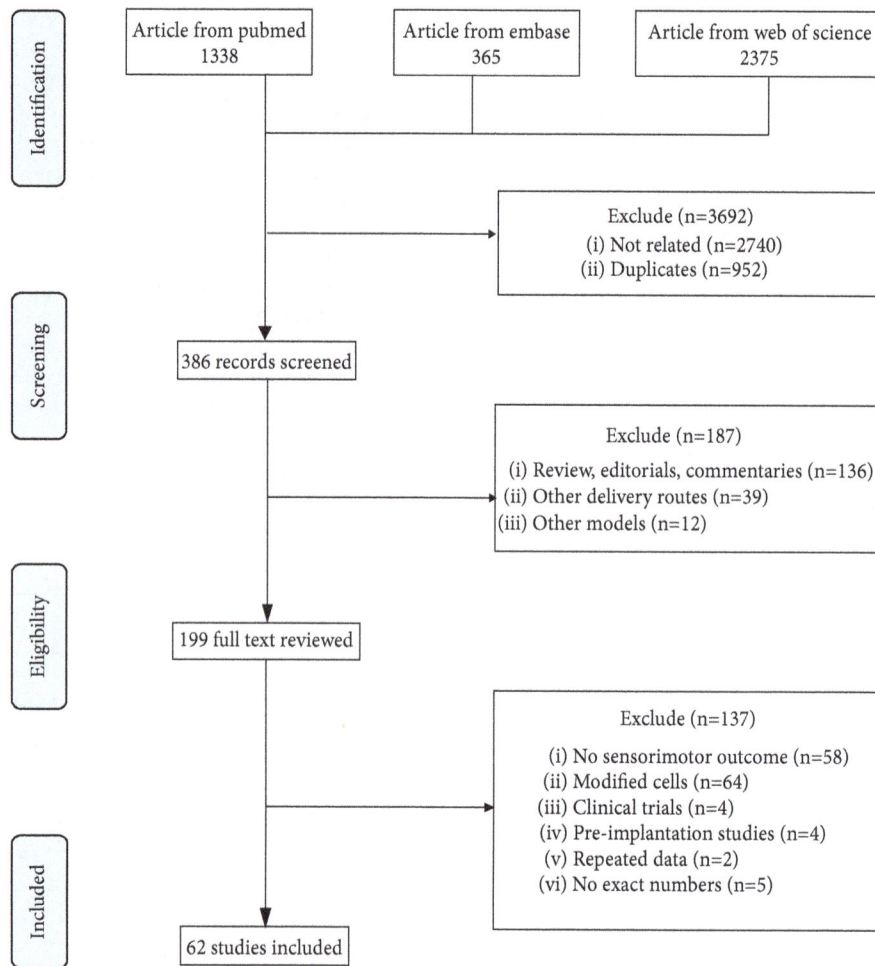

FIGURE 1: PRISMA flow diagram of including studies for this meta-analysis.

>0.8 as a large effect [19]. If heterogeneity defined by the I^2 metric exists among different studies, with a value of 25%, 50%, and 75% considered to be low, moderate, and considerable heterogeneity, sensitivity analysis was used for heterogeneity analysis. Subgroup analysis and metaregression with the following clinical parameters were used for further evaluation.

Univariate metaregression analysis was carried out according to 12 variables, including (1) timing of NSPC intervention after stroke onset, (2) NSPC dose, (3) ischemic stroke models (transient, permanent), (4) graft sites (focal or global), (5) degree of NSPC immunogenicity (allogeneic or xenogeneic), (6) species of NSPC recipients, (7) species of NSPC donors, (8) state of donor NSPCs (pluripotent stem cell derivatives or primary cells), (9) administration of immunosuppressive drugs, (10) design in blindness, (11) randomization, and (12) study quality score. Afterwards, funnel plots were used to check the potential of publication bias for a visual impression. The data of significant publication bias was reassessed using a 2-tailed Egger regression intercept method. If publication bias existed, trim and fill analysis was used to adjust the bias and check whether the effect size affects the final results.

3. Results

3.1. Selection and Description of Involved Studies.
The search procedure and strategies are described in Figure 1. A total of 4078 potentially relevant studies were extracted from three databases. After excluding 3692 irrelevant studies and 187 nonstandard papers, 199 studies with full text were reviewed. According to the inclusion and exclusion criteria, 137 studies dissatisfying the eligibility criteria were excluded. Finally, 62 studies containing 73 treatment arms without duplicate data description were included in this meta-analysis (Table S3 in Supplementary Materials available online). Among these identified studies, the ischemic stroke models were made transiently (46 of 62 studies) or permanently (16 of 62 studies). Rats (40 of 62 studies) and mice (19 of 62 studies) were used as recipient species, while three studies used Mongolian gerbil [20, 21] and pig [22]. The gender of all included animals was mainly male, except for seven studies with no statements [22–28], one study using female rats [29], and one study stating nonsex difference [30]. Meanwhile, human (28 of 62 studies), rat (14 of 62 studies), and mouse (20 of 62 studies) cells were chosen as the NSPC donors. The transplanted NSPCs were either from primary

cultures (45 of 73 comparisons) or from pluripotent stem cell derivatives (28 of 73 comparisons). There were also 21 studies stating the usage of immunosuppression drugs and 24 studies without it; the rest did not make a clear statement.

For SAEs related to intraparenchymal NSPC transplantation, tumor formation was most reported in 30 of the 62 studies (shown with an asterisk symbol in Table S3 in Supplementary Materials available online), but with no quantitative data.

3.2. Study Quality Assessment. The mean quality score across all studies was 5.10, ranging from 2 to 8 (Table S4 in Supplementary Materials available online). After being standardized by CAMARADES checklists, all the included studies were published in peer-reviewed journals and had claimed compliance with animal welfare regulations. No animals with relevant comorbidities were used for any of the studies. In addition, only thirteen studies did not describe the control of temperature, three studies had allocation concealment stressed, about 27 studies declared randomization to treatment, 39 studies described blinded assessment of outcomes, 38 studies avoided ketamine as anesthetics, and 35 studies stated conflict of interest (Table 1).

3.3. Meta-Analysis and Effect Size. Random-effects meta-analysis was performed for four considered measurements, and the pooled effect sizes ranged from 0.73 to 2.02 (2.02 (95% CI: 1.50–2.55) for mNSS, 1.54 (95% CI: 0.92–2.15) for the rotarod test, 0.73 (95% CI: 0.44–1.03) for the cylinder test, and 1.24 (95% CI: 0.83–1.65) for infarct volume) (Figure S1 in Supplementary Materials available online). However, the heterogeneity between studies for mNSS was large ($\chi^2 = 84.74$, $p \leq 0.001$, $I^2 = 75.2\%$, df = 21) (Figure S1(a) in Supplementary Materials available online). By sensitivity analysis, seven treatment arms whose effect size was greater than 3.0 were removed and the heterogeneity decreased ($\chi^2 = 20.82$, $p = 0.106$, $I^2 = 32.8\%$), with the corrected effect size of 1.27 (95% CI: 0.94–1.60) (Figure 2(a)). For the rotarod test, the heterogeneity among studies was big ($\chi^2 = 169.97$, $p \leq 0.001$, $I^2 = 87.1\%$, df = 22) (Figure S1(b) in Supplementary Materials available online). When sensitivity analysis was performed, the heterogeneity went down ($\chi^2 = 25.97$, $p = 0.038$, $I^2 = 42.2\%$) (Figure 2(b)) after three treatment arms with effect size greater than 3.0 and four other inadaptable comparisons were removed (Table S5 in Supplementary Materials available online). The corrected effect size was 1.69 (95% CI: 1.34–2.04) (Figure 2(b)). The heterogeneity among studies for the cylinder test was moderate ($\chi^2 = 19.38$, $p = 0.197$, $I^2 = 22.6\%$, df = 15) (Figure S1(c) in Supplementary Materials available online; Figure 2(c)). As for the infarct volume, the heterogeneity among studies was high ($\chi^2 = 135.19$, $p \leq 0.001$, $I^2 = 77.1\%$, df = 31) (Figure S1(d) in Supplementary Materials available online). After four inadaptable comparisons were removed by sensitivity analysis, the heterogeneity was slightly altered ($\chi^2 = 107.27$, $p \leq 0.001$, $I^2 = 74.8\%$), with the corrected effect size of 1.11 (95% CI: 0.73–1.50) (Figure 2(d)).

Effect sizes for cellular mechanisms related to NSPC transplantation in ischemic stroke animals, including apoptosis inhibition, immunomodulation, neurotrophic factor release, angiogenesis, neurogenesis, gliosis reduction, white matter function, enzyme supplementation, and axonal function, were evaluated (Table 2). Among these mechanisms, apoptosis reduction and axonal function were the most obvious effects following NSPC intraparenchymal transplantation (Table 2).

3.4. Subgroup Analysis and Metaregression Analysis. Following the effect size evaluation and sensitivity analysis, the heterogeneity in infarct volume effect size was still detected. Then, subgroup analysis and metaregression analysis based on the 12 clinically related parameters were chosen to analyze their contribution to statistical heterogeneity for infarct volume effect size. We found that administration time poststroke was negatively related to the infarct volume effect size (Adj $R^2 = 26.92\%$, $p = 0.008$), with an earlier NSPC transplantation and a bigger effect size (Table 3, Figure 3(a)). NSPC donor species also had a close correlation with infarct volume effect size (Adj $R^2 = 20.00\%$, $p = 0.025$), with mouse donors having more infarct volume reduction, indicating a preference for homologous transplantation (Table 3, Figure 3(b)). In addition, the transplantation immunity was correlated with the infarct volume reduction, with allograft indicating more reserved tissue (Adj $R^2 = 15.24\%$, $p = 0.044$) (Figure 3(c)). Meanwhile, for the cylinder test effect size, the NSPC dosage was discovered to be a negative correlative variable, with low dose for a better behavioral function (Adj $R^2 = 100.00\%$, $p = 0.063$) (Figure 3(d)).

3.5. Publication Bias. From the funnel plots (Figure 4), an approximately symmetrical distribution for mNSS and infarct volume was visualized, which means no publication bias. This was further confirmed by the Egger test in which the relative p values were 0.185 and 0.110 for mNSS and infarct volume, respectively, both of which exceeded 0.1. Although publication bias existed for the rotarod test and the cylinder test, with p values related to the Egger test equal to 0.094 and 0.073, respectively, these two recalibrated effect sizes were still larger than 1 (1.63 for the rotarod test and 0.71 for the cylinder test) after trim and fill analysis.

4. Discussion

This meta-analysis includes 62 controlled animal studies published from year 2004 to 2018. We found that intraparenchymal NSPC transplantation benefits neurobehavioral (mNSS, rotarod test, and cylinder test) and histological (infarct volume) outcomes poststroke with large effect sizes. The effect size of infarct volume reduction is correlated closely with administration time poststroke, NSPC donor species, and transplantation immunogenicity. The cylinder test effect size is correlated with NSPC donor dosage. No correlation was found between neurobehavioral or histological changes and other variables, such as stroke models, graft sites, species of NSPC recipients, state of donor NSPCs, immunosuppressive drugs, blinding and

TABLE 1: Distribution of included studies according to CAMARADES checklists.

Criteria	Number of studies	Per (%)
Publication on a peer-reviewed journal	62	100
Control of temperature	49	79.0
Randomization to a treatment group	27	43.5
Allocation concealment	3	4.8
Blinded assessment of outcome	39	62.9
Avoidance of neuroprotective anesthetics	38	61.3
Use of animal with relevant comorbidities	0	0
Sample size calculation	0	0
Compliance with animal welfare regulations	62	100
Statement of conflict of interest	35	56.5

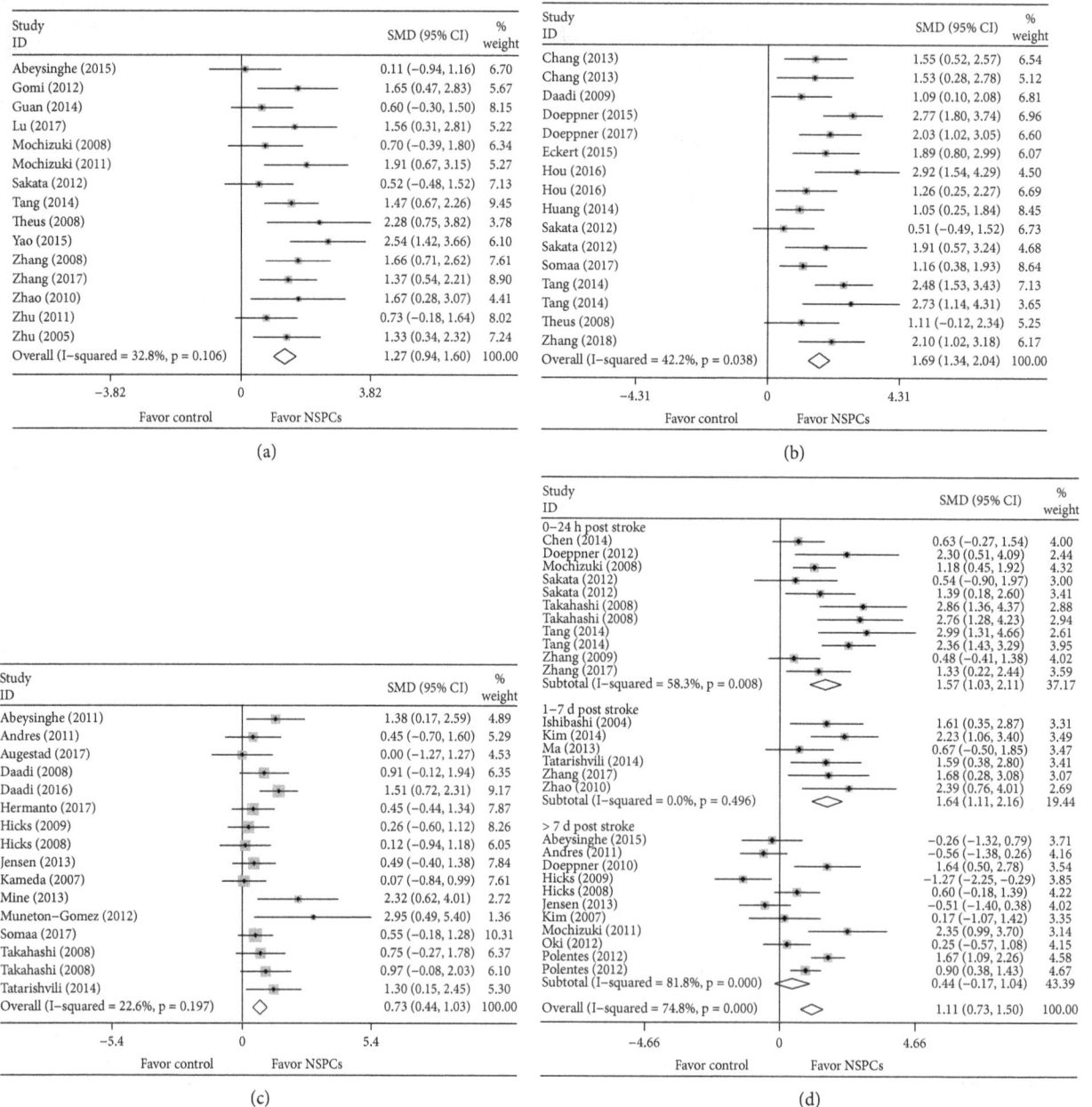

FIGURE 2: Effect sizes for intraparenchymal NPSC transplantation across related studies. Forest plot shows the mean effect sizes and 95% CI for (a) mNSS, (b) rotarod test, (c) cylinder test, and (d) infarct volume. SMD: standardized mean difference; CI: confidence interval; W: weight.

TABLE 2: Effect sizes for cellular treatment effects.

Treatment effects	Effect size	95% CI	Treatment arms
Apoptosis inhibition	3.09	1.94–4.25	13
Immunomodulation	1.47	0.34–2.61	13
Growth factors (BDNF)	1.37	0.57–2.17	14
Growth factors (VEGF)	1.15	0.47–1.84	13
Angiogenesis	1.18	0.42–1.94	11
Neurogenesis	1.23	0.40–2.07	13
Gliosis reduction	2.35	0.22–4.49	5
White matter function	1.00	0.40–1.61	3
Enzyme supplementation	0.81	−0.36–1.97	6
Axonal function	2.47	1.36–3.57	1

TABLE 3: Subgroup meta-analysis and metaregression of variants correlated with infarct volume reduction.

Clinical variants	Effect size (95% CI)	I^2, p value	df	Univariate analysis (Adj R^2, p)
Administration time poststroke				26.92%, 0.008
≤24 h	1.57 (1.03–2.21)	58.3%, 0.008	10	
1–7 d	1.64 (1.11–2.16)	0.0%, 0.496	5	
≥7 d	0.44 (−0.17–1.04)	81.8%, ≤0.001	10	
Cell dosage				1.27%, 0.261
≤1×10^6 cells/kg	1.45 (0.99–1.91)	57.4%, 0.012	9	
$1-5 \times 10^6$ cells/kg	0.82 (0.06–1.59)	83.1%, ≤0.001	10	
>5×10^6 cells/kg	0.99 (0.25–1.73)	61.5%, 0.016	6	
Animal model				0.79%, 0.280
Transient	1.24 (0.82–1.67)	68.9%, ≤0.001	19	
Permanent	0.78 (−0.07–1.64)	82.7%, ≤0.001	7	
Graft sites				
Global	0.24 (−0.59–1.08)	40.1%, 0.196	1	2.06%, 0.201
Focal	1.19 (0.78–1.60)	75.2%, ≤0.001	25	
Cell donor species				20.00%, 0.025
Mouse	1.46 (0.84–2.08)	54.7%, 0.031	7	
Rat	1.73 (1.15–2.31)	45.7%, 0.075	7	
Human	0.51 (−0.08–1.10)	81.0%, ≤0.001	11	
Cell recipient species				−4.82%, 0.761
Mouse	0.98 (0.40–1.56)	31.2%, 0.201	5	
Rat	1.12 (0.64–1.60)	79.8%, ≤0.001	20	
Others	1.61 (0.35–2.87)		0	
Immunoreactivity				15.24%, 0.044
No	1.52 (1.11–1.93)	30.9%, 0.136	12	
Yes	0.76 (0.21–1.31)	82.1%, ≤0.001	14	
State of donor cells				5.14%, 0.115
PSC-NSPCs	0.63 (−0.13–1.38)	84.1%, ≤0.001	7	
WT-NSPCs	1.33 (0.88–1.78)	68.2%, ≤0.001	19	
Immunosuppression drugs				−3.64%, 0.657
No	1.17 (0.22–2.12)	78.6%, ≤0.001	6	
Yes	0.95 (0.32–1.58)	83.2%, ≤0.001	11	
Unknown	1.28 (0.82–1.74)	26.9%, 0.205	8	
Blinding				−5.59%, 0.758
No	1.32 (0.17–2.46)	85.8%, ≤0.001	6	
Yes	1.06 (0.67–1.46)	69.1%, ≤0.001	20	
Randomization				−3.47%, 0.483
No	1.33 (0.61–2.05)	77.1%, ≤0.001	10	
Yes	0.99 (0.53–1.46)	74.6%, ≤0.001	16	

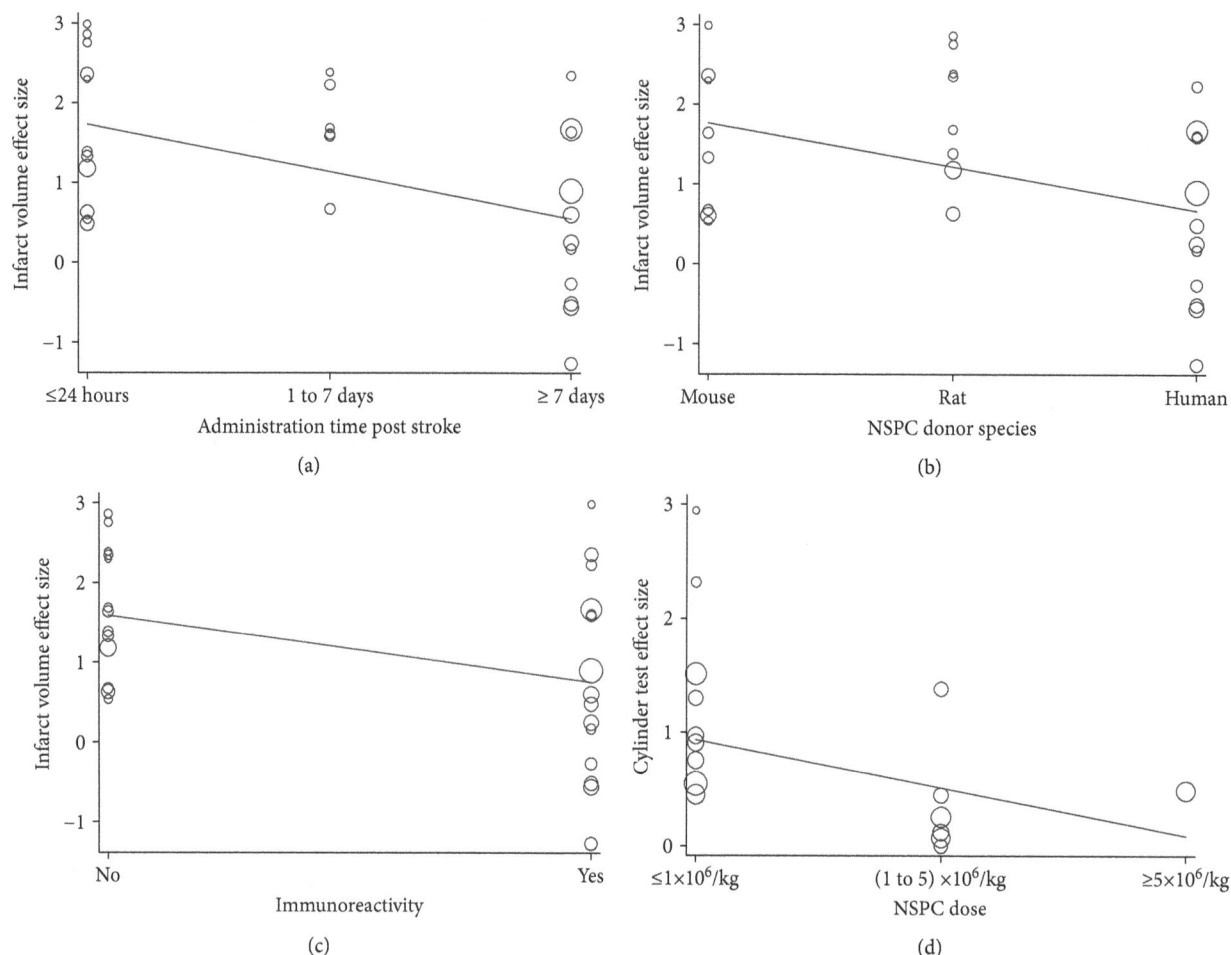

FIGURE 3: Metaregression analysis for related variables and effect sizes of infarct volume reduction and cylinder test. (a) An earlier intraparenchymal NSPC transplantation was associated with a smaller tissue loss (Adj $R^2 = 26.92\%$, $p = 0.008$). (b) Rodent cell donors were associated with greater residual tissue (Adj $R^2 = 20.00\%$, $p = 0.030$). (c) Allograft benefited the infarct volume reduction more (Adj $R^2 = 15.24\%$, $p = 0.044$). (d) A relatively lower NSPC dosage was associated with larger cylinder test performance (Adj $R^2 = 100.00\%$, $p = 0.063$). Values for effect sizes are Hedges' g.

randomization design, and study quality. The main mechanism by which intraparenchymal NSPC transplantation benefits ischemic stroke appears to lie in apoptosis inhibition and axonal function.

According to the STAIR guidance for methodological quality estimation [31], a mean quality score of 5.10 in this meta-analysis is higher than previous reports [32, 33]. However, the methodological quality of animal studies should be improved because the overestimation effect of low-quality studies potentially influences the results [34, 35]. After further analysis, we could not find direct proof in study quality score and neurobehavioral or histological effect size as was described in a similar study [36], and publication bias existed in neurobehavioral indices (rotarod and cylinder test), both of which encourage future research with rigorous design.

In this meta-analysis, the overall effect sizes for four considered indices are big, which would suggest an improvement in neurobehavioral and histological outcomes in adult ischemic stroke animals after intraparenchymal NSPC transplantation. However, because of the existence of heterogeneity among studies for mNSS, rotarod test, and infarct volume,

the output results should be interpreted with care. It also should be mentioned that there were several comparisons with an effect size more than 3.0, which contributes to the heterogeneity significantly [7, 17, 33]. After examining these studies, we found that there are some defects in the experimental design, including no blinding, no randomization, nonstatistical animal numbers, low-quality study, nonnormative procedure for assessments without pretraining, and low reliability for gained results. By sensitivity analysis to exclude inadequate comparisons, we obtained more homogenous data to draw a reliable conclusion for effect sizes of mNSS (1.27 SMD), rotarod test (1.63 SMD), and infarct volume.

The parameters used in this meta-analysis, including NSPC administration time, dosage, donor species, and transplantation immunogenicity, may be useful for future clinical application of stem cell therapy. Our metaregression analysis reveals that an earlier NSPC transplantation, that is, at the acute or subacute stage (within a period of 7 days), results in a greater reduction in infarct volume. This is partially consistent with the conclusions of a recent meta-analysis

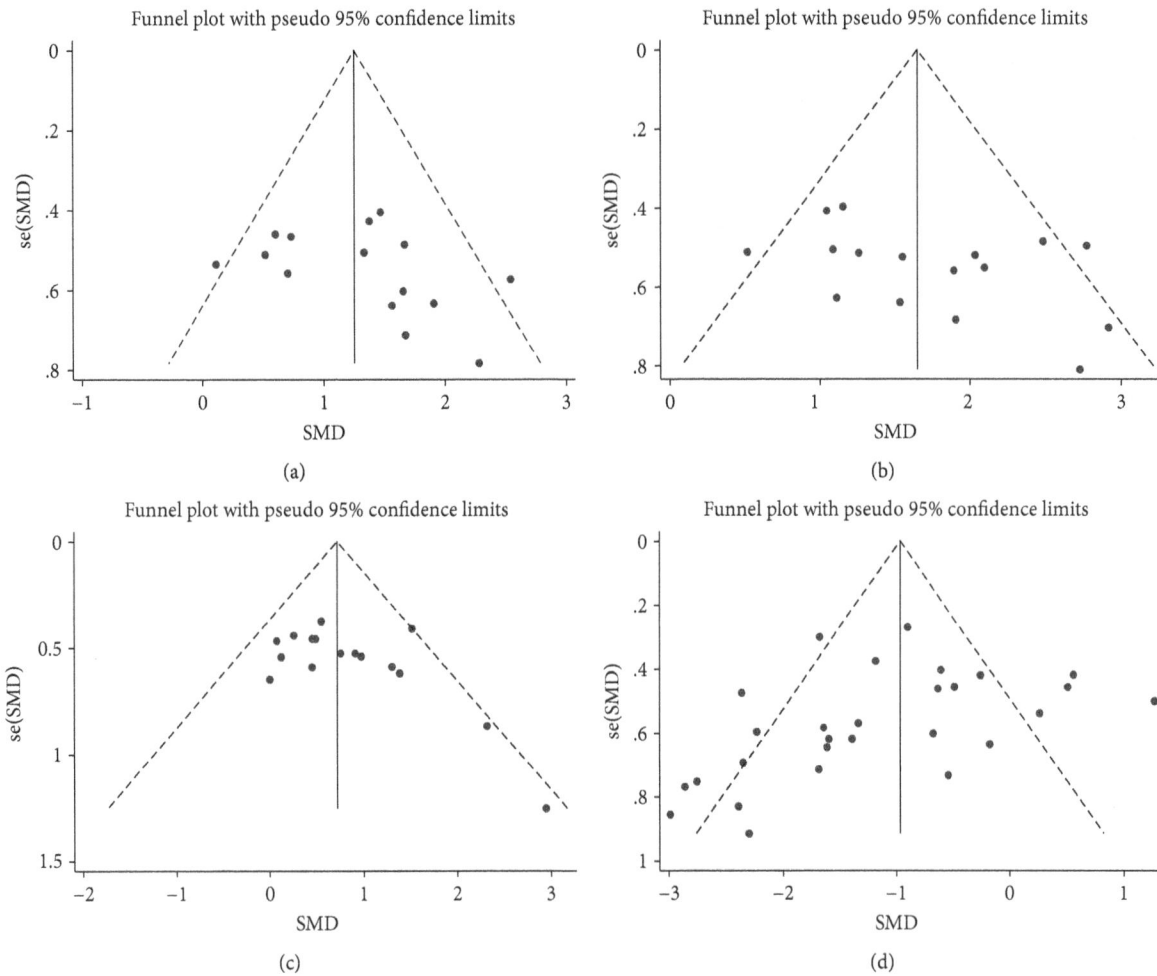

FIGURE 4: Funnel plots for publication bias of (a) mNSS, (b) rotarod test, (c) cylinder test, and (d) infarct volume. SMD: standardized mean difference.

[33]. Compared with the late NSPC transplantation, the early delivery may spare secondary damage to the brain tissue and preserve neural circuits more by neuroprotection effects [37, 38]. Interestingly, we found that a relatively low amount of NSPCs for intraparenchymal transplantation could improve the cylinder test more than the high-dose groups. The effective cell dose is less than 1×10^6 cells/kg. This appears to contradict the perceived understanding that a better neurobehavioral outcome results from a higher cell dose. A relatively low dose of NSPCs delivered intraparenchymally could migrate to the lesion area directly without exacerbating the ischemic brain injury by a high dose (volume) of grafted cells and tumor formation. Our subgroup meta-analysis and metaregression analysis also suggest that NSPCs from mouse donors contribute to a larger effect size of infarct volume reduction than those from rats and humans. And a more favorable lesion reduction effect is achieved through allogeneic transplantation rather than xenotransplantation, that is, rodent NSPCs to rodents, consistent with the results of Chen et al. [33] and Yousefifard et al. [39] in NSPC transplantation for spinal cord injury. This is likely related to the immunological reactions. For human NSPC grafts, the transplantation paradigm of mouse-mouse was within species, with low immune response to host tissue or cell grafts [40]. Finally, another factor that determines clinical translation is tumorigenesis. In our meta-analysis, about half of the included studies have claimed no malignant neoplasm formation from cell grafts. Since most of the NSPCs in the included studies are derived from pluripotent stem cells, this suggests that the cells used for transplantation are a reasonably appropriate source for stroke therapy [41].

The mechanisms underlying stem cell transplantation for ischemic stroke are not clear. Meta-analysis on MSC transplantation for stroke animal studies [7, 36, 42] suggests the involvement of apoptosis inhibition, immuno-modulation, neurotrophic factors, angiogenesis, neurogenesis, gliosis reduction, white matter function, enzyme supplementation, and axonal function. We found that apoptosis inhibition is the main contributor to neurobehavioral and histological improvement in intraparenchymal NSPC transplantation. Axonal function also has a significant role in behavioral and histological amelioration. Thus, neuroprotection and cell replacement underlie the therapeutic effect of intraparenchymal NSPC transplantation in ischemic stroke animals.

5. Conclusions

This study suggests that intraparenchymal delivery of NSPCs is a promising candidate for ischemic stroke therapy, improving the functional deficits and histopathology in animal models of ischemic stroke. The possible cellular mechanisms associated with intraparenchymal NSPC transplantation include apoptosis inhibition and axonal function.

Authors' Contributions

H.L.H. is responsible for the conception and design, collection and/or assembly of the data, and manuscript writing. K.Q. is responsible for the collection and/or assembly of the data and data analysis and interpretation. X.H.H. is responsible for the data analysis and interpretation. X.L. and Y.F.Z. are responsible for the collection and/or assembly of the data. Z.S.C. is responsible for the administrative support. X.L.H. and H.C. are responsible for the conception and design, financial support, and data analysis and interpretation. H.L.H. and K.Q. contributed equally to this study. And all the authors approved the final version of this manuscript.

Acknowledgments

This study was supported by the National Natural Science Foundation of China (NSFC) (81471302 and 81572238) and Huazhong University of Science and Technology Innovation Fund (2015ZDTD067 and 2015MS027). We thank Dr. Su-Chun Zhang of the University of Wisconsin for critically reading the manuscript.

Supplementary Materials

Supplementary 1. Figure S1: effect sizes of all included studies for (a) mNSS, (b) rotarod test, (c) cylinder test, and (d) infarct volume.

Supplementary 2. Table S1: PRISMA 2009 checklist.

Supplementary 3. Table S2: extracted data associated with cellular mechanisms of NSPC intraparenchymal transplantation in ischemic stroke animals.

Supplementary 4. Table S3: characteristics for all included studies.

Supplementary 5. Table S4: study quality assessment referred to the CAMARADES checklists.

Supplementary 6. Table S5: reasons for excluding related comparisons.

References

[1] V. L. Feigin, G. A. Roth, M. Naghavi et al., "Global burden of stroke and risk factors in 188 countries, during 1990–2013: a systematic analysis for the Global Burden of Disease Study 2013," *The Lancet Neurology*, vol. 15, no. 9, pp. 913–924, 2016.

[2] L. Liu, D. Wang, K. S. L. Wong, and Y. Wang, "Stroke and stroke care in China: huge burden, significant workload, and a national priority," *Stroke*, vol. 42, no. 12, pp. 3651–3654, 2011.

[3] S. Hesse and C. Werner, "Poststroke motor dysfunction and spasticity: novel pharmacological and physical treatment strategies," *CNS Drugs*, vol. 17, no. 15, pp. 1093–1107, 2003.

[4] J. Aked, H. Delavaran, O. Lindvall, B. Norrving, Z. Kokaia, and A. Lindgren, "Attitudes to stem cell therapy among ischemic stroke survivors in the Lund Stroke Recovery Study," *Stem Cells and Development*, vol. 26, no. 8, pp. 566–572, 2017.

[5] O. Lindvall and Z. Kokaia, "Stem cells in human neurodegenerative disorders—time for clinical translation?," *The Journal of Clinical Investigation*, vol. 120, no. 1, pp. 29–40, 2010.

[6] M. A. Dimyan and L. G. Cohen, "Neuroplasticity in the context of motor rehabilitation after stroke," *Nature Reviews Neurology*, vol. 7, no. 2, pp. 76–85, 2011.

[7] Q. Vu, K. Xie, M. Eckert, W. Zhao, and S. C. Cramer, "Meta-analysis of preclinical studies of mesenchymal stromal cells for ischemic stroke," *Neurology*, vol. 82, no. 14, pp. 1277–1286, 2014.

[8] M. M. Lalu, L. McIntyre, C. Pugliese et al., "Safety of cell therapy with mesenchymal stromal cells (SafeCell): a systematic review and meta-analysis of clinical trials," *PLoS One*, vol. 7, no. 10, article e47559, 2012.

[9] Y. Li, J. Chen, L. Wang, M. Lu, and M. Chopp, "Treatment of stroke in rat with intracarotid administration of marrow stromal cells," *Neurology*, vol. 56, no. 12, pp. 1666–1672, 2001.

[10] C. Q. Doe, "Neural stem cells: balancing self-renewal with differentiation," *Development*, vol. 135, no. 9, pp. 1575–1587, 2008.

[11] M. M. Daadi, A. L. Maag, and G. K. Steinberg, "Adherent self-renewable human embryonic stem cell-derived neural stem cell line: functional engraftment in experimental stroke model," *PLoS One*, vol. 3, no. 2, article e1644, 2008.

[12] M. Modo, R. P. Stroemer, E. Tang, S. Patel, and H. Hodges, "Effects of implantation site of stem cell grafts on behavioral recovery from stroke damage," *Stroke*, vol. 33, no. 9, pp. 2270–2278, 2002.

[13] M. Bacigaluppi, S. Pluchino, L. P. Jametti et al., "Delayed post-ischaemic neuroprotection following systemic neural stem cell transplantation involves multiple mechanisms," *Brain*, vol. 132, no. 8, pp. 2239–2251, 2009.

[14] E. Giusto, M. Donega, C. Cossetti, and S. Pluchino, "Neuro-immune interactions of neural stem cell transplants: from animal disease models to human trials," *Experimental Neurology*, vol. 260, pp. 19–32, 2014.

[15] C. V. Borlongan, "Age of PISCES: stem-cell clinical trials in stroke," *Lancet*, vol. 388, no. 10046, pp. 736–738, 2016.

[16] D. Moher, A. Liberati, J. Tetzlaff, D. G. Altman, and The PRISMA Group, "Preferred reporting items for systematic reviews and meta-analyses: the PRISMA statement," *PLoS Medicine*, vol. 6, no. 7, article e1000097, 2009.

[17] M. Janowski, P. Walczak, and I. Date, "Intravenous route of cell delivery for treatment of neurological disorders: a meta-analysis of preclinical results," *Stem Cells and Development*, vol. 19, no. 1, pp. 5–16, 2010.

[18] M. J. Gardner and D. G. Altman, "Confidence intervals rather than P values: estimation rather than hypothesis testing,"

British Medical Journal (Clinical Research Ed.), vol. 292, no. 6522, pp. 746–750, 1986.

[19] J. R. Thomas, W. Salazar, and D. M. Landers, "What is missing in p less than. 05? Effect size," *Research Quarterly for Exercise and Sport*, vol. 62, no. 3, pp. 344–348, 1991.

[20] S. Ishibashi, M. Sakaguchi, T. Kuroiwa et al., "Human neural stem/progenitor cells, expanded in long-term neurosphere culture, promote functional recovery after focal ischemia in Mongolian gerbils," *Journal of Neuroscience Research*, vol. 78, no. 2, pp. 215–223, 2004.

[21] J. Yamane, S. Ishibashi, M. Sakaguchi et al., "Transplantation of human neural stem/progenitor cells overexpressing galectin-1 improves functional recovery from focal brain ischemia in the Mongolian gerbil," *Molecular Brain*, vol. 4, no. 1, p. 35, 2011.

[22] V. W. Lau, S. R. Platt, H. E. Grace, E. W. Baker, and F. D. West, "Human iNPC therapy leads to improvement in functional neurologic outcomes in a pig ischemic stroke model," *Brain and Behavior*, vol. 8, no. 5, article e00972, 2018.

[23] L. Chen, R. Qiu, L. Li et al., "The role of exogenous neural stem cells transplantation in cerebral ischemic stroke," *Journal of Biomedical Nanotechnology*, vol. 10, no. 11, pp. 3219–3230, 2014.

[24] M. Gomi, Y. Takagi, A. Morizane et al., "Functional recovery of the murine brain ischemia model using human induced pluripotent stem cell-derived telencephalic progenitors," *Brain Research*, vol. 1459, pp. 52–60, 2012.

[25] O. Mohamad, D. Drury-Stewart, M. Song et al., "Vector-free and transgene-free human iPS cells differentiate into functional neurons and enhance functional recovery after ischemic stroke in mice," *PLoS One*, vol. 8, no. 5, article e64160, 2013.

[26] K. Oki, J. Tatarishvili, J. Wood et al., "Human-induced pluripotent stem cells form functional neurons and improve recovery after grafting in stroke-damaged brain," *Stem Cells*, vol. 30, no. 6, pp. 1120–1133, 2012.

[27] F. A. Somaa, T. Y. Wang, J. C. Niclis et al., "Peptide-based scaffolds support human cortical progenitor graft integration to reduce atrophy and promote functional repair in a model of stroke," *Cell Reports*, vol. 20, no. 8, pp. 1964–1977, 2017.

[28] F. Zhang, X. Duan, L. Lu et al., "In vivo long-term tracking of neural stem cells transplanted into an acute ischemic stroke model with reporter gene-based bimodal MR and optical imaging," *Cell Transplant*, vol. 26, no. 10, pp. 1648–1662, 2017.

[29] Y. Zhao, S. T. Yao, and S. J. Wang, "Neural stem cell transplantation in the hippocampus of rats with cerebral ischemia/reperfusion injury activation of the phosphatidylinositol-3 kinase/Akt pathway and increased brain-derived neurotrophic factor expression," *Neural Regeneration Research*, vol. 5, pp. 1605–1610, 2010.

[30] B. Hou, J. Ma, X. Guo et al., "Exogenous neural stem cells transplantation as a potential therapy for photothrombotic ischemia stroke in Kunming mice model," *Molecular Neurobiology*, vol. 54, no. 2, pp. 1254–1262, 2017.

[31] M. Fisher, G. Feuerstein, D. W. Howells et al., "Update of the stroke therapy academic industry roundtable preclinical recommendations," *Stroke*, vol. 40, no. 6, pp. 2244–2250, 2009.

[32] J. S. Lees, E. S. Sena, K. J. Egan et al., "Stem cell-based therapy for experimental stroke: a systematic review and meta-analysis," *International Journal of Stroke*, vol. 7, no. 7, pp. 582–588, 2012.

[33] L. Chen, G. Zhang, Y. Gu, and X. Guo, "Meta-analysis and systematic review of neural stem cells therapy for experimental ischemia stroke in preclinical studies," *Scientific Reports*, vol. 6, no. 1, article 32291, 2016.

[34] M. R. Macleod, T. O'Collins, D. W. Howells, and G. A. Donnan, "Pooling of animal experimental data reveals influence of study design and publication bias," *Stroke*, vol. 35, no. 5, pp. 1203–1208, 2004.

[35] Z. Zhang, X. Xu, and H. Ni, "Small studies may overestimate the effect sizes in critical care meta-analyses: a meta-epidemiological study," *Critical Care*, vol. 17, no. 1, article R2, 2013.

[36] Y. Hu, N. Liu, P. Zhang et al., "Preclinical studies of stem cell transplantation in intracerebral hemorrhage: a systemic review and meta-analysis," *Molecular Neurobiology*, vol. 53, no. 8, pp. 5269–5277, 2016.

[37] H. Sakata, K. Niizuma, H. Yoshioka et al., "Minocycline-preconditioned neural stem cells enhance neuroprotection after ischemic stroke in rats," *The Journal of Neuroscience: The Official Journal of the Society for Neuroscience*, vol. 32, no. 10, pp. 3462–3473, 2012.

[38] A. Eckert, L. Huang, R. Gonzalez, H. S. Kim, M. H. Hamblin, and J. P. Lee, "Bystander effect fuels human induced pluripotent stem cell-derived neural stem cells to quickly attenuate early stage neurological deficits after stroke," *Stem Cells Translational Medicine*, vol. 4, no. 7, pp. 841–851, 2015.

[39] M. Yousefifard, V. Rahimi-Movaghar, F. Nasirinezhad et al., "Neural stem/progenitor cell transplantation for spinal cord injury treatment; a systematic review and meta-analysis," *Neuroscience*, vol. 322, pp. 377–397, 2016.

[40] K. Warfvinge, P. H. Schwartz, J. F. Kiilgaard et al., "Xenotransplantation of human neural progenitor cells to the subretinal space of nonimmunosuppressed pigs," *Journal of Transplantation*, vol. 2011, Article ID 948740, 6 pages, 2011.

[41] G. S. Mack, "ReNeuron and StemCells get green light for neural stem cell trials," *Nature Biotechnology*, vol. 29, no. 2, pp. 95-96, 2011.

[42] Q. Wu, Y. Wang, B. M. Demaerschalk, S. Ghimire, K. E. Wellik, and W. Qu, "Bone marrow stromal cell therapy for ischemic stroke: a meta-analysis of randomized control animal trials," *International Journal of Stroke*, vol. 12, no. 3, pp. 273–284, 2017.

The Effects of Platelet-Derived Growth Factor-BB on Bone Marrow Stromal Cell-Mediated Vascularized Bone Regeneration

Maolin Zhang [iD],[1,2,3] Wenwen Yu,[4] Kunimichi Niibe,[3] Wenjie Zhang,[1,2] Hiroshi Egusa,[3] Tingting Tang,[5] and Xinquan Jiang [iD][1,2]

[1]*Department of Prosthodontics, Ninth People's Hospital affiliated to Shanghai Jiao Tong University, School of Medicine, 639 Zhizaoju Road, Shanghai 200011, China*
[2]*Shanghai Key Laboratory of Stomatology & Shanghai Research Institute of Stomatology, National Clinical Research Center of Stomatology, 639 Zhizaoju Road, Shanghai 200011, China*
[3]*Division of Molecular and Regenerative Prosthodontics, Tohoku University Graduate School of Dentistry, 4-1 Seiryo-machi, Aoba-ku, Sendai, Miyagi 980-8575, Japan*
[4]*Department of Oral and Craniomaxillofacial Science & Sleep-disordered Breathing Center, Ninth People's Hospital affiliated to Shanghai Jiao Tong University, School of Medicine, 639 Zhizaoju Road, Shanghai, China*
[5]*Shanghai Key Laboratory of Orthopaedic Implants, Department of Orthopaedic Surgery, Shanghai Ninth People's Hospital, Shanghai Jiaotong University, School of Medicine, Shanghai 200011, China*

Correspondence should be addressed to Xinquan Jiang; xinquanj@aliyun.com

Academic Editor: Heng Zhu

Regenerative medicine for bone tissue mainly depends on efficient recruitment of endogenous or transplanted stem cells to guide bone regeneration. Platelet-derived growth factor (PDGF) is a functional factor that has been widely used in tissue regeneration and repair. However, the short half-life of PDGF limits its efficacy, and the mechanism by which PDGF regulates stem cell-based bone regeneration still needs to be elucidated. In this study, we established genetically modified PDGF-B-overexpressing bone marrow stromal cells (BMSCs) using a lentiviral vector and then explored the mechanism by which PDGF-BB regulates BMSC-based vascularized bone regeneration. Our results demonstrated that PDGF-BB increased osteogenic differentiation but inhibited adipogenic differentiation of BMSCs via the extracellular signal-related kinase 1/2 (ERK1/2) signaling pathway. In addition, secreted PDGF-BB significantly enhanced human umbilical vein endothelial cell (HUVEC) migration and angiogenesis via the phosphatidylinositol 3 kinase (PI3K)/AKT and ERK1/2 signaling pathways. We evaluated the effect of PDGF-B-modified BMSCs on bone regeneration using a critical-sized rat calvarial defect model. Radiography, micro-CT, and histological analyses revealed that PDGF-BB overexpression improved BMSC-mediated angiogenesis and osteogenesis during bone regeneration. These results suggest that PDGF-BB facilitates BMSC-based bone regeneration by enhancing the osteogenic and angiogenic abilities of BMSCs.

1. Introduction

Reconstruction of bony defects caused by infection, trauma, or tumor resection is still a substantial clinical challenge. Bone marrow stromal cells (BMSCs) possessing regenerative potential have been considered an ideal cell source for bone regeneration [1, 2]. In addition, the combination of BMSCs with particular growth factors, such as bone morphogenetic proteins (BMPs) and vascular endothelial growth factor (VEGF), has been considered a promising strategy for bone tissue regeneration [3].

Platelet-derived growth factor (PDGF), a two-chain polypeptide, was originally identified in platelets [4, 5], and there are five polypeptide isoforms: PDGF-AA, PDGF-AB, PDGF-BB, PDGF-CC, and PDGF-DD [5, 6]. Among these isoforms, PDGF-BB is a unique ligand that can interact with all three PDGF receptors, namely, PDGFR-$\alpha\alpha$, PDGFR-$\alpha\beta$, and PDGFR-$\beta\beta$ [4]. PDGF-BB is a potent mitogen [7, 8] and chemoattractant for many cell types [9, 10] and has the ability to promote angiogenesis [11]. Thus, PDGF-BB is considered a key regulatory factor in tissue repair and regeneration [12]. Previous studies have demonstrated that PDGF-BB can enhance stem cell-based bone regeneration [13, 14]. However, the mechanisms by which PDGF-BB contributes to stem cell-based bone regeneration still need to be further elucidated. In addition, the short half-life of PDGF within the blood (only a few minutes) limits its efficacy [15]. Therefore, sustained local delivery of PDGF-BB is likely important to achieve ideal results. Forced expression of PDGF-BB by lentiviral transduction may be a useful method to investigate the effects of PDGF-BB on the regulation of stem cell-based bone regeneration. In this system, lentiviral transduction would enable stable and efficient expression of the transgene in cells even after several passages, which can facilitate both *in vitro* and *in vivo* investigations of the mechanism underlying PDGF-BB regulation of stem cell-based bone regeneration.

In this study, we established a PDGF-B-modified BMSC line using a lentivirus gene delivery vector and then explored the mechanism by which PDGF-BB regulates BMSC osteogenic and adipogenic differentiation. We further investigated the mechanism of PDGF-BB-induced vascular endothelial cell migration and angiogenesis. Finally, PDGF-B-modified BMSCs were mixed with a porous calcium phosphate cement (CPC) scaffold and transplanted into a rat critical-sized calvarial defect. Bone regeneration was evaluated using micro-CT and histological analysis.

2. Materials and Methods

2.1. Isolation and Culture of Rat BMSCs. BMSCs were isolated from 4-week-old Fisher 344 rats as previously described [16–18]. Briefly, bone marrow in bilateral rat tibias and femurs was flushed out using Dulbecco's modified Eagle's medium (DMEM, Gibco BRL, Grand Island, NY) containing 10% fetal bovine serum (FBS, Gibco, USA) and antibiotics (penicillin 100 U/mL, streptomycin 100 U/mL), and then, the cells were cultured in DMEM at 37°C in a humidified 5% CO_2 incubator. After two days, the nonadherent cells were discarded. Cells at passages 2 and 3 were used for this study.

2.2. Lentiviral Vector Construction and Transduction. Lentiviral vectors containing the human PDGF-B gene and enhanced green fluorescent protein (eGFP, Lenti-PDGF) or LacZ and eGFP (Lenti-LacZ) were constructed by Cyagen Biosciences, Inc. (Guangzhou, China). Briefly, the target plasmids pLV.EX3d.P/puro-EF1A > PDGFB > IRES/eGFP and pLV.EX3d.P/puro-EF1A > Lacz > IRES/eGFP were constructed using Gateway technology (pLV.EX3d.P/puro-EF1A > Lacz > IRES/eGFP was used as the control), and then, 293FT cells were transfected with the target plasmid together with the helper plasmid (pLV/helper-SL3, pLV/helper-SL4, and pLV/helper-SL5) using Lipofectamine 2000 (Invitrogen) according to the manufacturer's instructions [19]. The supernatant containing the lentivirus particles was harvested and ultracentrifuged. For transduction, BMSCs were cultured for 24 h to reach 70–80% confluence

and then transduced with Lenti-PDGF or Lenti-LacZ at a multiplicity of infection of 20. The transduction efficiency was analyzed by flow cytometry to calculate the percentage of eGFP-expressing cells at day 3.

The expression of PDGF-BB in BMSCs was evaluated using real-time reverse transcription polymerase chain reaction (real-time RT-PCR) and Western blotting. The amount of PDGF-BB secreted by PDGF-B-modified BMSCs in the culture medium from each group was detected using a PDGF-BB ELISA kit (Abcam) according to the manufacturer's instructions [19]. All experiments were performed in triplicate.

2.3. Osteogenic Induction of BMSCs. For osteogenic differentiation, cells were seeded in 12-well plates and cultured in osteogenic medium (DMEM, 10% FBS, 1% penicillin/streptomycin, 50 μg/mL L-ascorbic acid, 10 mM glycerophosphate, and 100 nM dexamethasone) with or without PD98059 (10 μM), an extracellular signal-related kinase (ERK) inhibitor (Cell Signaling Technology, Inc.). The osteogenic medium was changed every two days. The expression of osteogenesis-related genes was determined after 3 or 7 days of culture using real-time PCR and Western blotting. Osteogenic differentiation was also evaluated via alkaline phosphatase (ALP) and Alizarin Red S (ARS) staining for calcium deposition. For ALP analysis, cells in each group were fixed with 4% paraformaldehyde on day 7 and then stained with an ALP kit (Beyotime, China). Semiquantitative analysis of ALP activity was performed by testing optical density (OD) values at 405 nm using p-nitrophenyl phosphate (pNPP, Sigma) as the substrate [20]. For ARS analysis, cells from each group were fixed with 95% alcohol for 10 min and then stained with 0.1% ARS solution (Sigma) for 30 min on day 21. For a further quantitative assay, the ARS staining was desorbed with 10% cetylpyridinium chloride (Sigma), and the OD values were determined at 590 nm. The total protein content in each group was measured using a Bio-Rad protein assay kit (Bio-Rad, USA), and ALP and ARS levels were calculated as optical density per microgram of protein. All experiments were performed in triplicate.

2.4. Adipogenic Induction of BMSCs. For adipogenic differentiation, cells in each group were seeded on 12-well plates, cultured in DMEM until they reached 100% confluence, and then cultured in adipogenic medium containing 0.5 mM isobutylmethylxanthine (Sigma), 0.5 mM hydrocortisone, and 60 mM indomethacin (Sigma) with or without PD98059 (10 μM). Intracellular lipid accumulation was stained with Oil Red O as previously described [21]. Briefly, the cells were fixed with 4% paraformaldehyde for 15 min and stained with diluted Oil Red O solution for 10 min. All samples were viewed with an inverted phase contrast microscope (Leica, Germany), and the stained fields were evaluated using Image pro 5.0 (Media Cybernetics, USA). The expression of peroxisome proliferator-activated receptor γ2 (PPARγ2) was analyzed via real-time RT-PCR and Western blotting. All experiments were performed in triplicate.

TABLE 1: Nucleotide sequences for real-time RT-PCR primers.

Gene	Primer sequence (5′-3′) (forward/reverse)	Product size (bp)	Accession number
PPAR-γ2	TGCAGGTGATCAAGAAGACG TGGAAGAAGGGAAATGTTGG	177	NM_013124
PDGF-BB	CTGCGACCTGTCCAGGTGAG GCACCGTCCGAATGGTCACC	199	NM_033016.2
OPN	CCAAGCGTGGAAACACACAGCC GGCTTTGGAACTCGCCTGACTG	165	NM_012881
OCN	GCCCTGACTGCATTCTGCCTCT TCACCACCTTACTGCCCTCCTG	103	NM_013414
COL-I	CTGCCCAGAAGAATATGTATCACC GAAGCAAAGTTTCCTCCAAGACC	198	NM_053304
GAPDH	GGCAAGTTCAACGGCACAGT GCCAGTAGACTCCACGACAT	76	NM_017008.3

2.5. Real-Time RT-PCR Analysis. Total RNA was extracted from cells using Trizol Reagent (Invitrogen). The total RNA concentration was measured with a Thermo Scientific NanoDrop™ 1000 ultraviolet-visible spectrophotometer (NanoDrop Technologies, Wilmington, DE) as previously described [22]. cDNA was synthesized according to the manufacturer's instructions using a Prime-Script™ RT reagent kit (Takara Bio, Shiga, Japan). Osteogenesis-related marker genes, including *type I collagen (Col-I), osteopontin (OPN),* and *osteocalcin (OCN)*, and the adipogenic marker gene *PPARγ2* were examined. *Glyceraldehyde-3-phosphate dehydrogenase (GAPDH)* was used as the housekeeping gene for normalization of RNA expression levels. All experiments were performed in triplicate. The PCR primer sequences are displayed in Table 1.

2.6. Western Blot Analysis. Protein lysates were harvested using a protein extraction reagent (Kangchen, China), and then, the protein concentration was determined using a BCA Protein Assay. Equal amounts of protein were separated on 10% or 15% SDS-polyacrylamide gel electrophoresis (PAGE) gels and transferred to polyvinylidene difluoride (PVDF, Pall, USA) membranes, and then, the membranes were blocked with 5% nonfat milk for 1 h. After that, the membranes were incubated with primary antibodies against p-AKT, AKT, ERK, p-ERK (dilution rate: 1 : 1000; all antibodies related to PI3K/AKT signaling or Erk1/2 signaling were bought from Cell Signaling Technology, Inc.), PDGF-BB (1 : 1000; Abcam, ab23914), Col-I (1 : 1000; Abcam, ab34710), OPN (1 : 1000; Abcam, ab8448), OCN (1 : 500; Abcam, ab93876), PPARγ2 (1 : 500; Abcam, ab209350), and β-actin (1 : 3000; Sigma). Then, the membranes were incubated with HRP-conjugated secondary antibodies (Sigma). Finally, the immunoblots were visualized using ECL Plus reagents (Amersham Pharmacia Biotech, USA) [23].

2.7. Human Umbilical Vein Endothelial Cell (HUVEC) Migration and Angiogenesis Assay. HUVECs were purchased from AllCells, Ltd. (Shanghai, China). HUVECs were cultured in endothelial basal medium (EBM, AllCells) devoid of growth factors [19]. To investigate the stimulation effects of PDGF-BB secreted by PDGF-B-modified BMSCs on HUVEC migration and angiogenesis, PDGF-B-modified BMSCs were cultured in six-well plates in DMEM (10^6 cells per 2 mL per well) for 24 h, and then, supernatants were collected for the following studies.

A transwell chemotactic migration model was used to examine the migration activity of HUVECs cultured in the supernatant from each group. HUVECs were seeded into the upper chambers of 24-well plates (10^4 cells per well) containing membranes with 8 μm pores (Corning Inc., Corning, NY). In the lower chambers, different media were added as follows: (a) supernatant from the Lenti-LacZ group, (b) supernatant from the Lenti-PDGF group supplemented with PD98059 (10 μM), (c) supernatant from the Lenti-PDGF group supplemented with LY294002 (10 μM), or (d) supernatant from the Lenti-PDGF group. After incubation for 12 h at 37°C, the migrated cells were fixed with 4% paraformaldehyde and stained with hematoxylin for 15 min at room temperature, and then, the cells that had migrated toward the lower side of the filter were observed using a fluorescence stereomicroscope (Leica, Germany). The number of migrated cells in each group was counted in 6 random fields per chamber.

To investigate whether phosphatidylinositol 3 kinase (PI3K)/AKT pathway and ERK1/2 signaling pathways were involved in PDGF-BB-mediated HUVEC migration and angiogenesis *in vitro*, HUVECs were preincubated with PD98059 (10 μM) or LY294002 (10 μM, PI3K/AKT inhibitor, Cell Signaling Technology) for 30 min, and then, the cells were incubated with the supernatants for 15 min. Protein lysates were harvested for Western blot analysis.

For the *in vitro* angiogenesis assay, HUVECs (3×10^4 cells/well) were seeded into 96-well culture plates, which were coated with Matrigel (BD Biosciences), and cultured with the following media: (a) supernatant from the Lenti-LacZ group, (b) supernatant from the Lenti-PDGF group supplemented with PD98059 (10 μM), (c) supernatant from the Lenti-PDGF group supplemented with LY294002 (10 μM), or (d) supernatant from the Lenti-PDGF group. After being cultured for 12 h, the cells were observed using an inverted light microscope (Leica, Germany). Five random microscopic fields were photographed in each group, and then, the mesh numbers in each field were quantified using the angiogenesis analyzer of ImageJ.

2.8. Preparation of the BMSC/CPC Complex.

Porous calcium phosphate cement (CPC) scaffolds (Rebone, China) were sterilized before use. BMSCs from each group were collected and resuspended in FBS-free medium, and then, a cell suspension (2×10^7 cells/mL) from each group was added to CPC scaffolds until saturated. A portion of these implants was used for *in vivo* animal studies, and the remainder was cultured for 1 or 3 days for scanning electron microscopy examination to observe BMSC spreading, adhesion, and proliferation on the CPC scaffold. After being cultured for 1 or 3 days *in vitro*, the samples were fixed in 2% glutaraldehyde, dehydrated in a series of graded ethanol solutions, sputter-coated with gold, and observed via scanning electron microscopy (SEM, Hitachi, Tokyo, Japan).

2.9. Animal Experiments.

All procedures were approved by the Animal Research Committee of the Ninth People's Hospital, Shanghai Jiao Tong University School of Medicine. All surgical procedures were performed as described previously [22, 24]. Ten-week-old male F344 rats were used in this study. Briefly, the animals were anaesthetized by intraperitoneal injection of pentobarbital, and then, a 1.5 cm sagittal incision was made on the scalp to expose the calvarium. Two 5 mm diameter critical-sized defects were created using a trephine bur. A total of 24 rats were randomly divided into four groups to receive one of the following implants: (1) CPC ($n = 6$), (2) CPC with BMSCs ($n = 6$), (3) CPC with BMSCs/Lenti-LacZ ($n = 6$), or (4) CPC with BMSCs/Lenti-PDGF ($n = 6$).

2.10. Microfil Perfusion.

Microfil (Flowtech, Carver, MA, USA) perfusion was used to identify blood vessel formation as previously described [25]. Briefly, the hair on the chest was shaved, and then, a long incision was made in the chest and abdomen (from the front limbs to the xiphoid process). The sternum was cut using scissors, and the rib cage was retracted laterally. The left ventricle was penetrated with an angiocatheter after the descending aorta was clamped. After the inferior vena cava was incised, 20 mL of heparinized saline was perfused, and then, 20 mL of Microfil was perfused at 2 mL/min, followed by perfusion with saline.

2.11. Radiography and Micro-CT Analysis.

At 8 weeks postsurgery, all the rats in each group were sacrificed with an intraperitoneal overdose injection of pentobarbital. The calvarial bones were fixed in 10% formalin solution, and X-ray images of the skulls were obtained with a dental X-ray machine (Trophy, France). The morphology of the reconstructed skulls was evaluated using a micro-CT system (mCT-80, Scanco Medical, Switzerland) as previously described [26]. Briefly, the calvarial bone was scanned in high-resolution scanning mode (pixel matrix, 1024×1024; voxel size, $20 \, \mu m$; slice thickness, $20 \, \mu m$) to measure the bone volume. After scanning, three-dimensional images were reconstructed with GEHC Micro View software. Both the parameters bone mineral density (BMD) and the

percentage of new bone volume relative to tissue volume were measured using auxiliary software (Scanco Medical AG, Switzerland).

2.12. Histological Analyses.

After radiography and micro-CT analysis, the calvarial bones were dehydrated in ascending alcohol concentrations from 70% to 100%, and then, the samples were embedded in polymethylmethacrylate (PMMA). Sagittal sections of the central segment were cut using a microtome (Leica, Germany) and polished to a final thickness of approximately $40 \, \mu m$. The sections were stained with Van Gieson's picro fuchsin to evaluate new bone formation. Red indicated new bone formation; residual CPC materials appeared black, and blue spots from the Microfil perfusion indicated blood perfusion. For hematoxylin and eosin (HE) staining, the calvarial bones were decalcified in 15% EDTA for 3 weeks and embedded with paraffin. A series of 5 mm sections were cut in the same manner as the hard tissue slices, and then, the sections were stained with HE for histological analysis. The area of newly formed bone (red area in both Van Gieson's picro fuchsin-stained sections and HE-stained sections) and blood vessels (blue spots indicated blood vessels filled with Microfil in the Van Gieson's picro fuchsin-stained sections; blood vessels were permeated with intraluminal red blood cells in the HE-stained sections) was quantitatively evaluated in four randomly selected sections from each group using Image pro 5.0 (Media Cybernetics, USA).

2.13. Statistical Analysis.

The experimental data are presented as the mean ± standard derivation (SD). Differences between groups were analyzed via ANOVA with Tukey's post hoc test. Values of $P < 0.05$ were considered statistically significant.

3. Results

3.1. Gene Transduction and PDGF-BB Expression.

Three days after gene transduction, inverted fluorescence microscopy observations and flow cytometry results showed that the transfection efficiency of the target gene PDGF-B was greater than 80% (Figure 1(a), Figure 1(b)). Both real-time RT-PCR and Western blotting results indicated that the expression of PDGF-BB in BMSCs was significantly upregulated after gene transduction in the Lenti-PDGF group (Figure 1(c), Figure 1(d)). ELISA results demonstrated that PDGF-B-modified BMSCs could stably and continuously secrete PDGF-BB at the protein level (Figure 1(e)).

3.2. Cell Differentiation Analysis.

Osteogenic differentiation analysis showed that the expression of Col-I and OPN at both the mRNA and protein levels was increased in the Lenti-PDGF group compared with that in the Lenti-LacZ group at days 3 and 7 (Figure 2(a), Figure 2(b)). OCN was also remarkably increased at both the mRNA and protein levels at day 7 (Figure 2(a), Figure 2(b)). By contrast, there was no significant distinction between the Lenti-LacZ group and Lenti-PDGF group on day 3 (Figure 2(a), Figure 2(b)). ALP staining was more intense in the Lenti-PDGF group than in the Lenti-LacZ group, and the semiquantitative

(a)

(b)

(c)

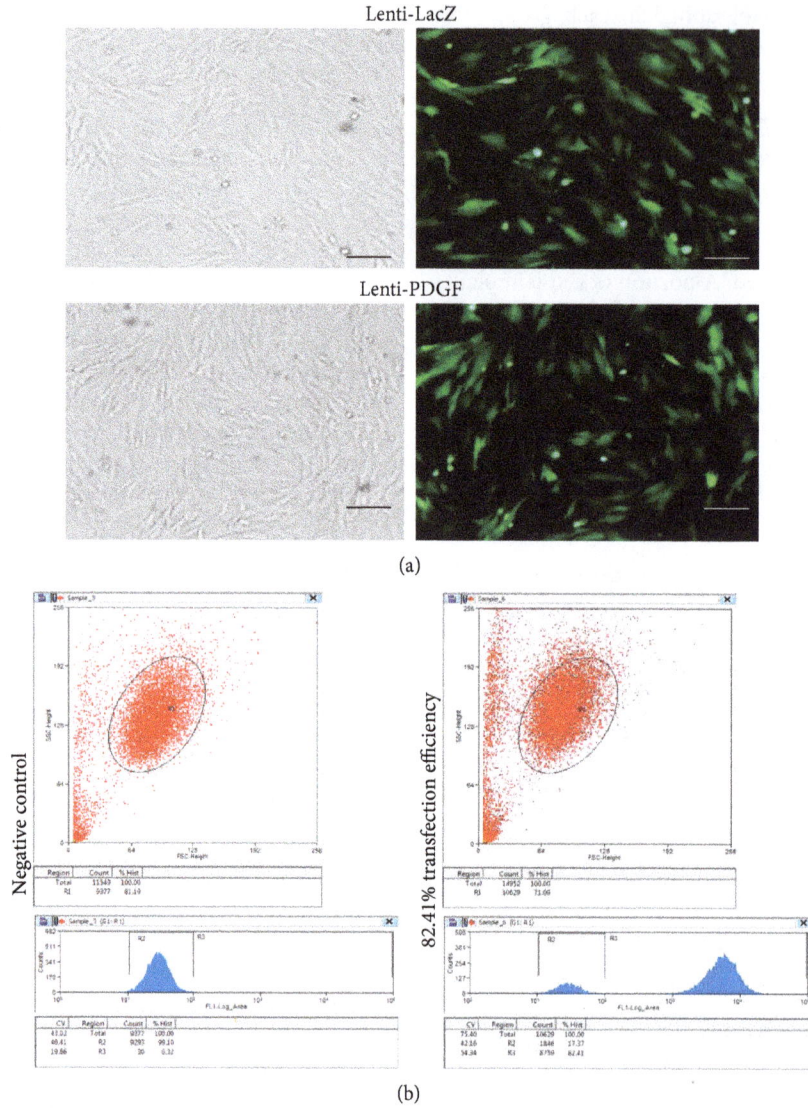

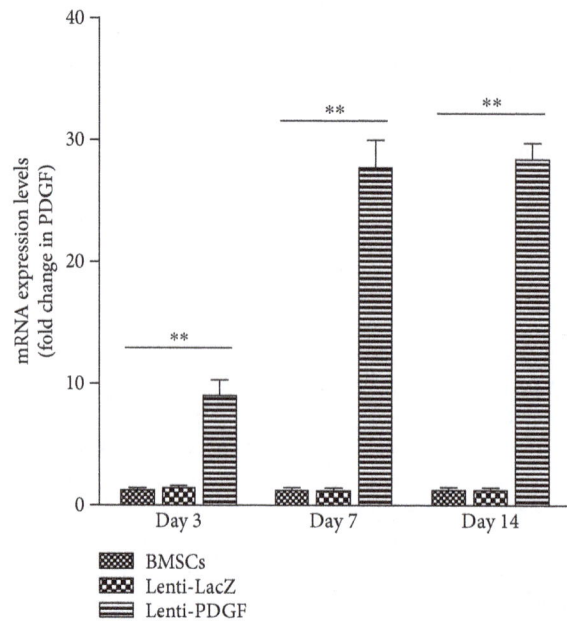

FIGURE 1: Continued.

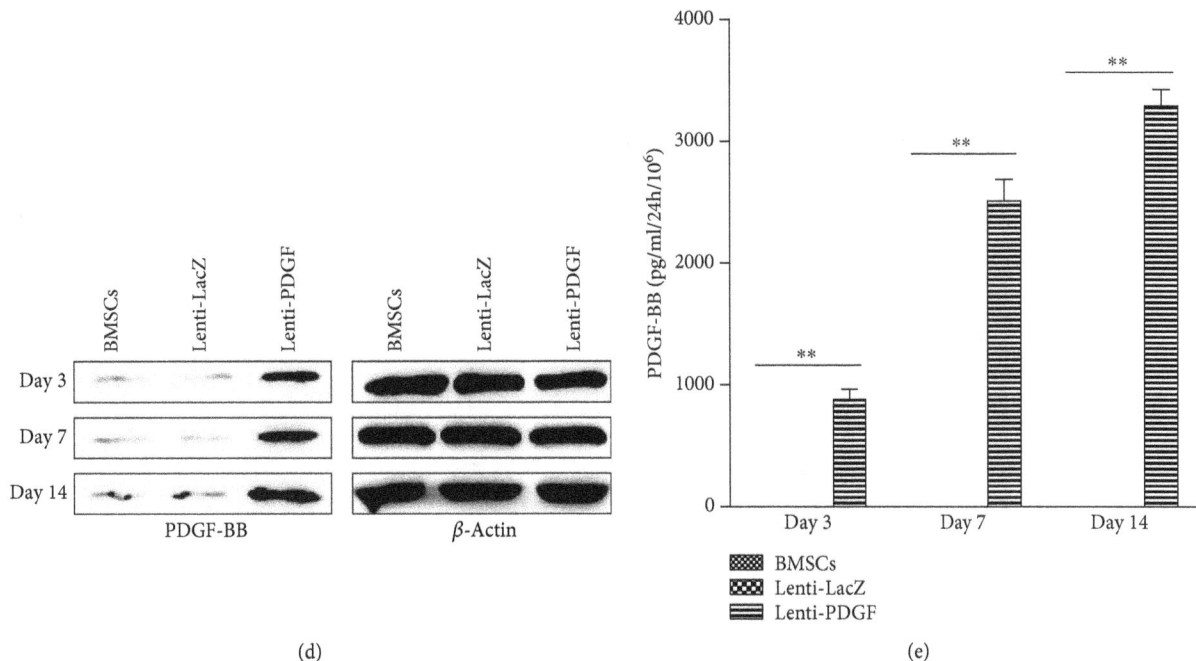

(d)

(e)

FIGURE 1: Detection of PDGF-BB expression. (a) At day 3 after gene transduction, both Lenti-LacZ-transfected and Lenti-PDGF-transfected BMSCs grew well and exhibited intense green fluorescence. (b) Flow cytometry assay showed 82.41% transfection efficiency. (c) *PDGF-B* mRNA expression in the BMSC, Lenti-LacZ, and Lenti-PDGF groups on days 3, 7, and 14. (d) PDGF-BB protein expression in the BMSC, Lenti-LacZ, and Lenti-PDGF groups on days 3, 7, and 14. (e) ELISA detection of PDGF-BB secretion *in vitro*. Scale bar: 100 μm; $^{**}P < 0.01$.

analysis showed a consistent result (Figure 2(c)). ARS staining revealed a significant increase in calcium deposition in the Lenti-PDGF group, and the quantitative analysis was consistent with the ARS staining results (Figure 2(d)).

Adipogenic differentiation analysis showed that lipid droplet accumulation was decreased significantly in the Lenti-PDGF group compared with that in the Lenti-LacZ group (Figure 3(a)). Oil Red O staining areas were remarkably decreased in the Lenti-PDGF group (Figure 3(b)). PPARγ2 mRNA and protein expression was significantly decreased in the Lenti-PDGF group compared with that in the Lenti-LacZ group (Figure 3(c), Figure 3(d)).

The ERK1/2 signaling pathway has been reported to be involved in mediating osteogenic and adipogenic differentiation of BMSCs [27, 28]. It is also known that PDGF-BB regulates the proliferation of several types of cells through the ERK1/2 signaling pathway [29, 30]. Therefore, we investigated whether this signaling pathway was activated in BMSCs by forcing PDGF-BB expression. Our results showed that the expression of phosphorylated ERK was significantly increased in PDGF-B-modified BMSCs (Figure 2(b)). The activation of the ERK1/2 signaling pathway was inhibited by administration of the inhibitor PD98059 (Figure 2(b)). The increased osteogenic differentiation and decreased adipogenic differentiation of BMSCs induced by PDGF-BB were also inhibited by administration of the inhibitor PD98059, which is an inhibitor of the ERK-MAPK signaling pathway (Figures 2 and 3). These results indicated that PDGF-BB enhances osteogenic differentiation and inhibits adipogenic differentiation of BMSCs via the ERK1/2 signaling pathway.

3.3. Effect of PDGF-BB on HUVEC Chemotactic Activity and Angiogenesis In Vitro.
PDGF is a chemoattractant and has the ability to promote angiogenesis. Thus, PDGF has been widely used for tissue regeneration and repair. As shown in Figure 4(a), PDGF-BB secreted by PDGF-modified BMSCs strongly stimulated the migration of HUVECs. An approximately 2.5-fold stimulatory effect was observed in the supernatant from the Lenti-PDGF group compared with that from the Lenti-LacZ group (Figure 4(b)). The PI3K/AKT and ERK1/2 signaling pathways are involved in PDGF-induced migration in various cell types [31–35]. To further confirm whether PDGF-BB secreted by PDGF-B-modified BMSCs activates the intracellular pathway of HUVECs, the cells were pretreated with supernatant from the Lenti-PDGF group. The results showed that the expression of phosphorylated AKT and phosphorylated ERK was significantly increased, and their activation was inhibited by the corresponding inhibitor LY294002 or PD98059 (Figure 4(c)). In addition, the inhibitors significantly reduced the chemotactic effect of PDGF-BB secreted by PDGF-B-modified BMSCs on HUVECs (Figure 4(a), Figure 4(b)). *In vitro* angiogenesis analysis revealed that a significantly increased number of mesh formed by HUVEC structures were present in the Lenti-PDGF group compared with that in the Lenti-LacZ group after 12 h of culture (Figure 4(d), Figure 4(e)). The stimulatory effects were inhibited by the addition of the inhibitor LY294002 or inhibitor PD98059 (Figures 4(d) and 4(e)).

3.4. Cell Attachment and Viability on a CPC Scaffold.
Cell attachment and growth of BMSCs seeded on porous CPC

(a)

(b)

(c)

(d)

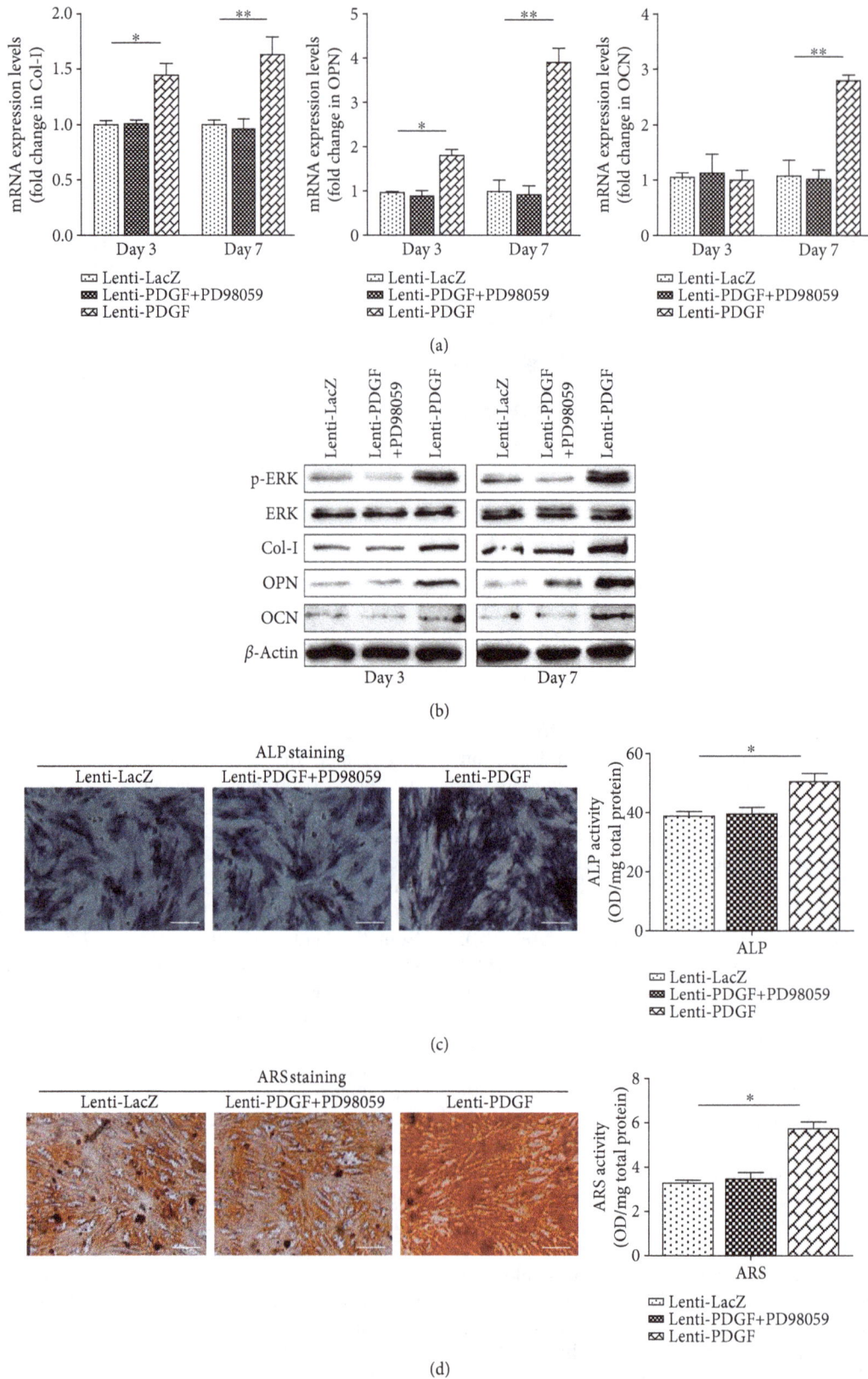

FIGURE 2: PDGF-BB enhanced BMSC osteogenic differentiation via ERK1/2 signaling pathways. (a) mRNA expression levels of *Col-I*, *OPN*, and *OCN* on days 3 and 7. (b) Protein expression levels of p-ERK, ERK, Col-I, OPN, and OCN on days 3 and 7. (c) ALP staining and semiquantitative analysis of ALP activity. (d) ARS staining and semiquantitative analysis of ARS staining. ALP: alkaline phosphatase; ARS: alizarin red S. Scale bar: 100 μm; $^{*}P < 0.05$; $^{**}P < 0.01$.

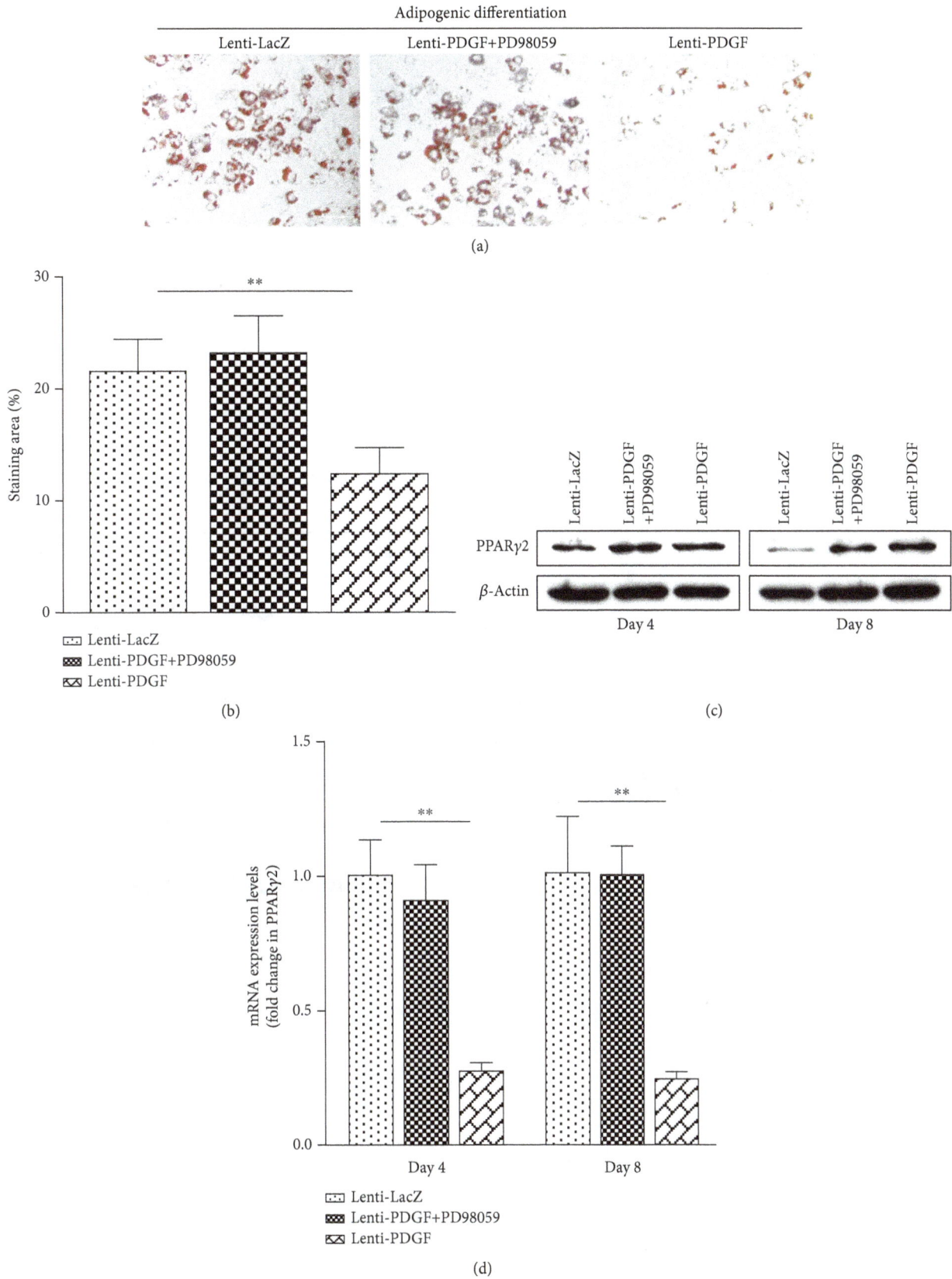

FIGURE 3: PDGF-BB inhibited BMSC adipogenic differentiation via ERK1/2 signaling pathways. (a) Oil Red O staining. (b) Oil Red O positively stained area in each group. (c) PPARγ2 protein expression. (d) *PPARγ2* mRNA expression. **$P < 0.01$; scale bar: $100\,\mu$m.

HUVEC migration

Lenti-LacZ

Lenti-PDGF

Lenti-PDGF
+LY294002

Lenti-PDGF
+PD98059

(a)

(b)

Lenti-LacZ
Lenti-PDGF+PD98059
Lenti-PDGF+LY294002
Lenti-PDGF

(c)

Lenti-LacZ   Lenti-PDGF   Lenti-PDGF+LY294002   Lenti-PDGF+PD98059

Super-
natant

Image J

(d)

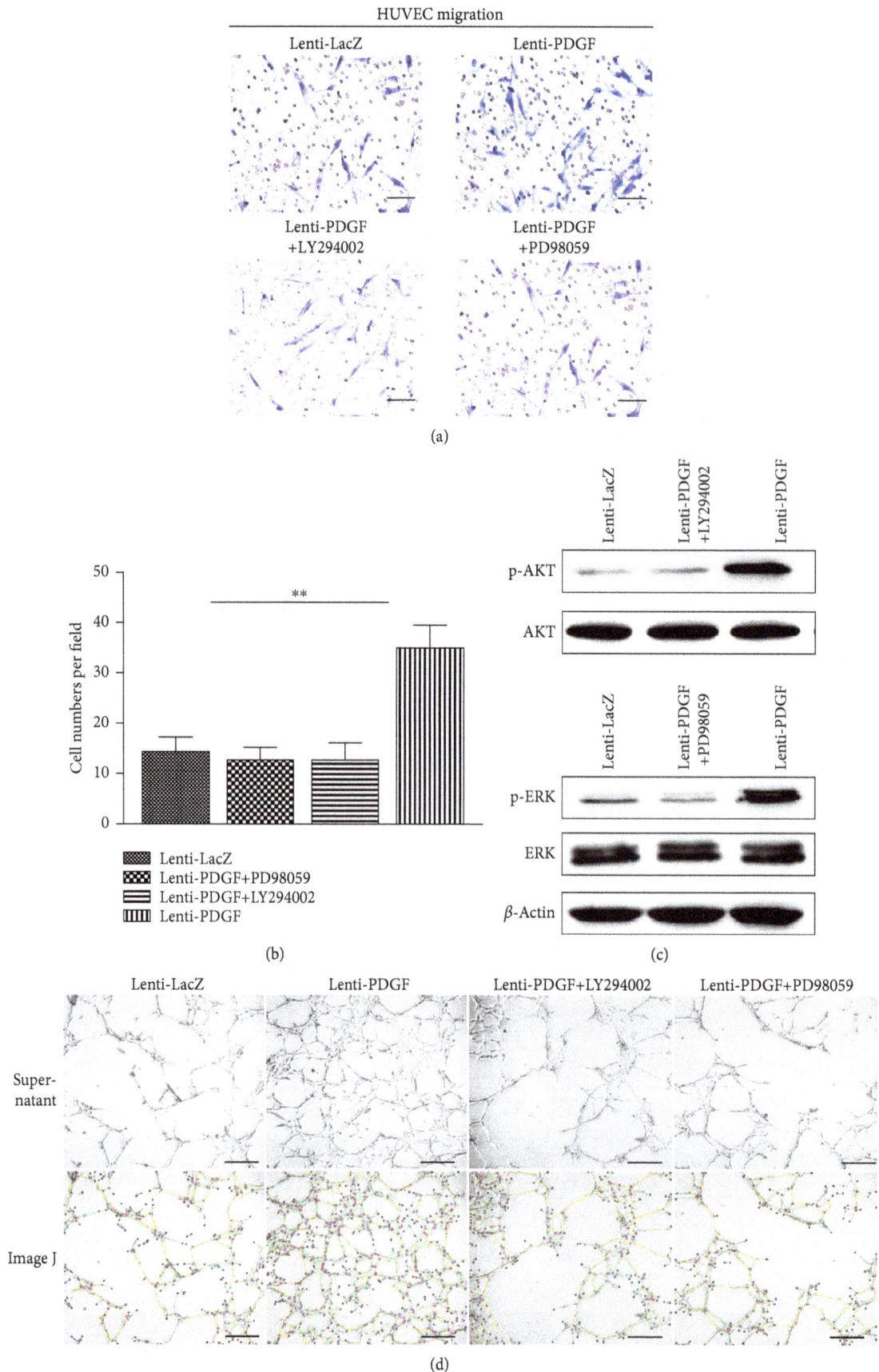

FIGURE 4: Continued.

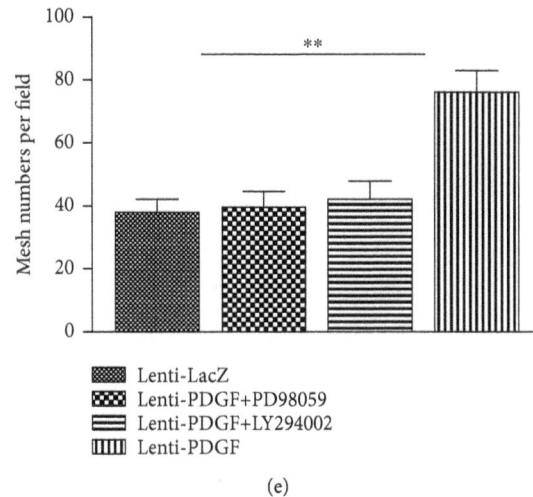

(e)

FIGURE 4: PDGF-BB secreted by Lenti-PDGF-B-modified BMSCs enhanced HUVEC migration and angiogenesis via the PI3K/AKT and ERK1/2 signaling pathways. (a) HUVECs on chemotaxis membranes stained with hematoxylin. (b) Cell numbers in each field. (c) PDGF-BB secreted by PDGF-B-modified-BMSCs induced ERK and AKT activation in HUVECs. (d) Optical images of HUVECs cultured on Matrigel with different supernatants after 12 h (upper panel); in the lower panel, ImageJ was used to measure the mesh number formed by HUVECs (green circle indicated mesh structure formed by HUVECs). (e) The mesh numbers in each group. $**P < 0.01$; scale bar: 100 μm. HUVECs: human umbilical vein endothelial cells.

scaffolds were examined via SEM. As shown in Figure 5(a), CPC scaffolds showed an average pore diameter of 300–500 μm. After being cultured for 1 day *in vitro*, BMSCs attached and spread well on the surface of the CPC scaffolds. When cultured for 3 days *in vitro*, the cells grew well and formed cellular connections (Figure 5(b)). These results demonstrate that porous CPC scaffolds possess good biocompatibility, making them suitable for the following *in vivo* study. Figure 5(c) shows the surgical procedure employed for the *in vivo* transplantation.

3.5. Radiography and Micro-CT Measurement. X-ray images were taken at 8 weeks after explantation of the skull, and representative photographs of each group are shown in Figure 6(a). In the Lenti-PDGF group, the implants were closely integrated with the surrounding bone tissue and more radiopaque. In contrast, more radiotransparent areas were observed in the CPC group, BMSC group, and Lent-LacZ group. The morphology of newly formed bone was also reconstructed using micro-CT, and the three-dimensional (3D) reconstruction images of the skulls showed results consistent with the X-ray images (Figure 6(b)). From the transverse view, there was more newly formed bone tissue in the Lenti-PDGF group than in the CPC group, BMSC group, and Lenti-LacZ group (Figure 6(b)). Quantitative analysis showed that the BMD in the BMSC group (0.81 ± 0.04) and Lenti-LacZ group (0.80 ± 0.08) was higher than that in the CPC group (0.06 ± 0.57). The Lenti-PDGF group showed the highest BMD value (1.04 ± 0.13) among all the groups (Figure 6(c)). The BV/TV percentage in all groups (CPC, 7.00 ± 1.32; BMSCs, 16.00 ± 3.00; Lenti-LacZ, 15.67 ± 3.79; and Lenti-PDGF, 26.33 ± 3.51) was consistent with the BMD levels (Figure 6(d)).

3.6. Histological Analysis of Bone Regeneration. The undecalcified calvarial bone specimens from each group were stained with Van Gieson's picro fuchsin, and the decalcified specimens were stained for histological analysis. The results showed that newly formed bone tissue was present in all groups. However, the amount of newly formed bone tissue varied among the groups. More new bone tissue formation was observed in the Lenti-PDGF group than in the CPC, BMSC, and Lenti-LacZ groups, which was consistent with the radiography and micro-CT results (Figure 7(a)). Histomorphometric analysis showed that the percentage of new bone area was $6.33 \pm 1.52\%$ in the CPC group, $12.33 \pm 2.51\%$ in the BMSC group, $12.50 \pm 2.78\%$ in the Lenti-LacZ group, and $22.66 \pm 2.08\%$ in the Lenti-PDGF group (Figure 7(b)). These results indicate that PDGF-B-modified BMSCs significantly enhanced bone regeneration capacity in the calvarial bone defect model. To assess vascularization, Microfil perfusion was performed. As shown in Figure 7(a), each blue spot (green arrow) represents a blood vessel. HE staining also showed that the newly formed bone tissue was infiltrated with blood vessels (green arrow) with intraluminal red blood cells (Figure 7(a)). The area of newly formed blood vessels stained by Microfil perfusion was $0.66 \pm 0.15\%$ in the CPC group, $1.46 \pm 0.25\%$ in the BMSC group, $1.48 \pm 0.36\%$ in the Lenti-LacZ group, and $2.70 \pm 0.26\%$ in the Lenti-PDGF group (Figure 7(c)).

4. Discussion

In this study, we established a PDGF-B-modified BMSC line using a lentivirus vector to investigate the mechanism underlying PDGF-BB regulation of stem cell-based bone regeneration. Several studies have demonstrated that the ERK1/2

CPC scaffold

(a)

Cell attachment

Day 1   Day 3

(b)

Surgical procedure

(c)

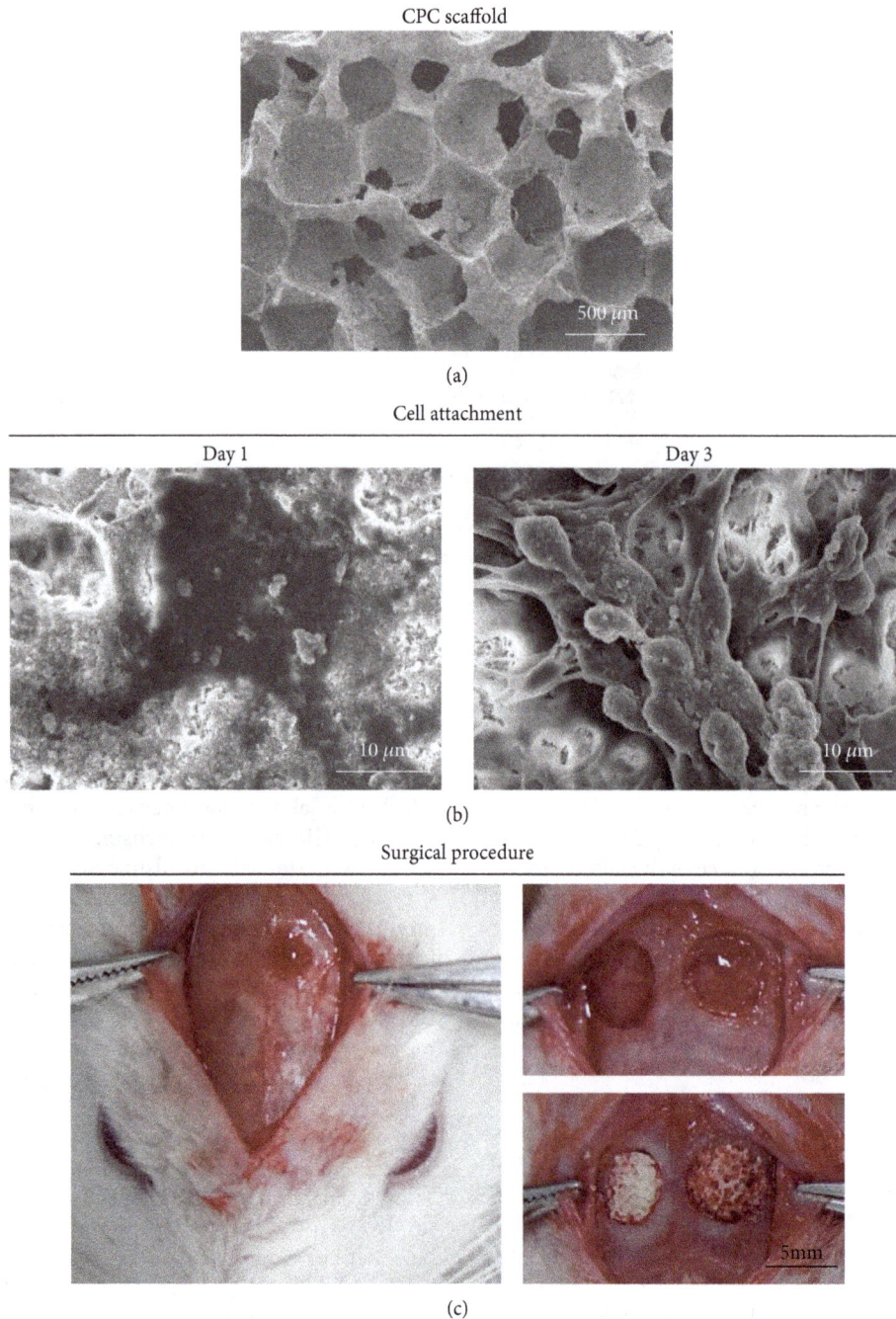

FIGURE 5: SEM analysis and surgical procedure. (a) SEM evaluation of porous CPC scaffold showing an average pore diameter of 300–500 μm. (b) BMSCs attached and spread well on CPC scaffolds. (c) Surgical procedure. CPC: calcium phosphate cement.

signaling pathway is involved in regulating osteogenic and adipogenic differentiation of MSCs [36]. Cell differentiation requires sustained activation of ERK, and transient activation of ERK leads to proliferation [37]. It is also known that PDGF-BB regulates the proliferation of several types of cells through the ERK1/2 signaling pathway [29, 30]. Thus, we speculated that continuous PDGF-BB expression may influence BMSC differentiation via the ERK signaling pathway. As we expected, forced expression of PDGF-BB in BMSCs activated the ERK signaling pathway, evidenced by the

significantly increased expression of phosphorylated ERK in PDGF-B-modified BMSCs. Osteogenic-related markers, such as Col-I, OPN, and OCN, were upregulated by PDGF-BB. ALP activity and calcium deposition were also significantly increased by PDGF-BB overexpression. However, the enhanced osteogenic differentiation of PDGF-B-modified BMSCs was inhibited by the addition of PD98059, an inhibitor of the ERK-MAPK signaling pathway. It is well known that increased adipogenesis in the bone marrow decreases osteogenesis, which results in osteoporosis. The balance

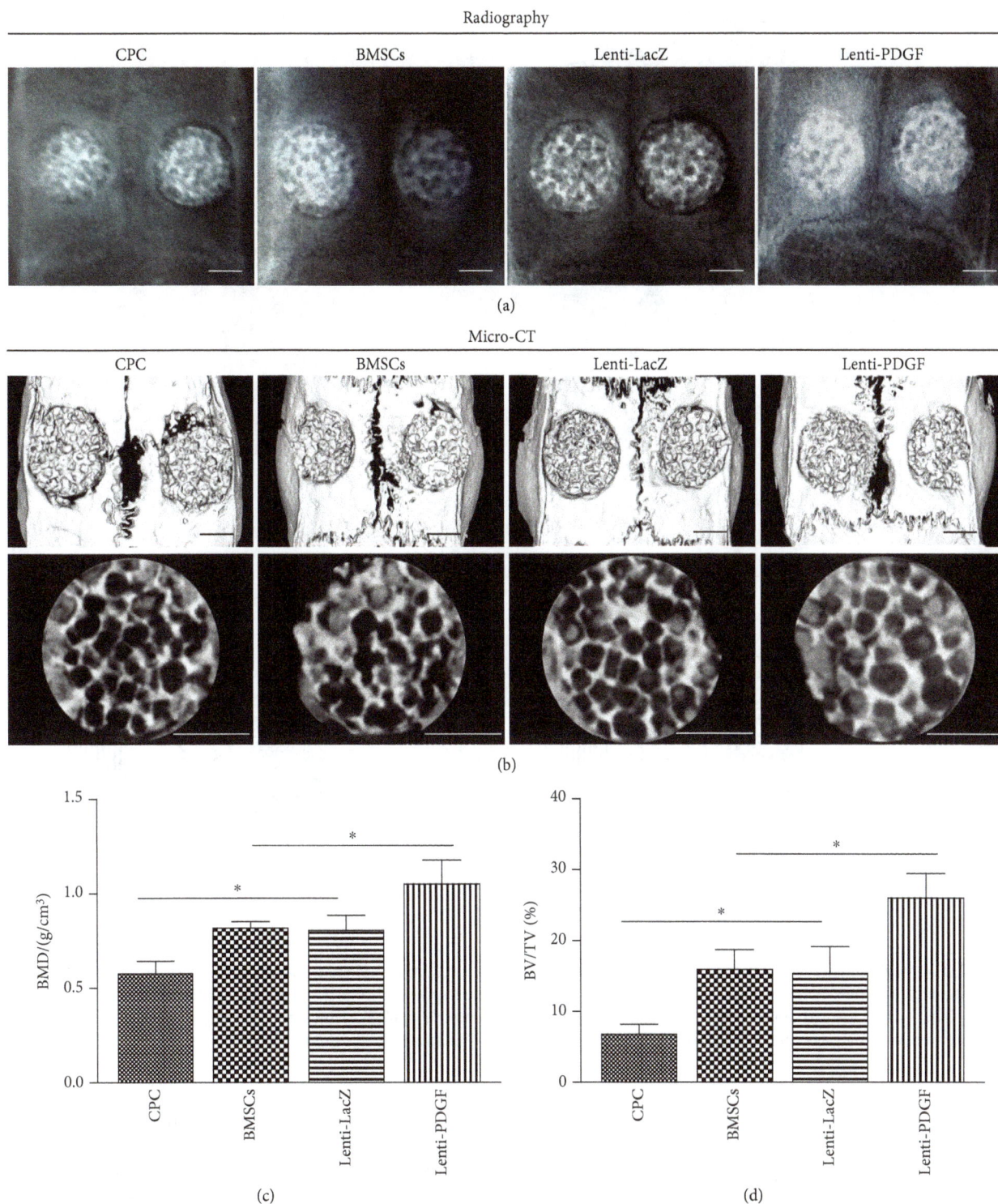

FIGURE 6: Radiography and micro-CT analysis. (a) Radiographic evaluation of the repaired skulls at 8 weeks. (b) 3D reconstruction images showing the reparative effect of the CPC, CPC with BMSCs, CPC with Lenti-LacZ-modified BMSCs, and CPC with PDGF-B-modified BMSCs. (c, d) Bone mineral density (BMD) and bone volume/total volume (BV/TV) analysis in each group. Scale bar: 2 mm; $^{*}P < 0.05$.

between osteogenic and adipogenic MSC differentiation is important for maintaining bone homeostasis [38]. Previous studies have demonstrated that PDGFRα signaling opposes adipogenesis of several types of cell [39, 40]. In this study,

adipogenic differentiation of PDGF-B-modified BMSCs was also evaluated. Oil Red O staining area and lipid droplet accumulation were significantly decreased in PDGF-B-modified BMSCs. The expression of PPARγ2, a nuclear

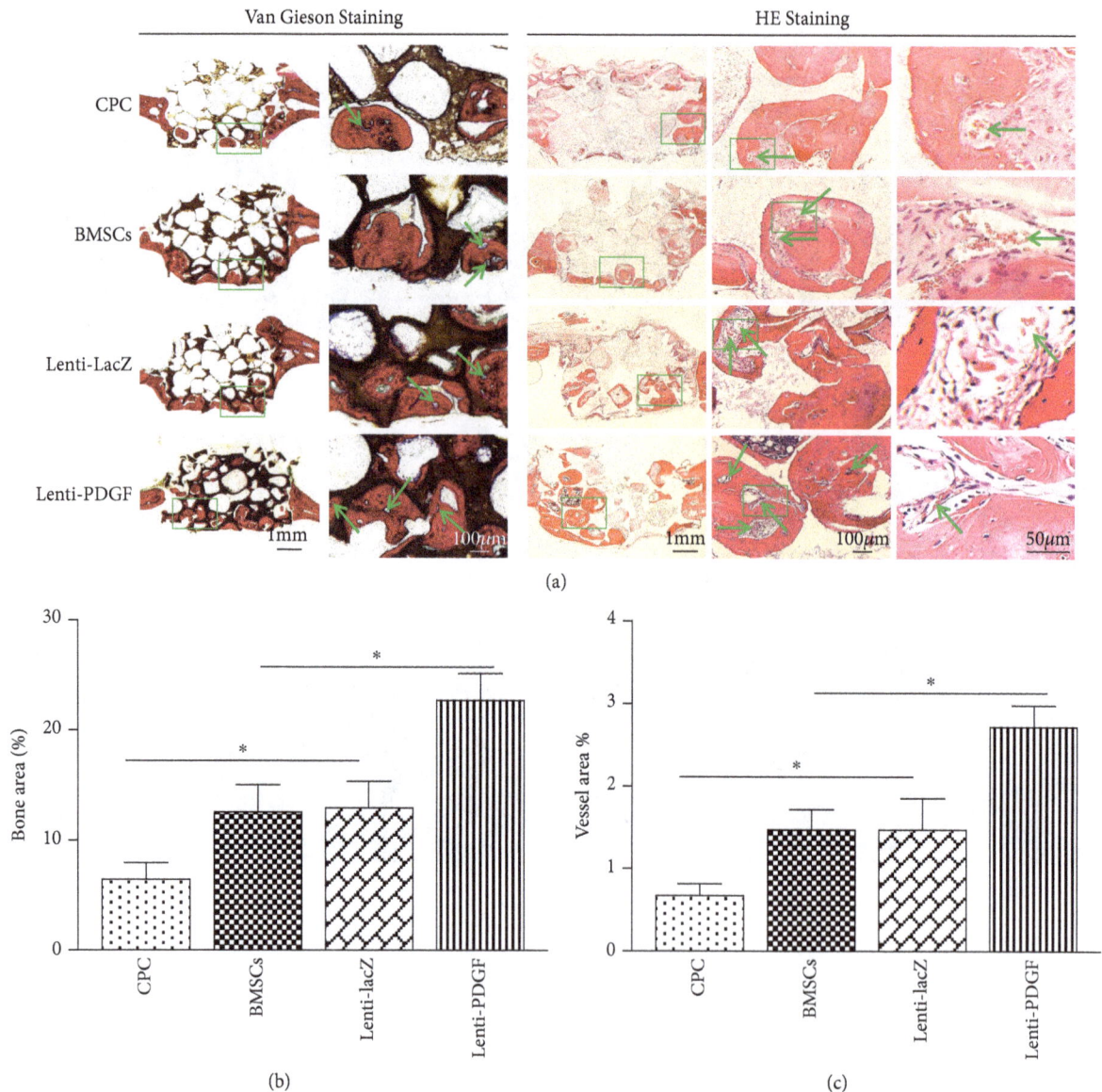

FIGURE 7: Histological analysis of newly formed bone and blood vessel in implants. (a) Histological images of each group. Left panel: Van Gieson staining, the new bone appears red, CPC appears black, and blue spots indicate blood vessels (green arrow); right panel: HE staining. The newly formed bone tissue was infiltrated with blood vessels (green arrow) with intraluminal red blood cells. (b) Histomorphometric analysis of the newly formed bone area. (c) Histomorphometric analysis of newly formed vessel area. $*P < 0.05$.

receptor that can activate the expression of adipocyte phenotype-specific genes [41, 42], in PDGF-B-modified BMSCs was significantly decreased both at mRNA and protein levels. However, the inhibitory effect of PDGF-BB on BMSC adipogenic differentiation was inhibited by the addition of PD98059. Taken together, our results indicate that PDGF-BB can increase osteogenic differentiation while inhibiting adipogenic differentiation of BMSCs via ERK1/2 signaling pathways.

One of the key mechanisms by which stem cells promote tissue regeneration is secretion of soluble growth factors [43–46]. Previous studies have shown that PDGF-BB secreted by preosteoclasts induces vessel formation during bone modeling and remodeling [47]. After the lentiviral gene

transduction, ELISA results showed that BMSCs stably and continuously secreted PDGF-BB. We further confirmed via HUVEC migration and angiogenesis assays that the secreted PDGF-BB protein possessed chemotactic activity and angiogenic activity. These results demonstrated that PDGF-BB secreted by PDGF-B-modified BMSCs stimulates the migration and angiogenic potential of HUVECs via the PI3K/AKT and ERK1/2 signaling pathways, which may further facilitate BMSC-based bone regeneration.

The effects of PDGF-BB on the regulation of BMSC-based bone regeneration *in vivo* were evaluated using a rat critical-sized calvarial defect model. Radiography and micro-CT measurements revealed that the implants were closely integrated with the surrounding bone tissue and more radiopaque in the PDGF-BB overexpression group. According to the transverse view of the micro-CT, more newly formed bone tissue was present in the Lenti-PDGF group than in the other groups. Quantitative analysis showed that the BMD and BV/TV values were higher in the Lenti-PDGF group than those in the other groups. Histomorphometric analysis showed results consistent with the above findings, and the percentage of new bone area was significantly higher in the PDGF-BB-overexpressing group. Bone formation is driven by the presence of vasculature, and the formation of new vasculature, which transports oxygen, nutrients, and soluble factors, is necessary for new bone regeneration [25]. The area of newly formed blood vessels stained by Microfil perfusion was remarkably increased in the PDGF-BB-overexpressing group compared with that in the other groups. HE staining also showed that the newly formed bone tissue was infiltrated with blood vessels with intraluminal red blood cells. As described above, PDGF-BB is well known for its ability to promote angiogenesis, and it also plays an important role in maintaining the stabilization of newly formed blood vessels [11, 48, 49]. Thus, PDGF-BB secreted by PDGF-B-modified BMSCs would likely promote angiogenesis to facilitate bone regeneration.

5. Conclusions

In summary, our results demonstrated that overexpression of PDGF-BB in BMSCs increases osteogenic differentiation while inhibiting adipogenic differentiation via the ERK1/2 signaling pathway. PDGF-BB secreted by the PDGF-B-modified BMSCs significantly enhanced the migration and angiogenesis of vascular endothelial cells via the PI3K/AKT and ERK1/2 signaling pathways. The enhanced angiogenesis and osteogenesis capacity of BMSCs induced by PDGF-BB overexpression could promote *in vivo* vascularized bone regeneration. These findings indicate that PDGF-BB would be a powerful therapeutic regulator of angiogenesis and osteogenesis during bone formation and repair.

Authors' Contributions

Maolin Zhang and Wenwen Yu have contributed equally to this work.

Acknowledgments

This work was jointly supported by The National Key Research and Development Program of China (2016YFC1102900), the National Natural Science Foundation of China (81620108006).

References

[1] S. P. Bruder, A. A. Kurth, M. Shea, W. C. Hayes, N. Jaiswal, and S. Kadiyala, "Bone regeneration by implantation of purified, culture-expanded human mesenchymal stem cells," *Journal of Orthopaedic Research*, vol. 16, no. 2, pp. 155–162, 1998.

[2] X. Jiang, J. Zhao, S. Wang et al., "Mandibular repair in rats with premineralized silk scaffolds and BMP-2-modified bMSCs," *Biomaterials*, vol. 30, no. 27, pp. 4522–4532, 2009.

[3] H. Hou, X. Zhang, T. Tang, K. Dai, and R. Ge, "Enhancement of bone formation by genetically-engineered bone marrow stromal cells expressing BMP-2, VEGF and angiopoietin-1," *Biotechnology Letters*, vol. 31, no. 8, pp. 1183–1189, 2009.

[4] M. Tallquist and A. Kazlauskas, "PDGF signaling in cells and mice," *Cytokine & Growth Factor Reviews*, vol. 15, no. 4, pp. 205–213, 2004.

[5] R. M. Manzat Saplacan, L. Balacescu, C. Gherman et al., "The role of PDGFs and PDGFRs in colorectal cancer," *Mediators of Inflammation*, vol. 2017, 9 pages, 2017.

[6] L. Fredriksson, H. Li, and U. Eriksson, "The PDGF family: four gene products form five dimeric isoforms," *Cytokine & Growth Factor Reviews*, vol. 15, no. 4, pp. 197–204, 2004.

[7] R. Gruber, F. Karreth, F. Frommlet, M. B. Fischer, and G. Watzek, "Platelets are mitogenic for periosteum-derived cells," *Journal of Orthopaedic Research*, vol. 21, no. 5, pp. 941–948, 2003.

[8] M. H. Lee, B.-J. Kwon, M.-A. Koo, K. E. You, and J.-C. Park, "Mitogenesis of vascular smooth muscle cell stimulated by platelet-derived growth factor-bb is inhibited by blocking of intracellular signaling by epigallocatechin-3-O-gallate," *Oxidative Medicine and Cellular Longevity*, vol. 2013, Article ID 827905, 10 pages, 2013.

[9] Y. Ozaki, M. Nishimura, K. Sekiya et al., "Comprehensive analysis of chemotactic factors for bone marrow mesenchymal stem cells," *Stem Cells and Development*, vol. 16, no. 1, pp. 119–130, 2007.

[10] C. H. Heldin and B. Westermark, "Mechanism of action and in vivo role of platelet-derived growth factor," *Physiological Reviews*, vol. 79, no. 4, pp. 1283–1316, 1999.

[11] J. Homsi and A. I. Daud, "Spectrum of activity and mechanism of action of VEGF/PDGF inhibitors," *Cancer Control*, vol. 14, no. 3, pp. 285–294, 2007.

[12] M. C. Phipps, Y. Xu, and S. L. Bellis, "Delivery of platelet-derived growth factor as a chemotactic factor for mesenchymal stem cells by bone-mimetic electrospun scaffolds," *PLoS One*, vol. 7, no. 7, article e40831, 2012.

[13] A. I. Caplan and D. Correa, "PDGF in bone formation and regeneration: new insights into a novel mechanism involving MSCs," *Journal of Orthopaedic Research*, vol. 29, no. 12, pp. 1795–1803, 2011.

[14] L. Xu, W. Zhang, K. Lv, W. Yu, X. Jiang, and F. Zhang, "Peri-implant bone regeneration using rhPDGF-BB, BMSCs, and β-TCP in a canine model," *Clinical Implant Dentistry and Related Research*, vol. 18, no. 2, pp. 241–252, 2016.

[15] D. F. Bowen-Pope, T. W. Malpass, D. M. Foster, and R. Ross, "Platelet-derived growth factor in vivo: levels, activity, and rate of clearance," *Blood*, vol. 64, no. 2, pp. 458–469, 1984.

[16] C. Zhu, Q. Chang, D. Zou et al., "LvBMP-2 gene-modified BMSCs combined with calcium phosphate cement scaffolds for the repair of calvarial defects in rats," *Journal of Materials Science: Materials in Medicine*, vol. 22, no. 8, pp. 1965–1973, 2011.

[17] W. Zhang, X. Zhang, S. Wang et al., "Comparison of the use of adipose tissue-derived and bone marrow-derived stem cells for rapid bone regeneration," *Journal of Dental Research*, vol. 92, no. 12, pp. 1136–1141, 2013.

[18] W. Zhang, C. Zhu, D. Ye et al., "Porous silk scaffolds for delivery of growth factors and stem cells to enhance bone regeneration," *PLoS One*, vol. 9, no. 7, article e102371, 2014.

[19] M. Zhang, F. Jiang, X. Zhang et al., "The effects of platelet-derived growth factor-BB on human dental pulp stem cells mediated dentin-pulp complex regeneration," *Stem Cells Translational Medicine*, vol. 6, no. 12, pp. 2126–2134, 2017.

[20] L. Xia, M. Zhang, Q. Chang et al., "Enhanced dentin-like mineralized tissue formation by AdShh-transfected human dental pulp cells and porous calcium phosphate cement," *PLoS One*, vol. 8, no. 5, article e62645, 2013.

[21] Y. Jin, W. Zhang, Y. Liu et al., "rhPDGF-BB via ERK pathway osteogenesis and adipogenesis balancing in ADSCs for critical-sized calvarial defect repair," *Tissue Engineering Part A*, vol. 20, no. 23-24, pp. 3303–3313, 2014.

[22] K. Lin, L. Xia, H. Li et al., "Enhanced osteoporotic bone regeneration by strontium-substituted calcium silicate bioactive ceramics," *Biomaterials*, vol. 34, no. 38, pp. 10028–10042, 2013.

[23] Y. Zhao, D. L. Zeng, L. G. Xia et al., "Osteogenic potential of bone marrow stromal cells derived from streptozotocin-induced diabetic rats," *International Journal of Molecular Medicine*, vol. 31, no. 3, pp. 614–620, 2013.

[24] D. Zou, Z. Zhang, D. Ye et al., "Repair of critical-sized rat calvarial defects using genetically engineered bone marrow-derived mesenchymal stem cells overexpressing hypoxia-inducible factor-1α," *Stem Cells*, vol. 29, no. 9, pp. 1380–1390, 2011.

[25] D. Zou, Z. Zhang, J. He et al., "Blood vessel formation in the tissue-engineered bone with the constitutively active form of HIF-1α mediated BMSCs," *Biomaterials*, vol. 33, no. 7, pp. 2097–2108, 2012.

[26] Y. Deng, H. Zhou, D. Zou et al., "The role of miR-31-modified adipose tissue-derived stem cells in repairing rat critical-sized calvarial defects," *Biomaterials*, vol. 34, no. 28, pp. 6717–6728, 2013.

[27] L. Fu, T. Tang, Y. Miao, S. Zhang, Z. Qu, and K. Dai, "Stimulation of osteogenic differentiation and inhibition of adipogenic differentiation in bone marrow stromal cells by alendronate via ERK and JNK activation," *Bone*, vol. 43, no. 1, pp. 40–47, 2008.

[28] Y. Zhao, S. Zhang, D. Zeng et al., "rhPDGF-BB promotes proliferation and osteogenic differentiation of bone marrow stromal cells from streptozotocin-induced diabetic rats through ERK pathway," *BioMed Research International*, vol. 2014, 9 pages, 2014.

[29] K. Kingsley, J. L. Huff, W. L. Rust et al., "ERK1/2 mediates PDGF-BB stimulated vascular smooth muscle cell proliferation and migration on laminin-5," *Biochemical and Biophysical Research*, vol. 293, no. 3, pp. 1000–1006, 2002.

[30] E. J. Battegay, J. Rupp, L. Iruela-Arispe, E. H. Sage, and M. Pech, "PDGF-BB modulates endothelial proliferation and angiogenesis in vitro via PDGF beta-receptors," *The Journal of Cell Biology*, vol. 125, no. 4, pp. 917–928, 1994.

[31] J. Fiedler, G. Röderer, K. P. Günther, and R. E. Brenner, "BMP-2, BMP-4, and PDGF-bb stimulate chemotactic migration of primary human mesenchymal progenitor cells," *Journal of Cellular Biochemistry*, vol. 87, no. 3, pp. 305–312, 2002.

[32] X. Sun, X. Gao, L. Zhou, L. Sun, and C. Lu, "PDGF-BB-induced MT1-MMP expression regulates proliferation and invasion of mesenchymal stem cells in 3-dimensional collagen via MEK/ERK1/2 and PI3K/AKT signaling," *Cellular Signalling*, vol. 25, no. 5, pp. 1279–1287, 2013.

[33] L. J. Yuan, C. C. Niu, S. S. Lin et al., "Additive effects of hyperbaric oxygen and platelet-derived growth factor-BB in chondrocyte transplantation via up-regulation expression of platelet-derived growth factor-beta receptor," *Journal of Orthopaedic Research*, vol. 27, no. 11, pp. 1439–1446, 2009.

[34] Y. J. Kang, E. S. Jeon, H. Y. Song et al., "Role of c-Jun N-terminal kinase in the PDGF-induced proliferation and migration of human adipose tissue-derived mesenchymal stem cells," *Journal of Cellular Biochemistry*, vol. 95, no. 6, pp. 1135–1145, 2005.

[35] D. Gentilini, M. Busacca, S. di Francesco, M. Vignali, P. Viganò, and A. M. di Blasio, "PI3K/Akt and ERK1/2 signalling pathways are involved in endometrial cell migration induced by 17β-estradiol and growth factors," *Molecular Human Reproduction*, vol. 13, no. 5, pp. 317–322, 2007.

[36] R. K. Jaiswal, N. Jaiswal, S. P. Bruder, G. Mbalaviele, D. R. Marshak, and M. F. Pittenger, "Adult human mesenchymal stem cell differentiation to the osteogenic or adipogenic lineage is regulated by mitogen-activated protein kinase," *The Journal of Biological Chemistry*, vol. 275, no. 13, pp. 9645–9652, 2000.

[37] C. J. Marshall, "Specificity of receptor tyrosine kinase signaling: transient versus sustained extracellular signal-regulated kinase activation," *Cell*, vol. 80, no. 2, pp. 179–185, 1995.

[38] J. Dragojevič, D. B. Logar, R. Komadina, and J. Marc, "Osteoblastogenesis and adipogenesis are higher in osteoarthritic than in osteoporotic bone tissue," *Archives of Medical Research*, vol. 42, no. 5, pp. 392–397, 2011.

[39] T. Iwayama, C. Steele, L. Yao et al., "PDGFRα signaling drives adipose tissue fibrosis by targeting progenitor cell plasticity," *Genes & Development*, vol. 29, no. 11, pp. 1106–1119, 2015.

[40] C. Sun, W. L. Berry, and L. E. Olson, "PDGFRα controls the balance of stromal and adipogenic cells during adipose tissue organogenesis," *Development*, vol. 144, no. 1, pp. 83–94, 2017.

[41] E. D. Rosen, P. Sarraf, A. E. Troy et al., "PPAR gamma is required for the differentiation of adipose tissue in vivo and in vitro," *Molecular Cell*, vol. 4, no. 4, pp. 611–617, 1999.

[42] Y. Barak, M. C. Nelson, E. S. Ong et al., "PPAR gamma is required for placental, cardiac, and adipose tissue development," *Molecular Cell*, vol. 4, no. 4, pp. 585–595, 1999.

[43] B. Parekkadan, D. van Poll, K. Suganuma et al., "Mesenchymal stem cell-derived molecules reverse fulminant hepatic failure," *PLoS One*, vol. 2, no. 9, article e941, 2007.

[44] A. I. Caplan and J. E. Dennis, "Mesenchymal stem cells as trophic mediators," *Journal of Cellular Biochemistry*, vol. 98, no. 5, pp. 1076–1084, 2006.

[45] S. Aggarwal and M. F. Pittenger, "Human mesenchymal stem cells modulate allogeneic immune cell responses," *Blood*, vol. 105, no. 4, pp. 1815–1822, 2005.

[46] T. Kinnaird, E. Stabile, M. S. Burnett et al., "Local delivery of marrow-derived stromal cells augments collateral perfusion through paracrine mechanisms," *Circulation*, vol. 109, no. 12, pp. 1543–1549, 2004.

[47] H. Xie, Z. Cui, L. Wang et al., "PDGF-BB secreted by preosteoclasts induces angiogenesis during coupling with osteogenesis," *Nature Medicine*, vol. 20, no. 11, pp. 1270–1278, 2014.

[48] G. D. Yancopoulos, S. Davis, N. W. Gale, J. S. Rudge, S. J. Wiegand, and J. Holash, "Vascular-specific growth factors and blood vessel formation," *Nature*, vol. 407, no. 6801, pp. 242–248, 2000.

Radiation Induces Apoptosis and Osteogenic Impairment through miR-22-Mediated Intracellular Oxidative Stress in Bone Marrow Mesenchymal Stem Cells

Zhonglong Liu,[1] Tao Li,[2] Si'nan Deng,[3] Shuiting Fu,[1] Xiaojun Zhou◉,[2] and Yue He◉[1]

[1]Department of Oral Maxillofacial & Head and Neck Oncology, Shanghai Ninth People's Hospital Affiliated to Shanghai Jiao Tong University School of Medicine, Shanghai 200011, China
[2]Department of Orthopedics, Shanghai Ninth People's Hospital Affiliated to Shanghai Jiao Tong University School of Medicine, Shanghai 200011, China
[3]Department of Stomatology, Central Hospital of Min-Hang District, Shanghai 201109, China

Correspondence should be addressed to Xiaojun Zhou; xjz362@163.com and Yue He; eddielew@sjtu.edu.cn
Zhonglong Liu and Tao Li contributed equally to this work.

Academic Editor: Giuseppe Mandraffino

Bone marrow mesenchymal stem cells (BMSCs) were characterized by their multilineage potential and were involved in both bony and soft tissue repair. Exposure of cells to ionizing radiation (IR) triggers numerous biological reactions, including reactive oxygen species (ROS), cellular apoptosis, and impaired differentiation capacity, while the mechanisms of IR-induced BMSC apoptosis and osteogenic impairment are still unclear. Through a recent study, we found that 6 Gy IR significantly increased the apoptotic ratio and ROS generation, characterized by ROS staining and mean fluorescent intensity. Intervention with antioxidant (NAC) indicated that IR-induced cellular apoptosis was partly due to the accumulation of intracellular ROS. Furthermore, we found that the upregulation of miR-22 in rBMSCs following 6 Gy IR played an important role on the ROS generation and subsequent apoptosis. In addition, we firstly demonstrated that miR-22-mediated ROS accumulation and cell injury had an important regulated role on the osteogenic capacity of BMSCs both in vitro and in vivo. In conclusion, IR-induced overexpression of miR-22 regulated the cell viability and differentiation potential through targeting the intracellular ROS.

1. Introduction

The delivery of radiotherapy is often required in oral and maxillofacial regions to serve as a major or an adjuvant therapy for malignancies. In addition to the effective control of local disease, damaging normal bone and soft tissues within the radiation field is inevitable. Radiation-induced skeletal system injury is characterized by the destruction of osteocytes, a deficiency of osteoblasts and osteoid, bone marrow fibrosis, a lack of bone marrow mesenchymal stem cells (BMSCs), and even osteoradionecrosis [1, 2]. This complication may contribute to the loss of metabolic equilibrium in bone formation.

Ionizing radiation (IR) may sensitize the bone marrow cells and osteoblasts to apoptogens and induce the apoptotic process, thus causing profound ramifications for osteogenic function and further bone formation [3]. BMSCs are one of the major types of progenitor cell, which hold the capability to differentiate into multilineage cells, including osteoblasts, and maintain the homeostasis with osteogenesis. The topic of whether mesenchymal stem cells (MSCs) are radiosensitive or radioresistant is still controversial. Some scholars supported that MSCs show considerably high radioresistance both in vitro and in vivo [4–7], while these MSCs may be different from those derived from bone. Others verified that BMSCs were sensitive to X-ray or γ-radiation, and a small portion of these cells developed apoptosis following exposure to different dosages [8–10]. Accordingly, radiation response of MSCs is a complicated biological process, and it may depend on cell-to-cell variations and resource of radiation, thus triggering different signals or mechanisms to determine the cell fate.

IR leads to the production of oxygen-derived free radicals and reactive nonradical molecules, so-called reactive oxidative species (ROS), which may impose indirect damage onto cells when this excessive oxidative stress is beyond the scavenge ability of antioxidant detoxification systems [11, 12]. Radiation-induced ROS generation has also been proven both in vitro and in vivo studies [13, 14]. IR and UV are the most important physical factors that trigger the generation of prooxidant compounds and the production of oxidative stress [15]. Moderate ROS is deemed as an indispensable stress or molecules involved in the normal physiological reaction, whereas enhanced or excessive ROS may influence the cell survival or death fate, including proliferation and apoptosis [16]. ROS participates in cellular signal transduction and acts as the main regulator in the pathways mediating apoptosis, such as mitochondrial pathway, death receptor pathway, and endoplasmic reticulum pathway [17].

MicroRNAs (miRNAs) belong to noncoding RNAs, which are initially transcribed in the nucleus by RNA polymerase II, and have negative regulation of mRNA through degradation or posttranscriptional inhibition via binding to the $3'$-untranslated region ($3'$-UTR) of target mRNAs [18]. In recent years, miRNAs have been verified as multifunctional genes involved in the cell cycle, survival and death, proliferation, differentiation, and so on [19]. By using miRNA microarrays, several publications have validated the upregulation of miR-22 after UV or IR within hours, suggesting that gene regulation of miRNAs occurred before the transcriptional responses of mRNA [20–23]. Other scholars found that the expression of miR-22 in the human lymphoblast cell line TK6 following radiation (2 Gy) exhibited two peaks of induction (8 h and 24 h post-IR) and was fluctuant with crests and troughs [24]. However, the biological function of this expression change has not been elucidated.

Through a review of the literature, miR-22 is defined as a multifunctional biomolecule involved in proliferation, cell survival, cell cycle, tumor invasiveness, and cardioprotection [22, 25–27]. Recent studies also demonstrated that miR-22 participated in the regulation of total intracellular ROS or mitochondrial ROS regeneration [28–30]. However, it is not clear whether radiation-induced miR-22 expression has a role on the regulation of IR-induced production of ROS and cellular apoptosis and subsequently osteogenic impairment. The current study was designed to elucidate the relationship of miR-22 with ROS and apoptosis, as well as the osteogenesis of BMSCs following radiation.

2. Material and Methods

2.1. Reagents and Chemicals. Annexin V-FITC/PI detection kit was purchased from BD Biosciences (San Jose, CA, USA). Fluorometric Intracellular ROS Kit and N-acetyl-L-cysteine (NAC) were from Sigma-Aldrich (St. Louis, USA). Information of primary antibodies is listed as follows: anti-Runx2 (1:500, Abcam), anti-Osterix (1:500, Abcam), anti-OPN (1:1000, Abcam), anti-BSP (1:1000, CST), anti-

OCN (1:500, Abcam), anti-NADPH oxidase 4 (NOX4) (1:500, Abcam), anti-SOD2 (1:500, Abcam), anti-Caspase-3 (1:1000, CST), and anti-GAPDH (1:5000, Bioworld Technology Inc., USA). ALP staining and alizarin red were both from Cyagen (Guangzhou, China). For semiquantitative analysis, p-nitrophenyl phosphate (p-NPP) and 10% cetylpyridinium chloride were from Sigma-Aldrich (St. Louis, USA). Alexa Fluor 488 conjugated was from Jackson ImmunoResearch (USA). DAPI was from Sigma-Aldrich (St. Louis, USA). For scaffold fabrication, gelatin, carboxymethyl chitosan, 1-ethyl-3-(3-dimethylaminopropyl)carbodiimide hydrochloride (EDC), and N-hydroxysuccinimide (NHS) were all purchased from Aladdin (Shanghai, China). Calcein AM (4 mM) and Lipofectamine 3000 were from Thermo Fisher Scientific (USA).

2.2. Rat BMSC (rBMSC) Isolation and In Vitro Culture. The current study was approved by the Ethics Committee of Shanghai Ninth People's Hospital. Male 4-week-old Sprague-Dawley rats were obtained from the Department of Experimental Animals in our institution. The SD rats were sacrificed through cervical dislocation and then were sterilized in 75% ethanol for approximately 10 min. The bilateral tibias were dissected free of muscle and connective tissue and were immersed into sterile PBS immediately. Both ends of the tibia were cut to expose the marrow cavity. A 1 ml syringe (BD Biosciences, San Jose, CA, USA) was used to repeatedly flush the bone marrow into a 10 cm dish with complete media. The cell suspension was then centrifuged at 1000 rpm for 5 min. We resuspended the cell sedimentation with complete medium containing 10% fetal bovine serum (Gibco, Thermo Fisher Scientific, USA), α-modified Eagle's medium (HyClone, USA), and 1% penicillin-streptomycin (HyClone, USA). This suspension was then filtered with a 70 μm cell strainer (BD Biosciences, San Jose, CA, USA) and was seeded into a 25 cm² flask for incubation at the condition of 37°C and 5% CO₂. After 48 h incubation, floating cells were removed, and fresh complete medium was added. Medium change was performed every 3 days. Once the cell confluence reached 80%–90%, cell expansion (1:3) was taken into consideration. Briefly, cells were treated with 1 ml of 0.25% EDTA-trypsin (Gibco, Thermo Fisher Scientific, USA) for 1 min. Then, complete medium was added to neutralize the trypsin. The novel cell suspension was cultured in three flasks of 25 cm². For osteogenic differentiation, cells at passage 3 with 80% confluence were induced under α-MEM supplemented with 10% FBS, 10 nM dexamethasone, 10 mM β-glycerol phosphate, and 50 μg/ml ascorbic acid. Osteogenic induction medium was changed every 3 days.

2.3. Cellular Exposure to Ionizing Radiation (IR). rBMSCs of the third passage were cultured in 6 cm φ dishes with complete medium and then were moved to a radiotherapy room when cells reached confluence at 80%. IR was performed in cells using 6 MeV (Precise Treatment System, Elekta, Swedish) with a dosage of 6 Gy and a dose rate of 600 Mu. Cells were then moved back to the incubator for continuous culture before collecting samples.

2.4. miRNA Isolation and Real-Time PCR Analysis. Total miRNA was extracted using the miRcute miRNA Isolation Kit (Tiangen Biotech, Beijing, China), and total miRNA was reverse-transcribed using miRcute miRNA First-Strand cDNA Synthesis Kit (Tiangen Biotech, Beijing, China). Briefly, Poly(A) was added to the 3′ end of miRNA, and then this production was reverse-transcribed using the oligo(dT)-universal tag to produce the first-strand cDNA. The relative miR-22 gene expression level was analyzed using miRcute miRNA qPCR Detection Kit (SYBR Green) (Tiangen Biotech, Beijing, China) in a 7300 Real-Time PCR system. U6 served as the endogenous normalization control. The fold change in miR-22 expression was determined by the comparative CT method $2^{-\Delta\Delta CT}$.

2.5. Lentiviral Vector Construction and Transduction. Plasmid vectors (pLenti-hU6-MSC-ubiquitin-EGFP-IRES-puromycin) were composed of rno-miR-22-NC, rno-miR-22, rno-miR-22-inhibitor-NC, and rno-miR-22-inhibitor and were obtained from GeneChem Technology Co., Ltd., China. Then, we transfected the 293T cells with plasmids shown above and Lipofectamine 3000 to produce the lentiviruses and collected the supernatant at 48 h after transfection. This supernatant with lentiviruses was then filtered and concentrated by using ultrafiltration. For the transfection procedure, rBMSCs were immersed in medium containing lentiviruses with 50 MOI, Opti-MEM, and 5 μg/ml polybrene for 24 h. The transfected efficiency was evaluated through RT-PCR and fluorescence microscopy.

2.6. Cellular Apoptosis Assay. An Annexin V-FITC/PI detection kit was used to measure the apoptotic ratio of cells by flow cytometry according to the manufacturer's instruction. Briefly, 5×10^5 cells (24 h after radiation, 0 or 6 Gy) were collected by trypsinization, washed with ice-cold PBS, and then resuspended in 300 μl of 1x binding buffer containing 5 μl Annexin V FITC, followed by dark incubation for 10 min at room temperature. PI (5 μl) was added to each sample for coincubation for another 5 min. After incubation, 200 μl of 1x binding buffer was added to further resuspend the cells, and at least 10,000 cells were measured on a BD FACS flow cytometer (FL1 and FL2 emission filter).

2.7. Measurement of Intracellular ROS Levels. rBMSCs were seeded on a 12-well plate in triplicates with a density of 2×10^4 cells. After routine culture (with or without NAC) or lentiviral transfection, cells were exposed to 0 or 6 Gy IR, and analysis was performed at 24 h after X-ray treatment. For ROS staining, cells were incubated with a Fluorometric Intracellular ROS Kit for 45 min (5% CO2, 37°C), gently washed with PBS 3 times, and then imaged with the fluorescence microscope. For ROS level detection, the fluorescence intensity (λex = 640/λem = 675 nm) of incubated cells was measured with a microscope. The results are shown as the mean fluorescence intensity of 2×10^4 cells ± SEM.

2.8. Western Blot Analysis. Whole cell lysates were acquired using RIPA lysis buffer and PMSF (1 mM) (Beyotime, China) by incubation on ice for 30 min. The protein concentration was detected using a BCA Protein Assay Kit (Pierce™,

Thermo Fisher Scientific, MA, USA). Equal amounts (20 μg/well) of protein samples were separated by SDS-PAGE (10%, 15%) and then transferred to PVDF (0.45 or 0.22 μm) membranes (Millipore Corporation, MA, USA). The membranes were blocked in 5% BSA containing TBS for 1 h and then incubated with primary antibodies. After washing three times with TBST, the membranes were further incubated with HRP-tagged secondary antibodies for 1 h at room temperature. Finally, the protein bands were visualized by Odyssey V3.0 image scanning (LI-COR, Lincoln, NE, USA). The densitometric intensities of the individual protein bands were quantified using ImageJ software (Version 1.8.0), and the values were normalized to the GAPDH values for each sample.

2.9. Alkaline Phosphatase (ALP), Alizarin Red S (ARS) Staining, and Semiquantitative Analyses. rBMSCs were seeded onto 12-well plates at a density of 5.0×10^5 cells. After routine culture or lentivirus transfection, cells were exposed to 0 or 6 Gy. Six hours after radiation, culture medium was replaced by osteogenic medium. On day 14, the cells were fixed in 4% paraformaldehyde, and ALP staining was performed according to the manufacturer's instructions. On day 21, after fixation in 90% ethanol for 20 min, cells were stained with alizarin red for 30 min at room temperature to detect matrix mineralization. Each experiment was repeated in triplicate. For ALP semiquantitative analyses, p-NPP was used as substrate and absorbance was measured at 405 nm in a microplate reader (Tecan Infinite M200, Switzerland). ARS staining was dissolved using 10% cetylpyridinium chloride, and the absorbance was read at 590 nm in Tecan M200. Finally, these data were normalized to the protein concentration of each sample.

2.10. Cellular Immunofluorescence. Cells were seeded onto confocal dishes (20 mm in diameter) at a density of 1×10^4 cells/dish. Lentivirus transfections (miR-22-NC, miR-22, miR-22-inhibitor-NC, or miR-22-inhibitor) were performed when cells reached confluence at 30–50%. Twenty-four hours after transfection, cells were exposed to 6 Gy radiation. Osteogenic induction began at 6 h after X-ray treatment and lasted for 14 days. The samples were fixed in 4% paraformaldehyde for 30 min, permeabilized with 0.5% Triton X-100 for 20 min, and blocked with 2% BSA for 30 min, respectively. Next, primary antibodies of anti-Runx2 (10 μg/ml, Abcam) and anti-Osterix (1 : 200, Abcam) were added to samples for incubation at 4°C overnight. The cells were then immersed in Alexa Fluor 488-conjugated secondary antibody for 1 h at RT. DAPI (Sigma-Aldrich, St. Louis, USA) was used to label cell nuclei for 10 min. The immunoreactive cells were visualized and captured using confocal microscopy (Leica TCS SP8, Germany). The ratio of positive cells in each sample was determined by dividing the number of immune-positive cells by the number of nuclei stained with DAPI in three random fields for each group.

2.11. Fabrication of Gelatin (G) and Carboxymethyl Chitosan (CMC) Scaffold. We obtained the CMC solution by adding 100 mg of powder to ultrapure water, which was then dissolved at 40°C. Subsequently, gelatin powder (1000 mg) was added to CMC solution through stirring for at least 1 h to obtain the G-CMC solution. The compound was then poured into the mold with different sizes, followed by frozen overnight (−20°C) and lyophilized for 48 h. Next, dried scaffolds were cross-linked by using EDC and NHS in a mixed solvent of acetone and water (volume ratio = 4 : 1) for 24 h at 4°C. The scaffolds were lyophilized and stored at −20°C. The surface morphology of the 3D scaffold was visualized and captured by SEM (TM-1000; Hitachi, Tokyo, Japan). The verification of scaffold constitution was applied via Fourier transform infrared spectroscopy (FITR).

2.12. Cell Adhesion in CLSM and SEM Imaging. Gelatin-chitosan scaffolds were immersed into 75% ethanol for 6 h and transferred to a 48-well plate with additional ethanol disinfection for 3 h. Sterile PBS with 1% penicillin-streptomycin was used to wash the residual ethanol for another 6 h. Finally, scaffolds were incubated with basal culture medium overnight at 37°C and 5% CO_2. Cells with different treatments were seeded onto scaffolds at a density of 5×10^4/well and were cultured for 5 days. Samples were then labeled with 4 mM calcein AM for 20 min and were visualized by confocal microscopy (FITC channel) after rinsing with PBS. Scanning electron microscopy (SEM) imaging was performed as previously described. Briefly, cell-seeded scaffolds were fixed in 2.5% glutaraldehyde for 2 h, then dehydrated in a graded ethanol series (100%, 90%, 80%, 70%, and 50%), and finally air-dried for 1 h. Gold-sputtered specimens were prepared using a JFC-1200 fine coater (JEOL, Tokyo, Japan) at 30 mA under high vacuum for 70 sec. The morphology and adhesion of the cells were visualized through SEM (TM-1000; Hitachi, Tokyo, Japan), which was manipulated at 15 kV under high vacuum mode.

2.13. Animal Surgical Procedure. Sprague-Dawley (SD) rats (8-week-old, female, weight: 160–200 g) were anesthetized and were cut on the scalp to make a 2 cm sagittal incision. Two critical-sized calvarial defects (CSDs) were created bilaterally on the scalps using a 5 mm-diameter trephine (Nouvag AG, Goldach, Switzerland). G-CMC (thickness: 1 mm, diameter: 5 mm) with or without cell adhesion was implanted to repair defects. Twenty-four rats were randomly allocated into the following groups: (1) G-CMC/BMSCs/Lenti-miR-22-NC (n = 6), (2) G-CMC/BMSCs/Lenti-miR-22 (n = 6), (3) G-CMC/BMSCs/Lenti-miR-22-inhibitor-NC (n = 6), (4) G-CMC/BMSCs/Lenti-miR-22-inhibitor (n = 6). Additionally, experimental groups were implanted on the right side and the control group was placed at the left side.

2.14. Microcomputed Tomography (Micro-CT) Analysis. The SD rats were sacrificed at 8 weeks after surgical procedure. The skull samples pretreated with 4% paraformaldehyde were then scanned using micro-CT (μCT 80, Scanco Medical, Switzerland) with the slice thickness of 20 μm and pixel matrix of 1024 × 1024. Subsequently, auxiliary histomorphometric software (Scanco Medical AG, Switzerland) was used to assess the three-dimensional structure of bone tissue at surgical fields. Other assessments, such as new bone volume

relative to tissue volume (BV/TV) and the bone mineral density (BMD), trabecular number (Tb.N) were also concluded in the current study.

2.15. Histological Analysis. We dissected the skull and removed the brain tissue and soft tissues in the skull base. The samples were then fixed in 10% formalin for 7 days, further decalcified by incubation in ethylenediaminetetraacetic acid (EDTA) solution for 15 days, and finally embedded in paraffin wax. Specimens were sagittally resected into 5 μm-thick slices and stained with hematoxylin and eosin (HE) to distinguish the bone and soft tissues, especially regenerative bone. Digital images of each slide were visualized and captured using a transmission and polarized light Axioskop microscope, Olympus BX51 (Olympus Corp, Tokyo, Japan).

2.16. Statistical Analysis. All data in the current study were shown as the mean ± SD of different numbers of independent experiments. Data comparison among different groups was performed using the Student t-test or one-way analysis of variance (ANOVA) in SPSS (version 20, Chicago, IL, USA), and $p < 0.05$ was deemed as statistical significance.

3. Results

3.1. IR Induces Cellular Apoptosis and Intracellular ROS Production. rBMSCs treated with 6 Gy radiation had a much higher apoptotic ratio than the 0 Gy group (15.3 ± 2.67% versus 5.73 ± 1.19%) ($p \leq 0.001$) (Figure 1(a)). Subsequently, we investigated the intracellular ROS level of rBMSCs following X-ray exposure. Irradiation increased the ROS production of rBMSCs, which was verified by ROS-positive cell number and mean fluorescence intensity (Figures 1(b)–1(d)). Meanwhile, upregulation of NOX4 and downregulation of SOD2 after radiation also proved this ROS change (Figures 1(e) and 1(f)). Since radiation induced both cellular apoptosis and ROS production, we attempted to reveal the relationship between apoptosis and intracellular ROS.

3.2. IR-Induced Cellular Apoptosis Partly Contributed to the ROS Generation. N-Acetyl-L-cysteine (NAC) is a classical antioxidant, which performs its function on the basis of a sulfhydryl group. Pretreatment with NAC significantly reduced the mean fluorescence intensity by 29% and the ROS-positive cell number by 26.7% in irradiated rBMSCs. Similarly, upregulation of SOD2 and downregulation of NOX4 were also observed in the group with NAC pretreatment. However, this ROS inhibition was not found in nonirradiated cells. These data proved the antioxygenation of NAC in the radiation model of rBMSCs. Subsequently, we tried to validate whether this antioxygenation had a role in the inhibition of apoptosis of rBMSCs induced by irradiation. As shown in Figure 1(a), the apoptotic ratio decreased from 15.3 ± 2.67% to 9.23 ± 1.89% ($p \leq 0.01$) with NAC pretreatment following radiation, and this reduction was also observed in the apoptotic protein expression of Caspase-3, an important marker of apoptosis. However, this cell viability promotion was not seen in nonirradiated cells. These results

(a)

(b)

(c)

(d)

(e)

(f)

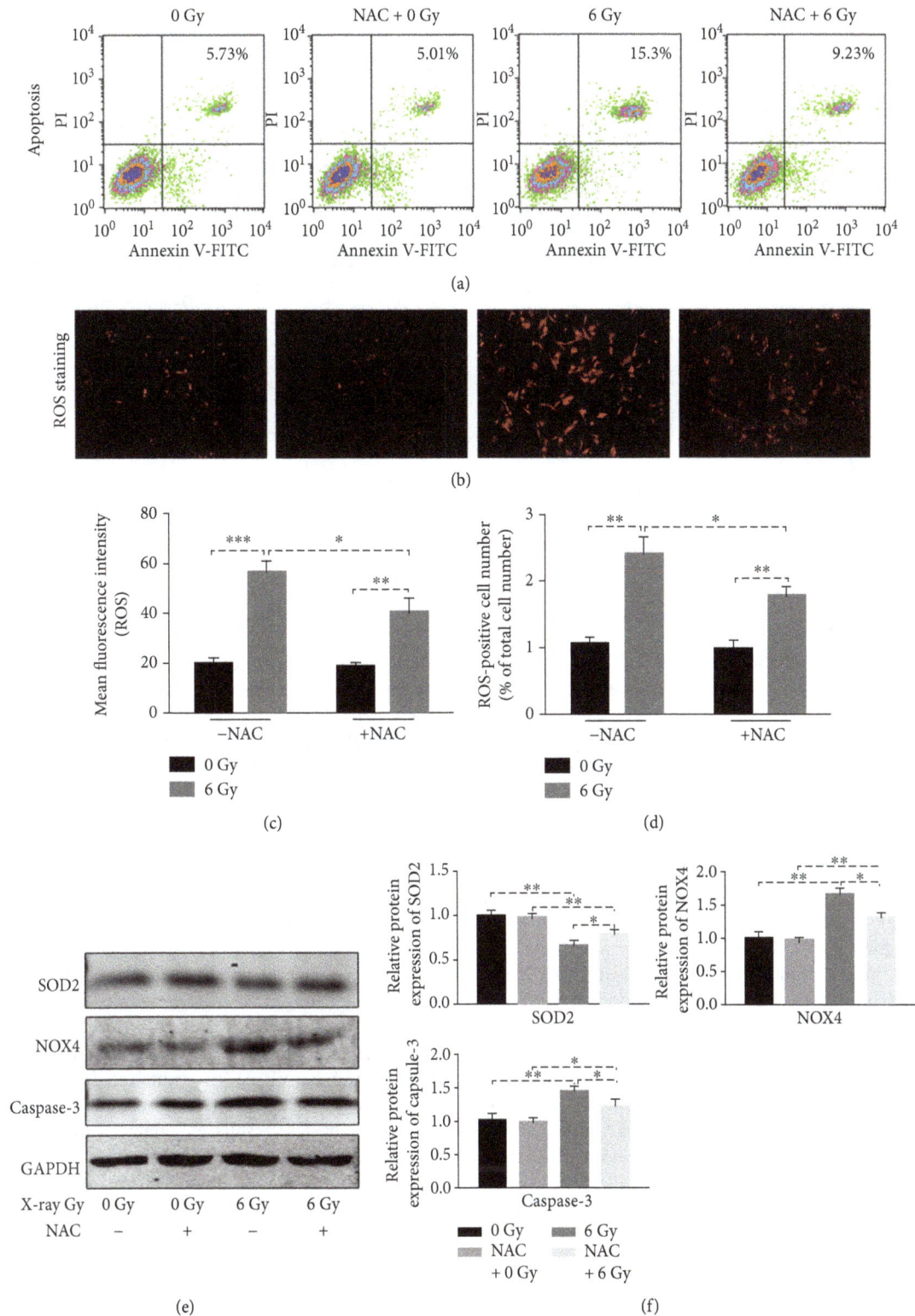

FIGURE 1: Cellular apoptosis and ROS generation following IR (0 or 6 Gy) in rBMSCs. N-Acetyl-L-cysteine (NAC) is a classical antioxidant, which was used to testify the relationship of ROS generation with apoptosis in our experiment. (a) Cellular apoptosis was measured at 24 h postradiation by using the Annexin V-FITC method. IR-induced apoptosis can be partly rescued by pretreatment with NAC ($n = 3$). (b–d) Detection of ROS level at 24 h postradiation, (b) ROS staining with Fluorometric Intracellular ROS Kit. (c) Mean fluorescent intensity was measured at 640/675 nm. (d) The ROS positive ratio (%) is shown as a percentage of the positive cells to the total cell number ($n = 3$, $^*p < 0.05$, $^{**}p < 0.01$, and $^{***}p < 0.001$). (e) Western blot showed the expression level of SOD2, NOX4, and Caspase-3 following IR; GAPDH served as endogenous reference. (f) The densitometric intensities were quantified using Photoshop. All bar graphs were shown as means ± SEM ($n = 3$, $^*p < 0.05$, $^{**}p < 0.01$, and $^{***}p < 0.001$).

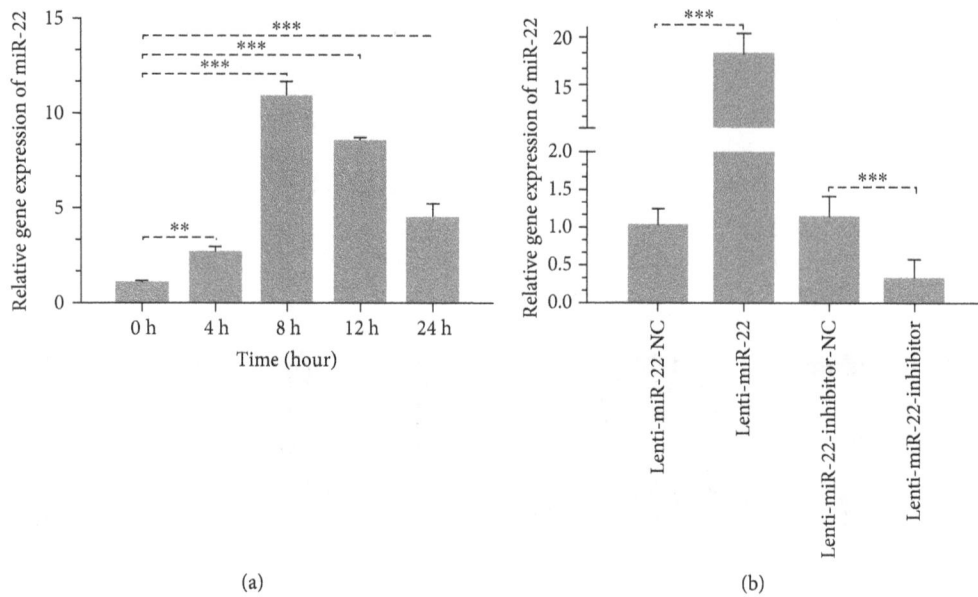

(a)

(b)

FIGURE 2: (a) miR-22 expression in rBMSCs following 6 Gy IR and transfection with miR-22 lentivirus. Upregulation of miR-22 showed a time-dependent manner with a peak induction at 8 h ($n = 3$, $^{**}p < 0.01$ and $^{***}p < 0.001$). (b) RT-PCR verification of miR-22 lentivirus transfection ($n = 3$, $^{***}p < 0.001$).

demonstrated that irradiation-induced cellular apoptosis may be partly due to ROS production stimulated by X-rays.

3.3. IR Induces the miR-22 Expression and Efficiency of Lentivirus Transfection in rBMSCs.

In an effort to explore the miR-22 expression change upon 6 Gy radiation, rBMSC samples were collected at different time points and detected by means of RT-PCR. A significant increase in the intracellular expression of miR-22 stimulated by radiation was observed in a time-dependent manner. This upregulation reached a peak at 8 h after radiation and lasted 24 h postradiation (Figure 2(a)). In addition, we probed into the expression of miR-22 following different dosages of X-ray radiation at 8 h post-IR (the peak time point), with the result that significant upregulation of miR-22 was detected among different groups (Figure S1). MiR-22 was reported to participate in ROS production through induction by butyrate, myocardial ischemia/reperfusion (I/R), and UV radiation. These investigations indicated that miR-22 may also have a regulatory role on the ROS production and apoptosis via induction by X-ray radiation.

To verify this hypothesis, we constructed a lentivirus of miR-22 (overexpression or downregulation) to perform a gain-and-loss experiment. This efficiency was also proven through RT-PCR analysis (18.235-fold upregulation and 0.311-fold downregulation, $p \leq 0.001$) (Figure 2(b)). As shown in Figure S2, fluorescence microscopy demonstrated positively stained cells with GFP emission in different groups at 24 h posttransfection. The transfection efficiency of rBMSCs at MOI of 100 was greater than 95.0% in four groups.

3.4. miR-22 Overexpression Increased the Intracellular ROS Level.

Twenty-four hours after lentivirus transfection, rBMSCs were exposed to 6 Gy IR. The ROS level was

estimated at 24 h postradiation using the methods mentioned above. The results showed that overexpression of miR-22 promoted the ROS release through both ROS-positive cell number (elevated 1.55-fold) and mean fluorescence intensity (elevated 2.3-fold), while cells transfected with the lentivirus miR-22 inhibitor had the capability to reverse the ROS regeneration (Figures 3(b)–3(d)). This regulated role of miR-22 in ROS intervention was further confirmed through detection of ROS-related protein expression (decreased by 25.6% in SOD2 and increased by 31.4% in NOX4) (Figures 3(e) and 3(f)).

3.5. Postradiation Survival of rBMSCs Was Rescued by Inhibition of miR-22.

We have verified that miR-22 participated in the regulation of IR-induced ROS production. To investigate whether ROS-mediated cellular apoptosis occurs through miR-22, the transfected cells were exposed to IR and further detected using flow cytometry at 24 h postradiation. The results elucidated a positive correlation between the overexpression of miR-22 and cellular apoptosis (Figure 3(a)). Furthermore, the expression of Caspase-3 increased 1.64-fold ($p < 0.01$) in the Lenti-miR-22 group and decreased 0.215-fold ($p < 0.05$) in the Lenti-miR-22-inhibitor group compared to NC-transfected cells (Figures 3(e) and 3(f)). These data confirmed the regulatory role of miR-22 on ROS-mediated cellular apoptosis of rBMSCs induced by IR.

3.6. Irradiation Impairs the Osteogenic Differentiation of rBMSCs.

The osteogenic capacity of rBMSCs following X-ray treatment was assessed by ALP/ARS staining and quantification. As shown in Figure 4, ALP staining on day 7 and day 14 indicated a lower density in the irradiated (6 Gy) and subsequent osteogenically differentiated rBMSCs

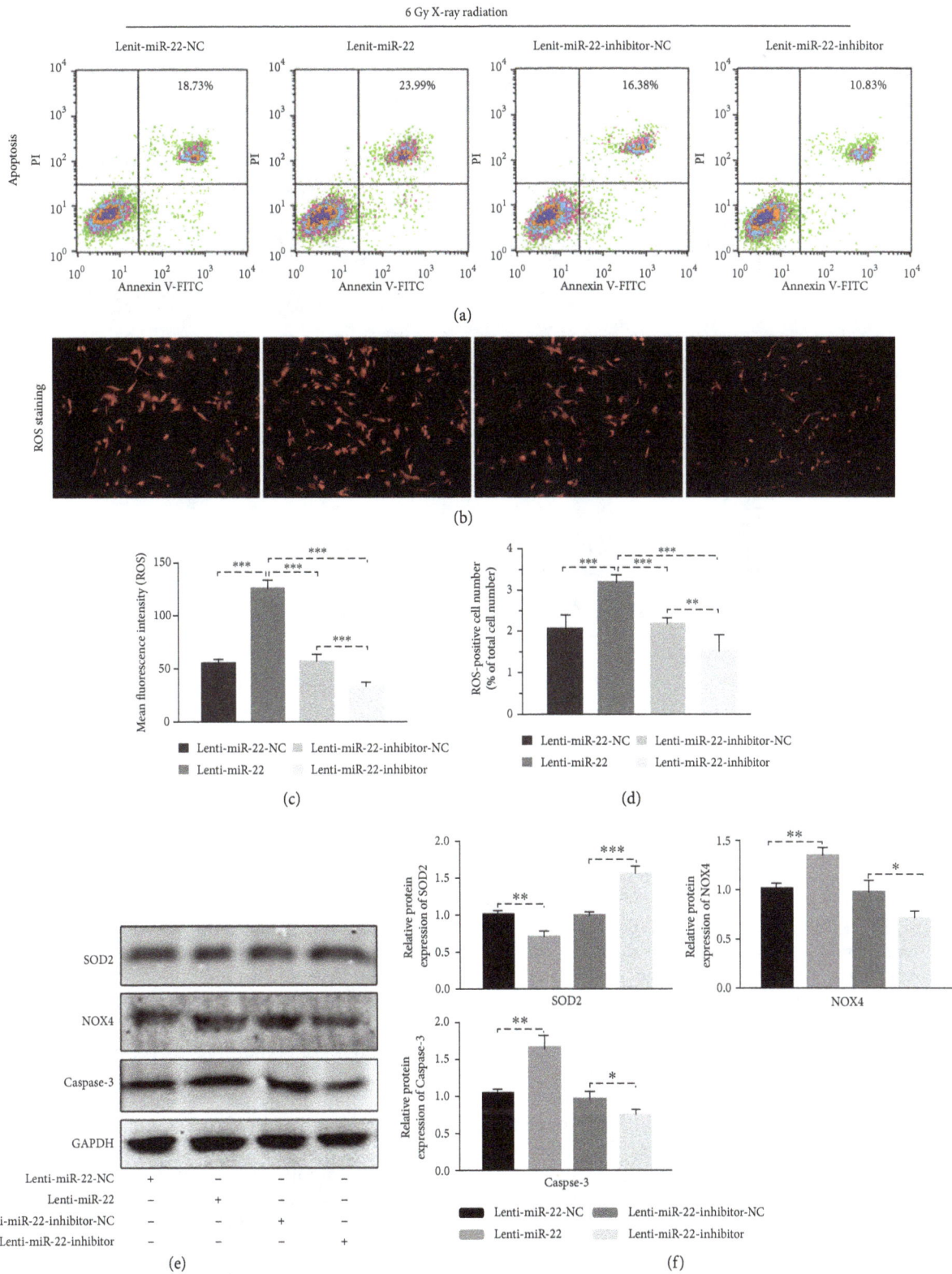

FIGURE 3: Cellular apoptosis and ROS generation in miR-22-modified rBMSCs following 6 Gy IR. After transfection of miR-22 lentivirus with 48 h, cells were than exposed to IR and samples were collected at 24 h postradiation. (a) Overexpression of miR-22 enhanced the apoptotic ratio of rBMSCs ($n = 3$). (b–d) Inhibition of miR-22 helps cells against the production of ROS. (b) ROS staining. (c, d) Mean fluorescent intensity and the ROS-positive ratio (%) ($n = 3$, $**p < 0.01$ and $***p < 0.001$). (e) Protein level of SOD2, NOX4, and Caspase-3 in miR-22-modified cells following IR. (f) The densitometric intensity analysis. Both showed that miR-22 played an important role on IR-induced ROS generation and apoptosis, vice versa. All bar graphs were shown as means ± SEM ($n = 3$, $*p < 0.05$, $**p < 0.01$, and $***p < 0.001$).

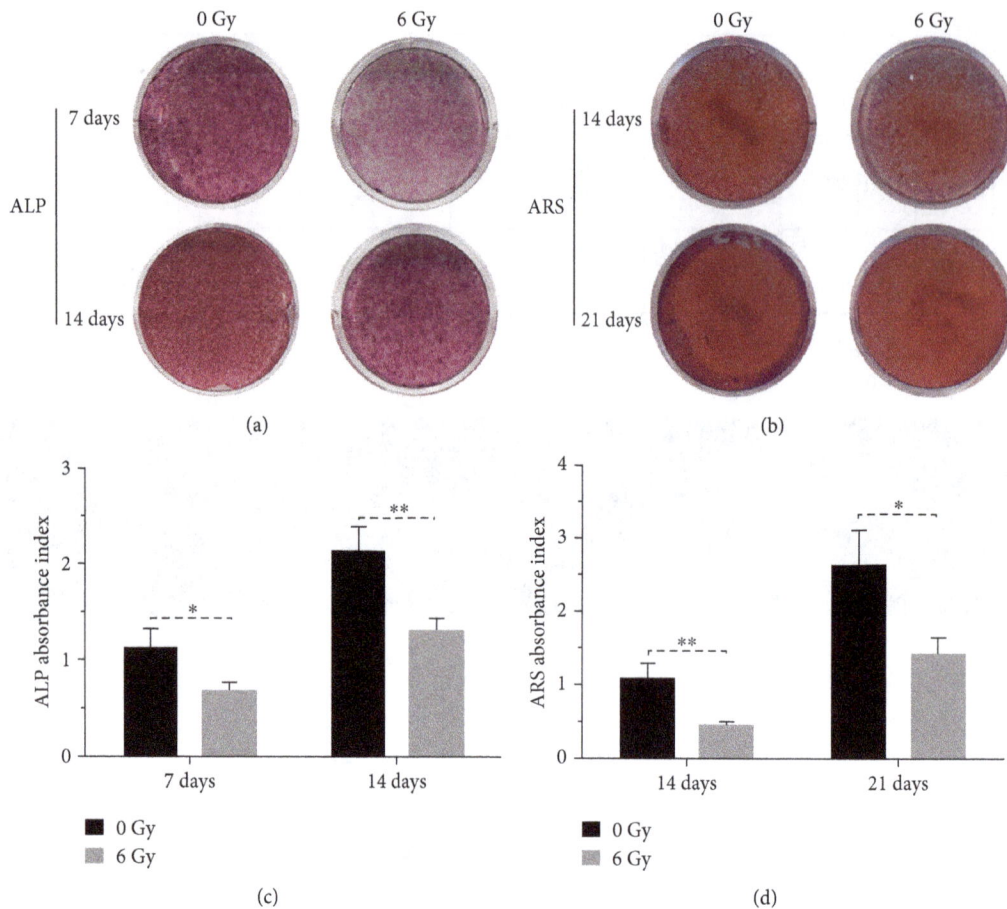

(a)

(b)

(c)

(d)

FIGURE 4: Impaired osteogenic capacity of rBMSCs with IR exposure. (a) ALP staining on days 7 and 14. (b) ARS staining on days 14 and 21. (c, d) The semiquantitative analysis of ALP and ARS staining ($n = 3$, * $p < 0.05$ and ** $p < 0.01$).

(Figure 4(a)). This qualitative evaluation was further confirmed by semiquantitative analysis using absorbance detection, which revealed that ALP activity in the control group was 1.94-fold ($p < 0.05$) and 1.65-fold ($p < 0.01$) higher than that in the irradiated group on days 7 and 14, respectively (Figure 4(c)). A similar phenomenon was seen in ARS assessment; a decrease in the density of mineralized deposits and nodules was seen in the irradiated group at both day 14 and day 21 (Figure 4(b)). Absorbance from calcium deposit staining was significantly lower in the 6 Gy sample than that in the 0 Gy group at different time points (Figure 4(d)). These data demonstrated a more pronounced osteogenic property in nonirradiated rBMSCs compared to that with 6 Gy exposure. This in vitro model revealed that osteogenic differentiation of rBMSCs was significantly inhibited by X-ray exposure with a dosage of 6 Gy.

3.7. Reverse of IR-Induced Apoptosis by miR-22 Inhibitor Promoted the Osteogenic Capability of rBMSCs In Vitro. To elucidate whether miR-22-mediated ROS-dependent apoptosis has a regulatory role on the osteogenesis of rBMSCs following IR exposure, transfected cells following IR were cultured in osteoinductive medium for 14 and 21 days. The protein expression level of osteogenic markers (Runx2, OSX, OPN, BSP, and OCN) were measured using

Western blot. As shown in Figures 5(a) and 5(b), these markers were repressed in the Lenti-miR-22 group but significantly promoted in the Lenti-miR-22-inhibitor group in comparison with the Lenti-miR-22-NC or Lenti-miR-22-inhibitor-NC group, respectively. Furthermore, cellular immunofluorescence was performed in 4 groups with osteogenic induction for 14 days to test the expression of Runx2 and Osterix (Figure 6). The results showed that $50.06 \pm 3.97\%$ of Lenti-miR-22-NC-tansduced cells and $53.17 \pm 2.86\%$ of Lenti-miR-22-inhibitor-NC-tansduced cells expressed Runx2, respectively. This expression percentage was much lower ($29.46 \pm 3.26\%$, $p < 0.01$) in the Lenti-miR-22 group and dramatically higher ($75.43 \pm 4.45\%$, $p < 0.01$) in the Lenti-miR-22 inhibitor group. The positive expression ratio of Osterix in four groups ($42.87 \pm 3.84\%$ in the Lenti-miR-22-NC group, $29.0 \pm 3.38\%$ in the Lenti-miR-22 group, $40.9 \pm 2.2\%$ in the Lenti-miR-22-inhibitor-NC group, and $57.0 \pm 3.2\%$ in the Lenti-miR-22-inhibitor group) had a similar pattern as the expression of Runx2.

ALP staining of 14-day samples was significantly attenuated in the Lenti-miR-22-transfected and irradiated groups but dramatically promoted in the Lenti-miR-22-inhibitor group (Figure 7(a)). This trend was also observed in ARS staining of 21-day-old samples (Figure 7(b)). The

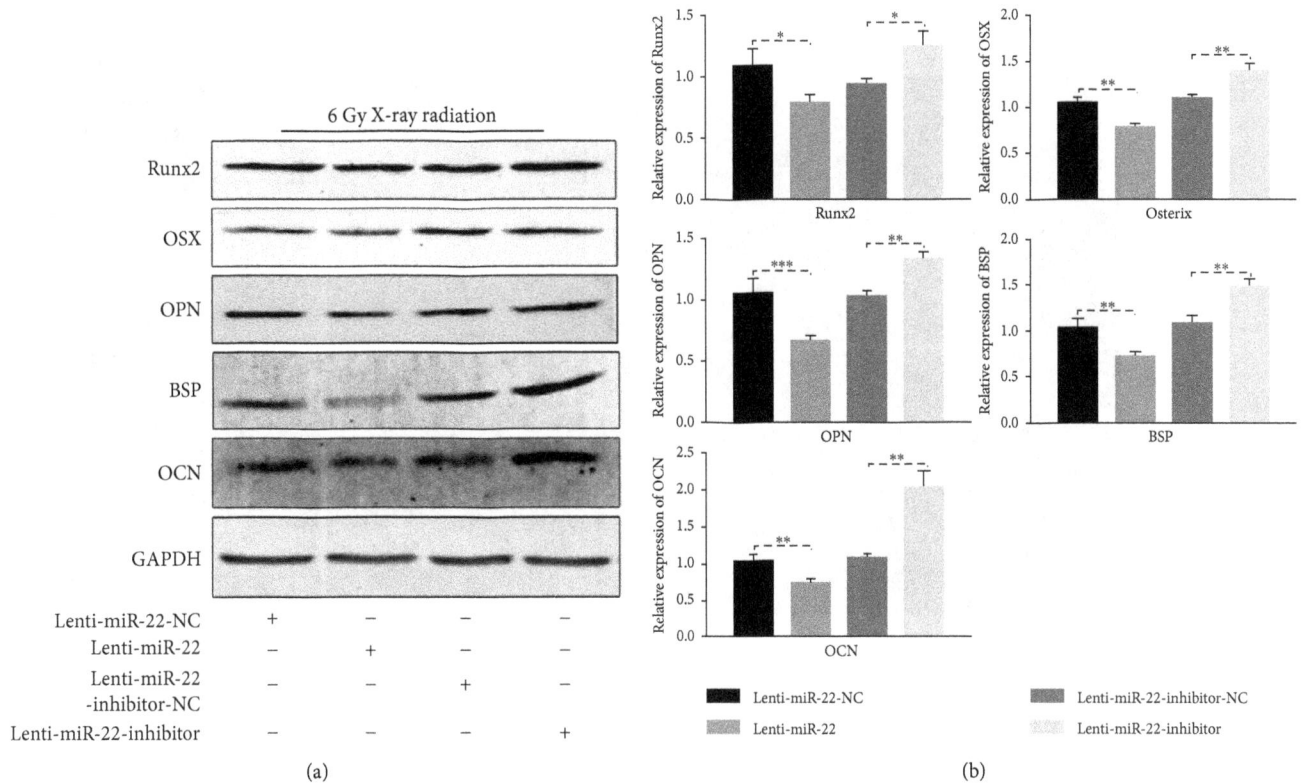

FIGURE 5: The protein level of osteogenic related markers (Runx2, Osx, OPN, BSP, and OCN) in miR-22-modified rBMSCs with 6 Gy IR exposure. (a) Protein bands. (b) The densitometric intensity analysis (normalized to GAPDH) ($n = 3$, $^*p < 0.05$, $^{**}p < 0.01$, and $^{***}p < 0.001$).

semiquantitative analysis of ALP showed a 33.3% lower expression level in the Lenti-miR-22-transfected and irradiated groups and a 73.3% higher expression level in the Lenti-miR-22-inhibitor group than in the Lenti-miR-22-NC and Lenti-miR-22-inhibitor-NC groups, respectively (Figures 7(c) and 7(d)). Similarly, the semiquantitative analysis of ARS staining was consistent with the trend of ALP staining (Figure 7(e)). To summarize, these findings, including protein expression, immunofluorescence, and ALP/ARS staining, demonstrated that miR-22-mediated ROS-dependent apoptosis has a regulatory role on the osteogenesis of rBMSCs following IR exposure.

3.8. In Vivo Estimation of Bone Regeneration by miR-22 Transfection and following Radiation. To evaluate the osteogenic capacity of rBMSCs with miR-22 transfection and following radiation, we fabricated the scaffold material composed of gelatin and carboxymethyl chitosan (CMC) by using the method of freeze-drying. SEM showed the microstructure of the G-CMC scaffold with different magnifications (Figures 8(a)–8(c)). FTIR analysis verified the existence of two different components (Figure 8(d)). After transfection with miR-22 lentivirus and following IR, rBMSCs were seeded onto the G-CMC scaffold that was presterilized for 7 days and then stained with calcein AM for 15 min. Confocal microscopy showed a sufficient surface of the G-CMC scaffold for cell attachment and proliferation. There was no significant difference in cell

number and morphology among the 4 groups with genetic modification (Figure 9(a)). A similar phenomenon was observed in SEM detection, which showed cell spreading (Figure 9(b)).

To validate whether miR-22 modified rBMSCs with subsequent IR exposure showed a distinct capacity of bone regeneration in vivo, we established a bilateral calvarial defect (5 mm) model in female rats and implanted the compounds, including rBMSCs/Lenti-miR-22-NC/IR/G-CMC (group 1), rBMSCs/Lenti-miR-22/IR/G-CMC (group 2), rBMSCs/Lenti-miR-22-inhibitor-NC/IR/G-CMC (group 3), rBMSCs/Lenti-miR-22-inhibitor/IR/G-CMC (group 4), into the defect areas. Experimental compounds were placed into the right defect and compared with G-CMC alone, which was placed on the left site.

The new bone formation in the defect area was measured using micro-CT at 8 weeks after the surgical procedure, which showed newly formed bone within the G-CMC area. As shown in Figure 10(a), group 2 produced a lower bone formation, and group 4 had significantly higher bone formation than group 1 and group 3, respectively. There was no obvious newly bone formation in G-CMC only group (right site in the figure). The quantitative analysis of newly formed bone tissue was performed using micro-CT assessment. The BV/TV in group 2 ($6.0 \pm 1.0\%$) was much lower than that in group 1 ($13.3 \pm 3.05\%$), while this ratio was dramatically higher in group 4 ($40.0 \pm 3.6\%$) than that in group 3 ($18.0 \pm 4.0\%$) (Figure 10(b)). Moreover, the BMD

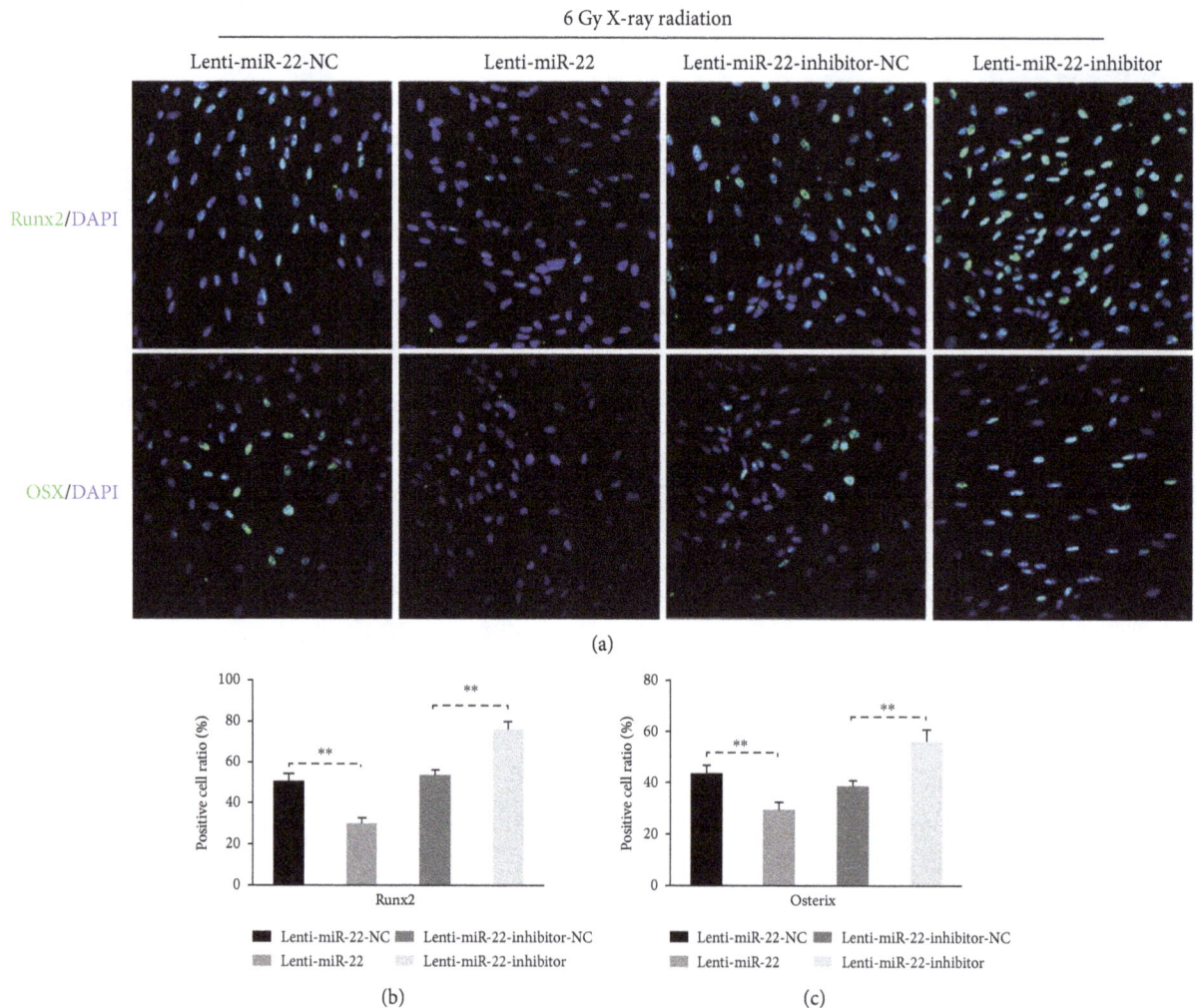

FIGURE 6: Immunofluorescence analysis of bone-specific markers (Runx2 and Osterix) in miR-22-modified rBMSCs with IR treatment. (a) Overexpression of miR-22 aggravated the osteogenic impairment induced by IR. (b, c) The ratio of immunoreactive cells was calculated by dividing the number of positive cells by the number of total cells stained with DAPI. We counted 800–1000 cells in random fields under microscopy for each group ($n = 3$, ** $p < 0.01$).

in group 2 ($0.076 \pm 0.016 \, \text{g/cm}^3$) and group 4 ($0.33 \pm 0.026 \, \text{g/cm}^3$) also had the same trend with the BV/TV compared to that in group 1 ($0.133 \pm 0.015 \, \text{g/cm}^3$) and group 3 ($0.156 \pm 0.15 \, \text{g/cm}^3$) (Figure 10(c)). The similar trend was also seen in Tb.N (Figure 10(d)). Thus, miR-22 overexpression may facilitate the osteogenic damage caused by IR exposure, while miR-22 inhibition seemed to have a role on the reverse of this biological damage. In addition, skull samples were fixed and cut in coronal direction to make HE slides, and this observation also supported the findings from micro-CT or in vitro study (Figure 11).

4. Discussion

Ionizing radiation (IR) characterized by X-ray exposure is frequently performed for medical applications. The typical influence of IR exposure on cells is composed of single- or double-strand DNA breaks, chromosomal destruction, cell cycle arrest, impairment of stemness (differentiation

capacity), production of ROS, and even cell death [14]. In the current study, we demonstrated that miR-22-mediated ROS regeneration had an important regulatory effect on cellular apoptosis and further osteogenic differentiation following IR exposure. We designated 6 Gy IR as the experimental treatment group and 0 Gy as the control group. The utilization of 6 Gy had an influence on DNA damage, cell cycle, and stemness, but no significant inhibition of the proliferation rate was proven through the colony formation assay [13].

Radiation, as well as other exogenous physical or chemical agents, can induce the production of ROS. This accumulation may lead to excessive oxidative stress and DNA damage, which are deemed as the main underlying mechanisms inducing cell injury. At 24 h after 6 Gy IR, increased intracellular ROS level was verified by ROS staining and mean fluorescence intensity measurements. The findings were consistent with the elevation of ROS in human keratinocyte HaCat cells at 24 h after X-ray

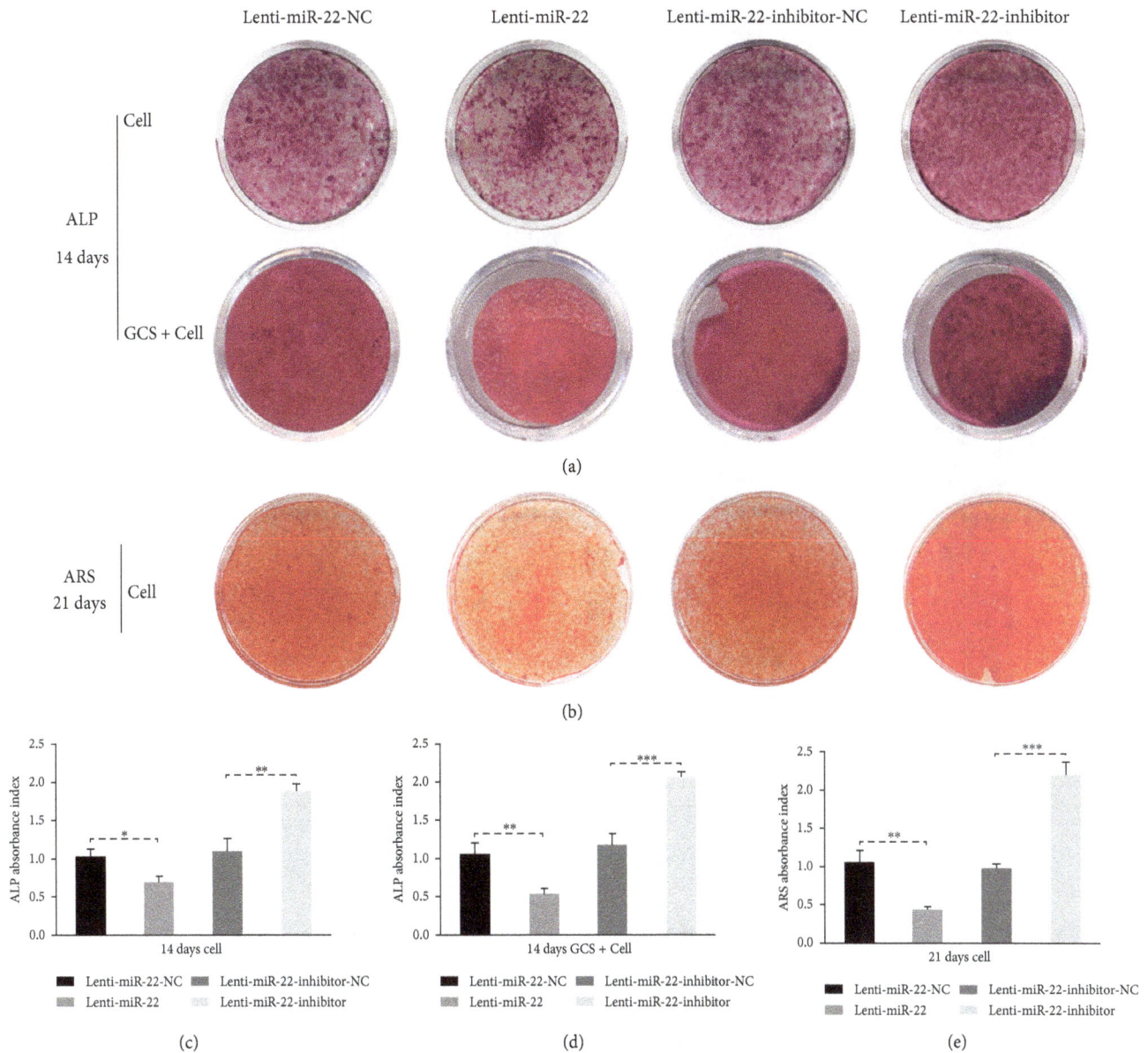

(a)

(b)

(c)

(d)

(e)

FIGURE 7: miR-22 negatively regulated the osteogenic capability of irradiated rBMSCs. (a) ALP staining of miR-22-modified cells and GCS scaffold combined with cells on day 14. (b) ARS staining of miR-22-modified cells on days 21. (c, d) The semiquantitative analysis of ALP in cell samples and GCS scaffold combined with cells samples. (e) The semiquantitative analysis of ARS in cell samples ($n = 3$, $^{*} p < 0.05$, $^{**} p < 0.01$, and $^{***} p < 0.001$).

radiation [31]. NOX4 belongs to the NOX/DUOX family and participates in the production of ROS in a wide range of cell types [32]. Superoxide dismutase 2 (SOD2) belongs to the iron/manganese superoxide dismutase family and allows cells to scavenge intracellular ROS. Furthermore, SOD2 also has an important role against cellular apoptosis induced by ROS, IR, and inflammatory cytokines [33]. Through establishment of a total body irradiation mouse model, scholars found that ROS regeneration was intimately correlated with the upregulation of NOX4 and downregulation of SOD2 in bone marrow injury [34]. This differential expression of NOX4 and SOD2, along with the

elevation of ROS, was also proven in our in vitro model of rBMSCs. To summarize, 6 Gy IR can induce the generation of ROS in rBMSCs.

IR-induced BMSC apoptosis has been extensively studied, but without coherent conclusion [4, 7–10, 13, 34–37]. We hold the view that the radiosensitivity of MSCs may depend to a large extent on several factors, such as the derivation of MSCs (bone or mesenchymal tissue), radiation resource (X-ray, γ-ray, or UV), dosage and dose rate, biological status of the cell at the time of IR, and the detection time (early or late). Rat BMSCs in our IR model showed a moderate radiosensitivity proven by the increase in the

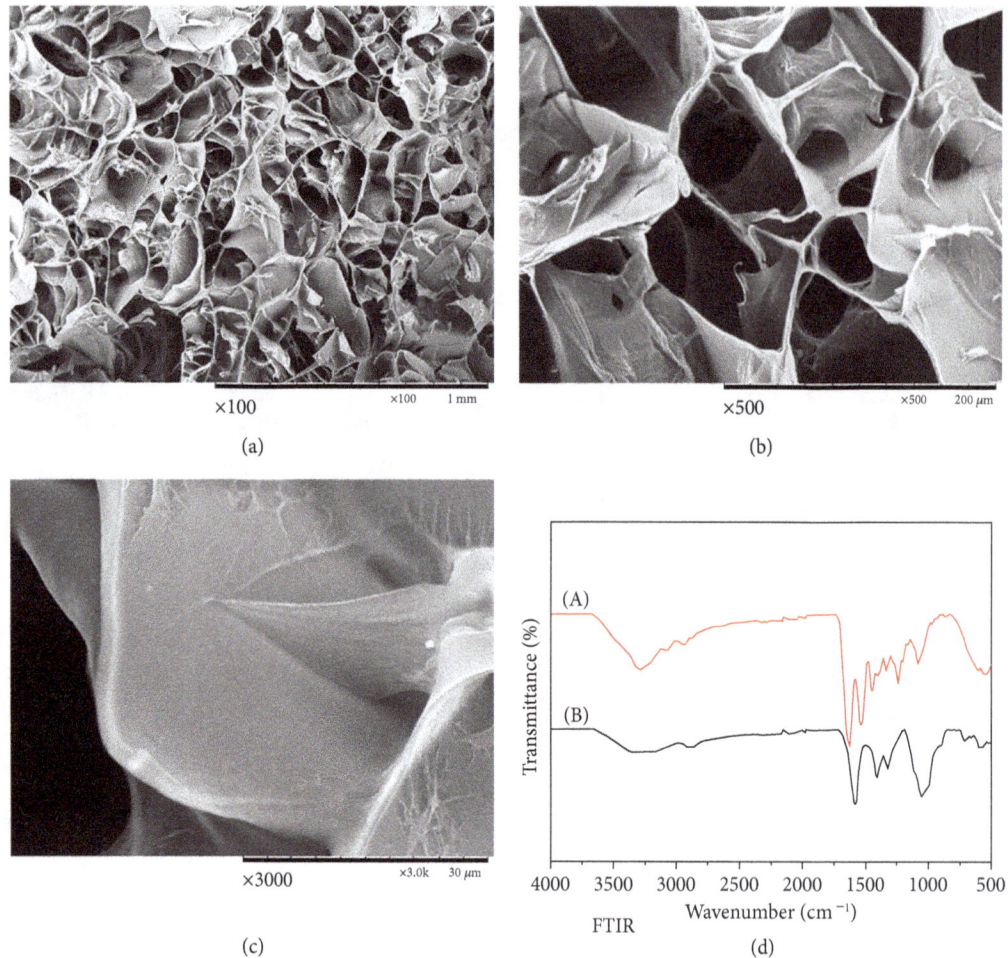

×100

×100   1 mm

(a)

×500

×500   200 μm

(b)

×3000

×3.0k   30 μm

(c)

FTIR

(d)

FIGURE 8: Evaluation of the GCS scaffold. (a–c) Surface structures of GCS were captured by SEM with different magnifications (×100, ×500, ×3000). (d) FTIR analysis. (A) Gelatin and (B) CMC ($n = 3$).

apoptotic ratio at 24 h postradiation both in Annexin V-FITC and Caspase-3 protein detection. To verify whether IR-induced ROS production participated in the regulation of IR-mediated apoptosis, we performed the intervention trial with N-acetyl-L-cysteine (NAC), a type of membrane-penetrating antioxidant that is widely used in the elimination or abatement of intracellular ROS. Through pretreatment with NAC for 2 h, a significant reduction in ROS level was detected following IR compared with the control group. Moreover, the inhibition of ROS had a protective effect on IR-induced apoptosis. This negative correlation of ROS and apoptosis was consistent with the findings of Banerjee et al., who investigated the IR-induced cell death and oxidative stress in mouse embryonic fibroblasts (MEFs) [38]. The initiation of apoptosis is mediated by the caspase family, and ROS can activate these enzymes through mitochondria injury, cytochrome c release, and other signaling pathway activation.

MicroRNAs (miRNAs) have a negative regulatory role on mRNA through degradation or inhibition of posttranslation via binding to the $3'$-untranslated region ($3'$-UTR) of target mRNAs and have been verified as multifunctional genes involved in cell cycle, survival and death, proliferation,

differentiation, and so on. Researchers have found that miRNA response following radiation may participate in the biological process of DNA damage, cell cycle, or proliferation. For this reason, more studies have focused on miRNA expression analysis through miRNA array profiles upon UV and IR exposure in different cell types, and they found that miR-22 was upregulated with statistically significant differences [20–24]. In our study, we also showed the upregulation of miR-22 following IR at different time points within 24 hours. miR-22 has been reported to participate in ROS-mediated apoptosis induced by butyrate, contributes to myocardial ischemia-reperfusion injury by affecting the mitochondrial function (ROS, ATP, and membrane potential), and has a neuroprotective role in a 6-hydroxydopamine-induced model of Parkinson's disease via regulation of ROS [28–30]. The role of miR-22 in ROS regeneration was not constant, and it may be involved in activation or inhibition according to the cell type and different stimuli. The issue of whether miR-22 is an indispensable regulator of ROS and apoptosis in rBMSCs following IR has not been elucidated. In the current research, we verified that the overexpression of miR-22 can enhance the ROS level and apoptotic ratio induced by IR and vice versa. Through this

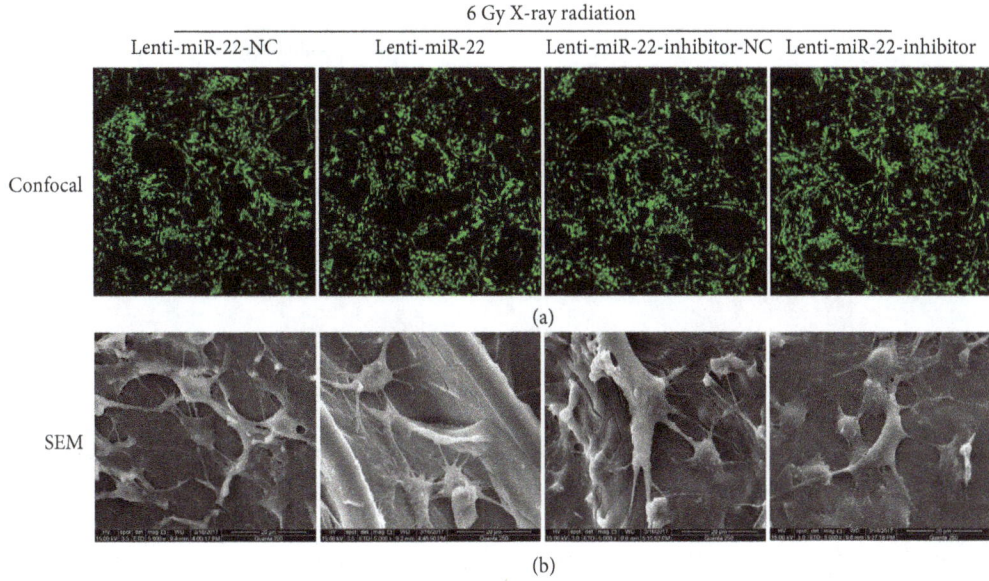

FIGURE 9: Biocompatibility and adhesion property of scaffold. (a) CLSM images showed a favorable cell morphology and proliferation of miR-22-modified rBMSCs ($n = 3$). (b) Cell adhesion was captured by using SEM scanning ($n = 3$).

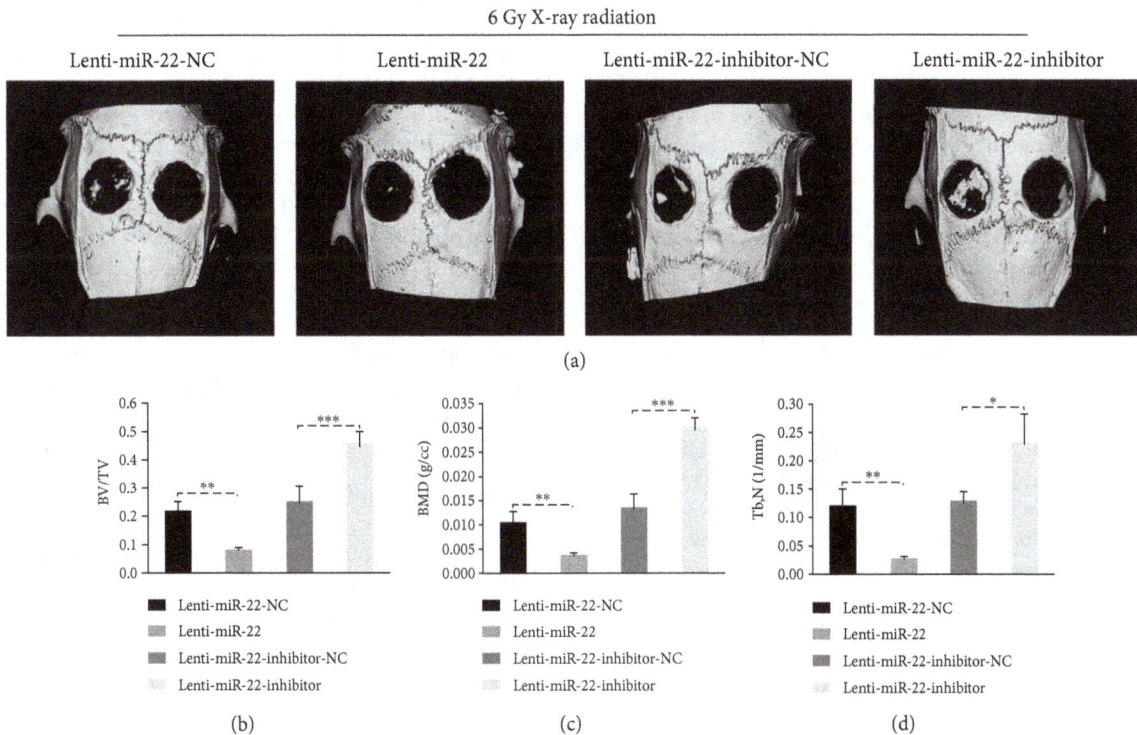

FIGURE 10: Micro-CT evaluation of the osteogenic capacity of miR-22-modified and irradiated rBMSCs in vivo. (a) Images with three-dimensional reconstruction revealed different restorative effects among four groups ($n = 6$). (b, c, d) Quantitative analysis, new bone volume relative to tissue volume (BV/TV), the bone mineral density (BMD) and trabecular number (Tb.N) ($n = 6$, $^*p < 0.05$, $^{**}p < 0.01$, and $^{***}p < 0.001$).

gain and loss analysis, we confirmed that IR-induced miR-22 expression participated in the process of ROS-mediated cellular apoptosis.

rBMSCs belong to the multipotential stem cell family and hold the capability to differentiate into multilineage cells, including osteoblasts, adipocytes, chondrocytes, and fibroblasts. Although IR, especially for X-rays, is deemed as a mainstream therapeutic method for malignancies, its side effects, such as decreased viability of bone tissues, osteomyelitis, osteoradionecrosis, and even IR induced

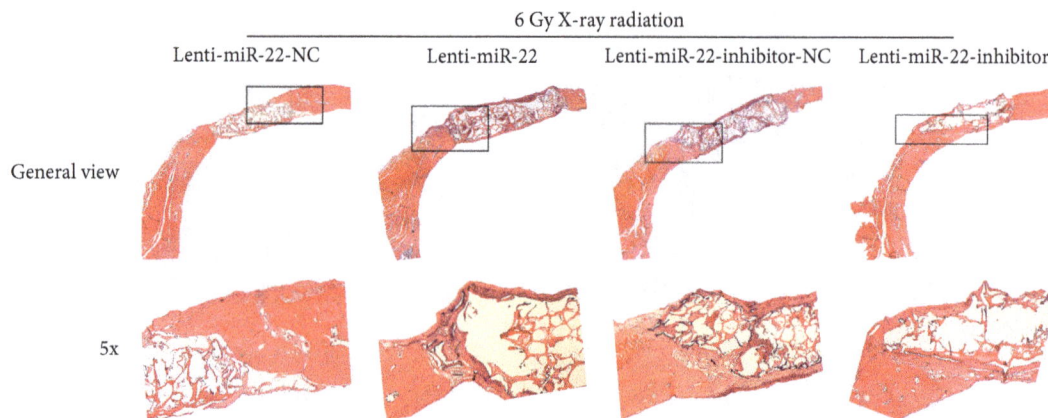

FIGURE 11: Histological analysis of the reparative effect among different groups. Samples were cut in coronal section to make HE slides ($n = 3$).

osteosarcoma, cannot be ignored. In the current investigation, we focused on the osteogenic influence of rBMSCs following IR and its relationship with miR-22-mediated ROS production and subsequent apoptosis. Previous publications have proven the impairment of osteogenesis of MSCs following IR in a dose-dependent manner [39–41]. In our findings, 6 Gy IR was sufficient to impair the osteogenic capacity of rBMSCs, which was proven by ALP/ARS analysis in vitro. BMSCs with higher resistance to apoptosis hold higher osteogenic potential. Wang et al. showed that the inhibition of dexamethasone-induced cytotoxicity and subsequent cellular apoptosis were dependent on the autophagy targeting the mTOR pathway, and this protection of cell viability correlated with new bone formation. In addition, BMSCs from the novel bone group showed a lower ratio of cell apoptosis and higher proportion of autophagy [42]. This relationship between apoptosis and osteogenic capacity was also verified in our findings. Oxidative stress induced by H_2O_2 has been linked to the decreased potential of osteogenic differentiation in MSCs by affecting the transcriptional programs and promoting the adipogenic differentiation [43]. However, the mechanism of ROS-mediated osteogenic impairment was undefined. With our verification, we suggest that IR-induced damage of osteogenesis may be partly due to ROS-mediated cellular apoptosis, which was regulated by the overexpression of miR-22.

As for the in vitro analysis of the impact of miR-22-mediated ROS and apoptosis on osteogenesis, we measured the ALP/ARS staining, protein expression, and immunofluorescence. To validate this regulatory function, we fabricated a gelatin/carboxymethyl chitosan scaffold for cell seeding and subsequent in vivo evaluation. Gelatin was chosen for its biocompatibility and fabrication capabilities, as it has been widely used to construct a 3D scaffold for bone regeneration. Carboxymethyl chitosan is a derivation of chitosan and demonstrates better water solubility and adhesive capacity than normal chitosan, and thus, it could be used for controlled release experiment and further tissue engineering [44]. Because we focused on the osteogenic capability of miR-22-modified rBMSCs following IR, this scaffold was suitable for the current study design in terms of its good

biocompatibility, cell adhesive capacity (proved by SEM and confocal microscopy), and most importantly, low promotion of osteogenesis for the scaffold alone. In vivo analysis, including the micro-CT and HE slide observation, also demonstrated that miR-22-modified rBMSCs following IR hold the same trend as that detected in vitro.

In conclusion, IR was an important exogenous stimulus to induce the production of ROS and further apoptosis in rBMSCs, and these biological processes may be conducted by the overexpression of miR-22. Furthermore, miR-22-mediated ROS regeneration and apoptosis were intimately correlated with the impairment of osteogenic capacity both in vitro and in vivo. However, the mechanism of miR-22 in the regulation of ROS and apoptosis was still unclear. Further study should be performed to determine which mechanism dominates the ROS production, such as mitochondrial pathway, death receptor pathway, or ER pathway, as well as to elucidate the role of autophagy on this biological process.

Authors' Contributions

Yue He and Xiaojun Zhou conceived the study design and contributed in manuscript revision; Si'nan Deng participated in radiotherapy analysis and data extraction; Zhonglong Liu, Tao Li, and Shuiting Fu participated in data collection, statistical analysis, and manuscript preparation and writing. All authors read and approved the final manuscript.

Acknowledgments

Current work was supported by the National Natural Science Foundation of China (81570949) and the Shanghai Municipal Education Commission Gaofeng Clinical Medicine Grant Support (20152222).

References

[1] C. G. Murray, J. Herson, T. E. Daly, and S. Zimmerman,

"Radiation necrosis of the mandible: a 10 year study. Part I. Factors influencing the onset of necrosis," *International Journal of Radiation Oncology, Biology, Physics*, vol. 6, no. 5, pp. 543–548, 1980.

[2] D. A. Costa, T. P. Costa, E. C. Netto et al., "New perspectives on the conservative management of osteoradionecrosis of the mandible: a literature review," *Head & Neck*, vol. 38, no. 11, pp. 1708–1716, 2016.

[3] K. H. Szymczyk, I. M. Shapiro, and C. S. Adams, "Ionizing radiation sensitizes bone cells to apoptosis," *Bone*, vol. 34, no. 1, pp. 148–156, 2004.

[4] N. H. Nicolay, R. Lopez Perez, R. Saffrich, and P. E. Huber, "Radio-resistant mesenchymal stem cells: mechanisms of resistance and potential implications for the clinic," *Oncotarget*, vol. 6, no. 23, pp. 19366–19380, 2015.

[5] J. S. Greenberger and M. Epperly, "Bone marrow-derived stem cells and radiation response," *Seminars in Radiation Oncology*, vol. 19, no. 2, pp. 133–139, 2009.

[6] T. Sugrue, N. F. Lowndes, and R. Ceredig, "Hypoxia enhances the radioresistance of mouse mesenchymal stromal cells," *Stem Cells*, vol. 32, no. 8, pp. 2188–2200, 2014.

[7] S. Singh, F. R. Kloss, R. Brunauer et al., "Mesenchymal stem cells show radioresistance *in vivo*," *Journal of Cellular and Molecular Medicine*, vol. 16, no. 4, pp. 877–887, 2012.

[8] Y. S. An, E. Lee, M. H. Kang et al., "Substance P stimulates the recovery of bone marrow after the irradiation," *Journal of Cellular Physiology*, vol. 226, no. 5, pp. 1204–1213, 2011.

[9] A. Meng, Y. Wang, G. Van Zant, and D. Zhou, "Ionizing radiation and busulfan induce premature senescence in murine bone marrow hematopoietic cells," *Cancer Research*, vol. 63, pp. 5414–5419, 2013.

[10] W. Su, Y. Chen, W. Zeng, W. Liu, and H. Sun, "Involvement of Wnt signaling in the injury of murine mesenchymal stem cells exposed to X-radiation," *International Journal of Radiation Biology*, vol. 88, no. 9, pp. 635–641, 2012.

[11] K. R. Brown and E. Rzucidlo, "Acute and chronic radiation injury," *Journal of Vascular Surgery*, vol. 53, no. 1, pp. 15S–21S, 2011.

[12] J. H. Kim, K. A. Jenrow, and S. L. Brown, "Mechanisms of radiation-induced normal tissue toxicity and implications for future clinical trials," *Radiation Oncology Journal*, vol. 32, no. 3, pp. 103–115, 2014.

[13] J. Hou, Z. P. Han, Y. Y. Jing et al., "Autophagy prevents irradiation injury and maintains stemness through decreasing ROS generation in mesenchymal stem cells," *Cell Death & Disease*, vol. 4, no. 10, article e844, 2013.

[14] Y. Wang, L. Liu, S. K. Pazhanisamy, H. Li, A. Meng, and D. Zhou, "Total body irradiation causes residual bone marrow injury by induction of persistent oxidative stress in murine hematopoietic stem cells," *Free Radical Biology & Medicine*, vol. 48, no. 2, pp. 348–356, 2010.

[15] J. P. Kehrer and L. O. Klotz, "Free radicals and related reactive species as mediators of tissue injury and disease: implications for health," *Critical Reviews in Toxicology*, vol. 45, no. 9, pp. 765–798, 2015.

[16] L. Covarrubias, D. Hernández-García, D. Schnabel, E. Salas-Vidal, and S. Castro-Obregón, "Function of reactive oxygen species during animal development: passive or active?," *Developmental Biology*, vol. 320, no. 1, pp. 1–11, 2008.

[17] M. Redza-Dutordoir and D. A. Averill-Bates, "Activation of apoptosis signalling pathways by reactive oxygen species,"

Biochimica et Biophysica Acta (BBA) - Molecular Cell Research, vol. 1863, no. 12, pp. 2977–2992, 2016.

[18] W. Filipowicz, S. N. Bhattacharyya, and N. Sonenberg, "Mechanisms of post-transcriptional regulation by micro-RNAs: are the answers in sight?," *Nature Reviews Genetics*, vol. 9, no. 2, pp. 102–114, 2008.

[19] S. Peng, D. Gao, C. Gao, P. Wei, M. Niu, and C. Shuai, "MicroRNAs regulate signaling pathways in osteogenic differentiation of mesenchymal stem cells (review)," *Molecular Medicine Reports*, vol. 14, no. 1, pp. 623–629, 2016.

[20] Y. Xu, B. Zhou, D. Wu, Z. Yin, and D. Luo, "Baicalin modulates microRNA expression in UVB irradiated mouse skin," *Journal of Biomedical Research*, vol. 26, no. 2, pp. 125–134, 2012.

[21] B. R. Zhou, Y. Xu, and D. Luo, "Effect of UVB irradiation on microRNA expression in mouse epidermis," *Oncology Letters*, vol. 3, no. 3, pp. 560–564, 2012.

[22] G. Tan, Y. Shi, and Z. H. Wu, "MicroRNA-22 promotes cell survival upon UV radiation by repressing PTEN," *Biochemical and Biophysical Research Communications*, vol. 417, no. 1, pp. 546–551, 2012.

[23] G. Chen, W. Zhu, D. Shi et al., "MicroRNA-181a sensitizes human malignant glioma U87MG cells to radiation by targeting Bcl-2," *Oncology Reports*, vol. 23, no. 4, pp. 997–1003, 2010.

[24] M. A. Chaudhry, R. A. Omaruddin, C. D. Brumbaugh, M. A. Tariq, and N. Pourmand, "Identification of radiation-induced microRNA transcriptome by next-generation massively parallel sequencing," *Journal of Radiation Research*, vol. 54, no. 5, pp. 808–822, 2013.

[25] Y. H. Su, W. C. Huang, T. H. Huang et al., "Folate deficient tumor microenvironment promotes epithelial-to-mesenchymal transition and cancer stem-like phenotypes," *Oncotarget*, vol. 7, no. 22, pp. 33246–33256, 2016.

[26] S. Dhar, A. Kumar, C. R. Gomez et al., "MTA1-activated Epi-microRNA-22 regulates E-cadherin and prostate cancer invasiveness," *FEBS Letters*, vol. 591, no. 6, pp. 924–933, 2017.

[27] S. Li, R. Hu, C. Wang, F. Guo, X. Li, and S. Wang, "miR-22 inhibits proliferation and invasion in estrogen receptor α-positive endometrial endometrioid carcinomas cells," *Molecular Medicine Reports*, vol. 9, no. 6, pp. 2393–2399, 2014.

[28] K. Pant, A. K. Yadav, P. Gupta, R. Islam, A. Saraya, and S. K. Venugopal, "Butyrate induces ROS-mediated apoptosis by modulating miR-22/SIRT-1 pathway in hepatic cancer cells," *Redox Biology*, vol. 12, pp. 340–349, 2017.

[29] J.-K. Du, B.-H. Cong, Q. Yua et al., "Upregulation of microRNA-22 contributes to myocardial ischemia-reperfusion injury by interfering with the mitochondrial function," *Free Radical Biology & Medicine*, vol. 96, pp. 406–417, 2016.

[30] C. P. Yang, Z. H. Zhang, L. H. Zhang, and H. C. Rui, "Neuroprotective role of MicroRNA-22 in a 6-hydroxydopamine-induced cell model of Parkinson's disease via regulation of its target gene TRPM7," *Journal of Molecular Neuroscience*, vol. 60, no. 4, pp. 445–452, 2016.

[31] J. Xue, C. Yu, W. Sheng et al., "The Nrf2/GCH1/BH4 sxis ameliorates radiation-induced skin injury by modulating the ROS cascade," *Journal of Investigative Dermatology*, vol. 137, no. 10, pp. 2059–2068, 2017.

[32] U. Weyemi, C. E. Redon, T. Aziz et al., "Inactivation of NADPH oxidases NOX4 and NOX5 protects human primary

fibroblasts from ionizing radiation-induced DNA damage," *Radiation Research*, vol. 183, no. 3, pp. 262–270, 2015.

[33] P. Becuwe, M. Ennen, R. Klotz, C. Barbieux, and S. Grandemange, "Manganese superoxide dismutase in breast cancer: from molecular mechanisms of gene regulation to biological and clinical significance," *Free Radical Biology & Medicine*, vol. 77, pp. 139–151, 2014.

[34] G. Xu, H. Wu, J. Zhang et al., "Metformin ameliorates ionizing irradiation-induced long-term hematopoietic stem cell injury in mice," *Free Radical Biology & Medicine*, vol. 87, pp. 15–25, 2015.

[35] N. Alessio, S. Capasso, G. di Bernardo et al., "Mesenchymal stromal cells having inactivated RB1 survive following low irradiation and accumulate damaged DNA: hints for side effects following radiotherapy," *Cell Cycle*, vol. 16, no. 3, pp. 251–258, 2017.

[36] X. Liang, Y. H. So, J. Cui et al., "The low-dose ionizing radiation stimulates cell proliferation via activation of the MAPK/ERK pathway in rat cultured mesenchymal stem cells," *Journal of Radiation Research*, vol. 52, no. 3, pp. 380–386, 2011.

[37] M. F. Chen, C. T. Lin, W. C. Chen et al., "The sensitivity of human mesenchymal stem cells to ionizing radiation," *International Journal of Radiation Oncology Biology Physics*, vol. 66, no. 1, pp. 244–253, 2006.

[38] S. Banerjee, N. Aykin-Burns, K. J. Krager et al., "Loss of C/EBPδ enhances IR-induced cell death by promoting oxidative stress and mitochondrial dysfunction," *International Journal of Radiation Oncology Biology Physics*, vol. 99, pp. 296–307, 2016.

[39] S. Cruet-Hennequart, C. Drougard, G. Shaw et al., "Radiation-induced alterations of osteogenic and chondrogenic differentiation of human mesenchymal stem cells," *PLoS One*, vol. 10, no. 4, article e0119334, 2015.

[40] Y. Wang, G. Zhu, J. Wang, and J. Chen, "Irradiation alters the differentiation potential of bone marrow mesenchymal stem cells," *Molecular Medicine Reports*, vol. 13, no. 1, pp. 213–223, 2016.

[41] J. Li, D. L. W. Kwong, and G. C.-F. Chan, "The effects of various irradiation doses on the growth and differentiation of marrow-derived human mesenchymal stromal cells," *Pediatric Transplantation*, vol. 11, no. 4, pp. 379–387, 2007.

[42] L. Wang, H. Y. Zhang, B. Gao et al., "Tetramethylpyrazine protects against glucocorticoid-induced apoptosis by promoting autophagy in mesenchymal stem cells and improves bone mass in glucocorticoid-induced osteoporosis rats," *Stem Cells and Development*, vol. 26, no. 6, pp. 419–430, 2017.

[43] C. H. Lin, N. T. Li, H. S. Cheng, and M. L. Yen, "Oxidative stress induces imbalance of adipogenic/osteoblastic lineage commitment in mesenchymal stem cells through decreasing SIRT1 functions," *Journal of Cellular and Molecular Medicine*, vol. 22, no. 2, pp. 786–796, 2017.

[44] Y. Tang, J. Sun, H. Fan, and X. Zhang, "An improved complex gel of modified gellan gum and carboxymethyl chitosan for chondrocytes encapsulation," *Carbohydrate Polymers*, vol. 88, no. 1, pp. 46–53, 2012.

MicroRNA-132, Delivered by Mesenchymal Stem Cell-Derived Exosomes, Promote Angiogenesis in Myocardial Infarction

Teng Ma, Yueqiu Chen, Yihuan Chen, Qingyou Meng, Jiacheng Sun ⓘ, Lianbo Shao ⓘ, Yunsheng Yu, Haoyue Huang, Yanqiu Hu, Ziying Yang ⓘ, Junjie Yang ⓘ, and Zhenya Shen ⓘ

Department of Cardiovascular Surgery of the First Affiliated Hospital & Institute for Cardiovascular Science, Soochow University, Suzhou, China

Correspondence should be addressed to Ziying Yang; skyinger@163.com, Junjie Yang; junjieyang2009@gmail.com, and Zhenya Shen; zhenyashen@sina.cn

Academic Editor: Marco Tatullo

Background. To cure ischemic diseases, angiogenesis needs to be improved by various strategies in ischemic area. Considering that microRNA-132 (miR-132) regulates endothelial cell behavior during angiogenesis and the safe and efficacious delivery of microRNAs *in vivo* is rarely achieved, an ideal vehicle for miR-132 delivery could bring the promise for ischemic diseases. As a natural carrier of biological molecules, exosomes are more and more developed as an ideal vehicle for miRNA transfer. Meanwhile, mesenchymal stem cells could release large amounts of exosomes. Thus, this study aimed to investigate whether MSC-derived exosomes can be used for miR-132 delivery in the treatment of myocardial ischemia. *Methods.* MSC-derived exosomes were electroporated with miR-132 mimics and inhibitors. After electroporation, miR-132 exosomes were labelled with DiI and added to HUVECs. Internalization of DiI-labelled exosomes was examined by fluorescent microscopy. Expression levels of miR-132 in exosomes and HUVECs were quantified by real-time PCR. The mRNA levels of miR-132 target gene RASA1 in HUVECs were quantified by real-time PCR. Luciferase reporter assay was performed to examine the targeting relationship between miR-132 and RASA1. The effects of miR-132 exosomes on the angiogenic ability of endothelial cells were evaluated by tube formation assay. Matrigel plug assay and myocardial infarction model were used to determine whether miR-132 exosomes can promote angiogenesis *in vivo*. *Results.* miR-132 mimics were effectively electroporated and highly detected in MSC-derived exosomes. The expression level of miR-132 was high in HUVECs preincubated with miR-132 mimic-electroporated exosomes and low in HUVECs preincubated with miR-132 inhibitor-electroporated exosomes. The expression level of RASA1, miR-132 target gene, was reversely correlated with miR-132 expression in HUVECs pretreated with exosomes. Luciferase reporter assay further confirmed that RASA1 was a direct target of miR-132. Exosomes loaded with miR-132, as a vehicle for miRNA transfer, significantly increased tube formation of endothelial cells. Moreover, subcutaneous injection of HUVECs pretreated with miR-132 exosomes in nude mice significantly increased their angiogenesis capacity *in vivo*. In addition, transplantation of miR-132 exosomes in the ischemic hearts of mice markedly enhanced the neovascularization in the peri-infarct zone and preserved heart functions. *Conclusions.* The findings suggest that the export of miR-132 via MSC-derived exosomes represents a novel strategy to enhance angiogenesis in ischemic diseases.

1. Introduction

In acute ischemic diseases such as myocardial ischemia, blood flow to the heart is impaired. Vessels need to be regenerated to rescue the ischemic cascade. Neoangiogenesis can be improved by activating endogenous progenitor cells, supplying exogenous stem cells and/or therapeutic molecules such as angiogenic mRNA or microRNAs [1, 2].

MicroRNAs, a class of small noncoding RNAs (containing about 18–22 nucleotides), regulate gene expression by direct binding to the $3'$-untranslated region ($3'$-UTR) of their target mRNAs and inducing their translational inhibition and/or degradation. MicroRNAs are recognized to participate in biological development, cell differentiation, apoptosis, and many other physiological and pathological processes [3]. Recently, multiple lines of evidence indicate that miR-132 regulate many processes in endothelial cells including angiogenic responses [1, 4, 5]. In 2010, Anand et al. demonstrated that upregulation of miR-132 positively controls pathological angiogenesis in response to vascular endothelial growth factor A (VEGF-A) by suppressing p120RasGap (RASA1) [4]. Recently, a study conducted by Katare et al. reported pericyte progenitor cells constitutively expressed and secreted miR-132 and promoted endothelial angiogenesis via modulation of methyl-CpG-binding protein 2 (MeCP2) [1]. Moreover, the potent proangiogenic effect of miR-132 has been confirmed in a mouse hind limb ischemia model. The study suggested that miR-132 may exert their proangiogenic effect by enhancing the Ras-mitogen-activated protein kinases (MAPK) signaling pathway through direct inhibition of RASA1 and Spred1 [5].

Exosomes are nanosized extracellular vesicles (30–100 nm in diameter) and are positive for CD9, CD63, and CD81. As a type of membrane vesicle, exosomes now have been recognized as a vehicle to facilitate intercellular communication and modulate the function of recipient cells though delivery of proteins, RNA, and other molecular constituents [6]. Exosomes have many remarkable attributes, such as stability, biocompatibility, and low immunogenicity, that delivery vehicles should have. The wide distribution of exosomes in the blood, urine, bronchoalveolar lavage fluid, breast milk, synovial fluid, pleural effusions, and ascites demonstrated that exosomes are well tolerated in biological fluids [7]. Another highly desired attribute of delivery vehicles is the ability to home to target location. Accumulating evidence suggests that depending on their cell source, surface antigen, and contents, exosomes could target specific cell types [8, 9]. These attributes provide a rationale for the applications of exosomes as therapeutic delivery vehicles in a wide spectrum of diseases such as cardiovascular disease, kidney injury, immune disease, neurological diseases, and cancer [9, 10–13].

The contents of exosomes are cell type specific and vary from different pathological conditions [14, 15]. Appropriate cell types need to be considered to obtain optimal and plentiful exosomes. Recently, mesenchymal stem cells (MSCs) are reported to be capable of secreting a large amount of functional exosomes. Studies have also demonstrated that MSC-derived exosomes have a significant proangiogenic function in myocardial infarction (MI) and hind limb ischemia model [10, 16].

In this study, we proposed that miR-132, delivered by MSC-derived exosomes, could exert the angiogenic effect in myocardial infarction. We investigated the angiogenic effect of miR-132-electroporated exosomes derived from MSCs *in vitro* and *in vivo*, as well as the underlying mechanisms. We treated HUVECs with miR-132 exosomes and found that miR-132 was upregulated in recipient cells, while the target gene RASA1 was downregulated in HUVECs. miR-132 exosomes promoted angiogenesis of HUVECs both *in vitro* and

in vivo. In addition, transplantation of miR-132 exosomes in the ischemic hearts of mice markedly enhanced the neovascularization in the peri-infarct zone and preserved heart functions. Our study represents a potential strategy for revascularization and has important implications for new therapeutic approaches to ischemic diseases.

2. Materials and Methods

2.1. Animals. The mice were purchased from the Laboratory Animal Center of Nanjing University (Nanjing, China). The animals were housed under specific pathogen-free conditions, with 12-hour light/dark cycles and free access to food and water. The animal experiment was approved by the Ethic Committee of Soochow University. All efforts were made to minimize animal suffering.

2.2. Cell Culture. Bone marrow-derived mesenchymal stem cells (BMSCs) were isolated based on a previously reported procedure [17]; bone marrow cells were flushed from the bone cavity of femurs and tibias using 1 ml syringe with low-glucose Dulbecco's modified eagle medium (DMEM). All bone marrow cells were passed through a 70 μm cell strainer. The obtained bone marrow cells were seeded onto a culture dish and incubated at 37°C in a humidified atmosphere containing 5% CO_2, with C57BL/6 mouse mesenchymal stem cell growth medium (Cyagen, Guangdong, China). The phenotype profile of BMSCs (P4–P6) was identified by flow cytometry, using antibodies against mouse CD31, CD44, and CD105 and Sca-1. Human umbilical venous endothelial cells (HUVECs; Cell Bank of Chinese Academy of Sciences, Shanghai, China) were cultured in EGM2 supplemented with 5% fetal bovine serum according to manufacturer's instructions. All experiments were performed before passage 7.

2.3. Isolation and Purification of MSC-Derived Exosomes. MSCs were cultured in DMEM/F12 supplemented with 10% exosome-free FBS. After 48 h, exosomes were isolated from BMSC supernatant as previously described [10]. Briefly, the supernatant was obtained and centrifuged at 200 ×g for 30 min at 4°C to remove cellular debris. Afterwards, the supernatants were mixed with total exosome isolation reagent (Invitrogen, USA) overnight at 4°C. After centrifuging at 10,000 ×g for 1 h, the pellet was then carefully resuspended in 200 μl of PBS and used immediately or stored at −80°C. To analyze these exosomes, the characteristic surface marker proteins of exosomes were analyzed by Western blot and the exosome morphologies were observed with a transmission electron microscope (TEM) (JEOL JEM-1230) as described previously in detail.

2.4. Loading miR-132 into Exosomes. Resuspended exosomes were diluted in the Gene Pulser electroporation buffer (Bio-Rad Laboratories, CA) in 1 : 1 ratio. 1 μmol of mouse miR-132 mimic (Ambion, NY) or inhibitor was added to 200 μl of exosome sample. The mixtures were transferred into cold 0.2 cm electroporation cuvettes and electroporated at 150 V/ 100 μF capacitance using a Gene Pulser II system (Bio-Rad Laboratories, CA) as described previously [18]. After removing the free-floating miRNA mimic, exosomes were reisolated using ultracentrifugation. The final pellet (exosome) was resuspended in PBS and stored at −80°C.

2.5. Exosome Labelling and Internalization. Exosomes (250 μg) were labelled with 1 μM of DiI lipophilic dye (Invitrogen). After incubating at 37°C for 30 min, excess dye was removed by washing with PBS, and labelled exosomes were reisolated by ultracentrifugation (described above). Recipient HUVECs (3×10^5) were incubated with DiI-labelled exosomes (10 μg) for 2 h, fixed in 4% paraformaldehyde (PFA) for 10 min at room temperature, washed with PBS for three times, incubated with DAPI (1 : 500, Invitrogen) for 5 minutes at room temperature, and subjected to confocal microscopy using a Zeiss LSM 780 confocal microscope with 100x magnification ($n = 3$).

2.6. Tube-Like Structure Formation Assay. 2×10^4/well HUVECs (three replicates per group) were seeded on top of Matrigel (BD Biosciences) in a 96-well plate and treated with the blank exosomes, miR-132 mimic electroexosomes, or miR-132 inhibitor electroexosomes, respectively. After incubation at 37°C for 6 h, tube formation was observed by an inverted microscope (Leica DMI6000B, Germany), and the cumulative tube length of the network structure was quantified (4x magnification) using ImageJ software.

2.7. Matrigel Plug Angiogenesis Assay. Matrigel plug angiogenesis assays were performed as previously described [19]; 2.5×10^5 HUVECs were treated with 30 μg of exosomes, or vehicle control (DMEM), premixed with Matrigel (1 mg/ml, BD Biosciences) and DMEM, and injected subcutaneously into SCID male mice (6-week-old, $n = 6$) in both inguinal regions. After 14 days, the animals were sacrificed using overdose of anesthetic. Plugs were excised and performed to the subsequent immunofluorescence assay.

2.8. Acute MI Model and Assessment of Heart Functions. An acute myocardial infarction (AMI) was generated in mice as described previously [20]. Briefly, C57BL/6J mice (female, ~20 g) were anesthetized with ketamine (80 mg/kg, IP) and mechanically ventilated. The left anterior descending artery (LAD) was ligated with a 6-0 suture, and the animals were divided into four groups: saline control, miR-132, Exo-null, and Exo-132. After LAD ligation, each mouse received an intramyocardial injection of PBS, miR-132, normal exosome, or miR-132-electroporated exosome, respectively. A total of 20 μl saline containing PBS, miR-132, or exosomes (600 μg) was transplanted by myocardial injection near the ligation site in the free wall of the left ventricle.

Cardiac function was determined by performing echocardiography on days 3, 7, and 28 after MI, using the Vevo 2100 system (VisualSonics Inc., Toronto, ON, Canada) with an 80 MHz probe. The left ventricular parameters were recorded from two-dimensional images using the M-mode interrogation in the short-axis view. Finally, the mice were sacrificed to harvest the heart tissue for immunohistochemical analysis.

2.9. Immunohistochemical Analysis. Immunohistochemistry staining was performed to detect vessel density of Matrigel plug and heart tissue as described previously [21]. The fresh tissue samples were fixed in 4% paraformaldehyde (PFA) and then embedded in OCT and cut into 6 μm thick slices. After blocking with 3% bovine serum albumin (BSA) for 30 min, the sections were subsequently incubated overnight at 4°C with the primary antibody against CD31. Secondary antibody goat anti-mouse Alexa 594 (1 : 500; Life Technologies) was used for detection. The nuclei were counterstained with 4,6-diamidino-2-phenylindole (DAPI). Images were observed by using a fluorescence microscope (Olympus).

2.10. Dual-Luciferase Reporter Assay. To elucidate whether RASA1 was a target gene of miR-132, TargetScan (http://targetscan.org) was used to predict miRNA molecules that may regulate RASA1, and miR-132 was identified as a potential regulator of RASA1. Wild-type (WT) and mutant seed regions of miR-132 in the 3′-UTR of RASA1 gene were cloned into pMIR-REPORT luciferase reporter plasmids (Invitrogen, USA). Plasmids with WT or mutant 3′-UTR DNA sequences were cotransfected with miR-132 mimic (100 nM; Sangon Biotech Co. Ltd., Shanghai, China) or negative control mimics into HEK293T cells (ATCC, Manassas, VA, USA). After cultivation at 37°C for 24 hours, cells were assayed using the dual-luciferase assay system (Promega, Madison, USA) according to the manufacturer's instructions. All assays were repeated at least three times.

2.11. Quantitative RT-PCR Assay. Total RNA was isolated from exosomes or HUVECs using TRIzol reagent (Invitrogen, USA) as described previously [22], and reverse transcription was performed using the microRNA reverse transcription system (GenePharma, Shanghai, China) or the PrimeScript RT reagent kit (TAKARA, Japan). The expression level of miR-132 was analyzed by SYBR Green assay following the manufacturer's instruction, using U6 as control. For RASA1, quantitative RT-PCR (Q-PCR) was performed using SYBR PCR master mix in the ABI Step One-Plus Detection system (Applied Biosystems, USA) according to the manufacturer's instructions. The primers used for RASA1 are as follows: sense, 5′-TTATGATGGGAGGCCG CTATT-3′, and antisense: 5′-CTGCATTGGTACAGGT TCCTT-3′. GAPDH was used as an internal control. The $2-\Delta\Delta CT$ method was employed to determine the relative mRNA expression. Each assay was performed in triplicate.

2.12. Western Blot Analysis. Western blotting was performed to quantify specific protein expression levels in BMSCs and BMSC-derived exosomes. Samples were lysed with RIPA buffer containing protease inhibitor cocktail (Roche, USA), and the protein concentration was determined by BCA assay (Roche, USA). Equal quantities of protein were loaded and run on 10% SDS-PAGE gels and then transferred to polyvinylidene difluoride (PVDF) membranes. Each membrane was blocked in 5% BSA and subsequently incubated overnight at 4°C with anti-CD9 and anti-CD63, respectively. After washing, the membranes were incubated with peroxidase-conjugated goat anti-mouse secondary antibody (Invitrogen, USA). Image analysis and blot quantification

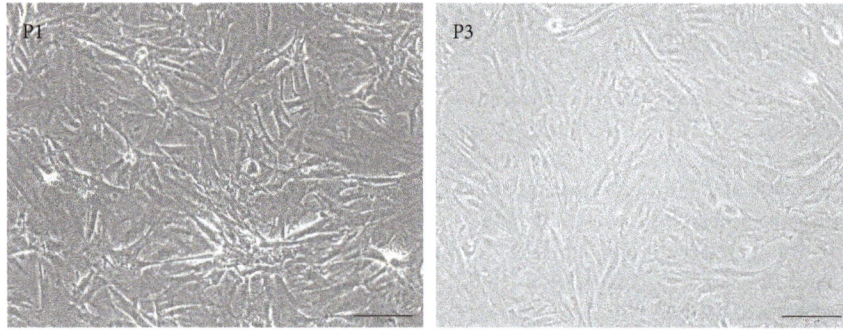

(a)

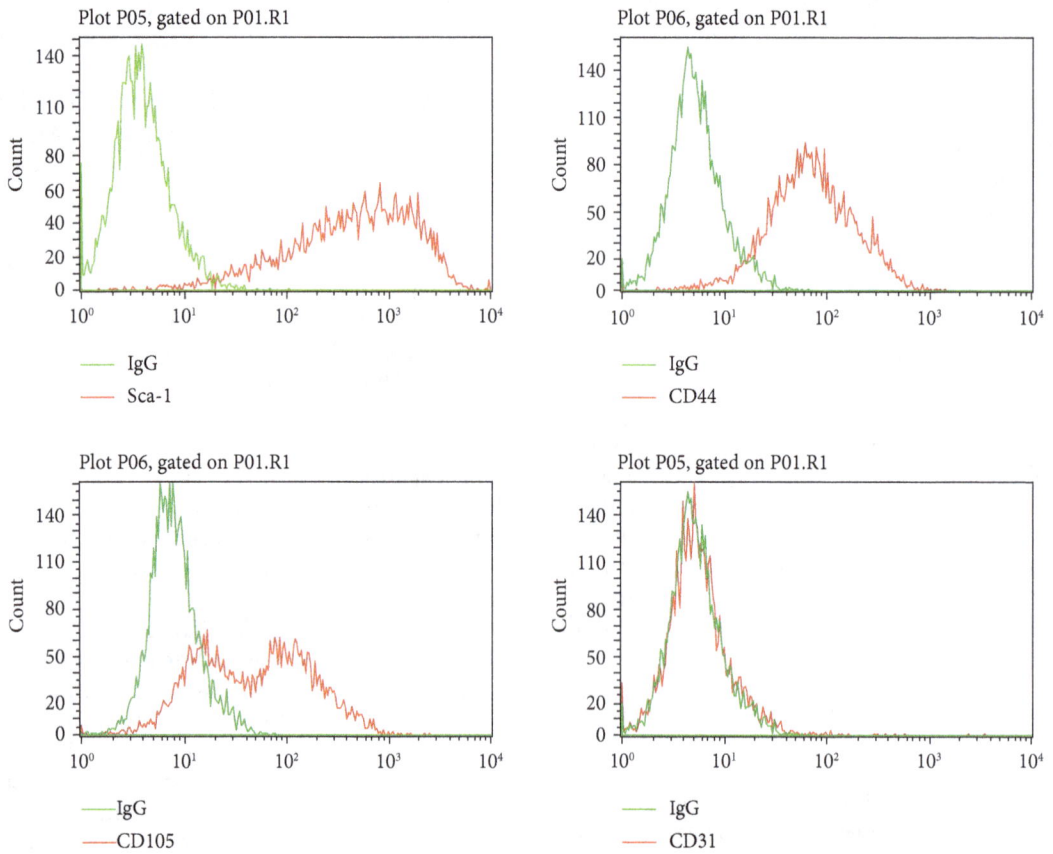

(b)

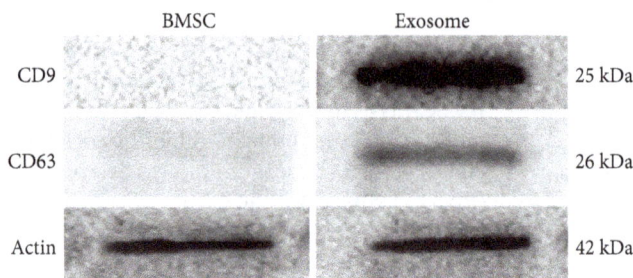

(c)

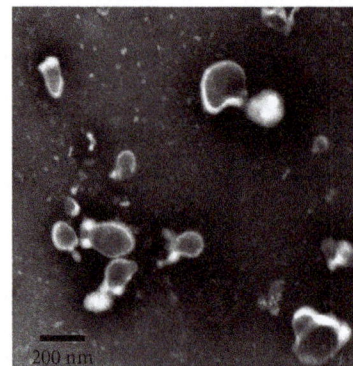

(d)

FIGURE 1: Continued.

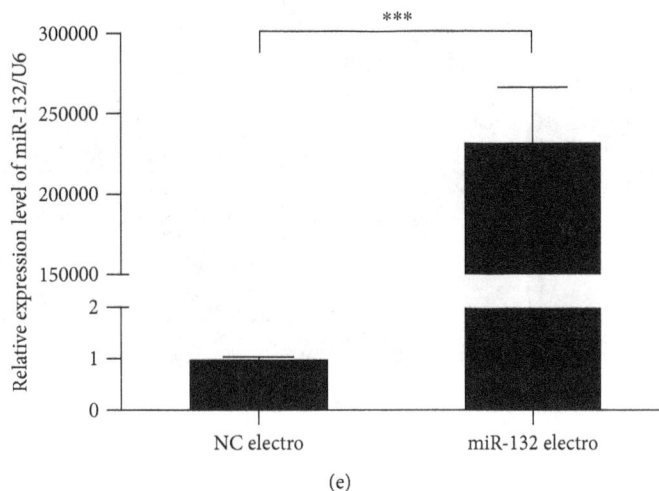

(e)

FIGURE 1: Characterization of BMSCs and BMSC-derived exosomes. (a) Morphology of MSCs (P1, P3) observed under an inverted fluorescence microscope. Scale bar: 100 μm. (b) Phenotypic analysis of cell surface antigens of MSCs by flow cytometry ($n = 3$). (c) Surface marker proteins of BMSCs and BMSC-derived exosomes analyzed by Western immunoblotting ($n = 3$). (d) Morphology of MSC-derived exosomes under transmission electron microscopy. Scale bar: 200 nm. (e) The expression level of miR-132 determined by Q-PCR ($n = 3$). ***$P < 0.001$. NC: negative control.

were performed with Image Quant LAS 4000 mini biomolecular imager (GE Healthcare, Uppsala, Sweden).

2.13. Statistical Analysis. All data of *in vitro* experiments were obtained from at least three independent experiments. In the *in vivo* study, more than 6 samples were used in each group. The results were presented as means ± SD unless otherwise indicated and were analyzed using GraphPad Prism 5 software. Statistical analyses were performed using a two-tailed Student *t*-test or one-way ANOVA with post hoc tests to determine significant differences between the groups. $P < 0.05$ was considered statistically significant.

3. Results

3.1. Characterization of BMSCs and BMSC-Derived Exosomes. MSCs were isolated from the bone marrow of C57BL/6 mice as described previously. MSCs were typically spindle-shaped and adherent to the plastic dishes (Figure 1(a)). Flow cytometry was used to identify the surface antigens of MSCs. Results showed that MSCs were negative for CD31, but positive for Sca-1, CD44, and CD105 (Figure 1(b)). The exosomes secreted from BMSCs were isolated as described in Materials and Methods and subjected to biochemical and biophysical analyses. Biochemical analysis of isolated exosomes showed the presence of the exosome proteins CD63 and CD9 (Figure 1(c)), while no expression of CD63 and CD9 was detected in BMSCs. Electron microscopy analysis of exosomes exhibited typical cup-shaped morphology and confirmed the size range of less than 150 nm (Figure 1(d)). Furthermore, a significant miR-132 overexpression was detected by qRT-PCR in electroporated MSCs with miR-132 (Figure 1(e)).

3.2. miR-132 Exosomes Are Efficiently Taken Up by HUVECs. Exosomes were labelled with CM-DiI dye and incubated

with HUVECs *in vitro*. Using an inverted fluorescence microscope, we provided qualitative evidence that HUVECs take up DiI-labelled exosomes derived from BMSCs (Figure 2(a)). Next, we performed qPCR to evaluate the expression of miR-132 in HUVECs. We observed a significant increase of miR-132 expression in HUVECs taking up miR-132 mimic electro-Exos, when compared with both blank HUVECs and HUVECs taking up miR-132 inhibitor electro-Exos (Figure 2(b)). It is worthy of note that the expression of RASA1, a target gene of miR-132, was significantly downregulated (Figure 2(c)). Luciferase reporter assay was used to further confirm the targeting relationship between miR-132 and RASA1. Results showed that miR-132 significantly decreased the relative luciferase reporter activity of the wild-type RASA1 3′-UTR, whereas that of the mutant RASA1 3′-UTR did not change significantly, which suggests that miR-132 could directly bind to the 3′-UTR of RASA1 (Figure 2(d)).

3.3. miR-132-Electroporated Exosomes Promote Angiogenesis In Vitro. We investigated whether miR-132 electroexosomes could enhance the angiogenic behavior of endothelial cells *in vitro*. The tube length and the number of meshes were increased in HUVECs treated with miR-132 mimic electroexosomes for 12 h, compared to those treated with blank exosomes and miR-132 inhibitor electroexosomes (Figures 3(a)–3(c)). As evidenced by tube formation assay, our study suggests that overexpressed miR-132 could enhance the proangiogenic effects of exosome on endothelial cells.

3.4. miR-132-Electroporated Exosomes Promote Angiogenesis In Vivo. Finally, we utilized Matrigel plug to examine *in vivo* angiogenic behavior. Matrigel containing HUVECs, HUVECs treated with blank exosome, or HUVECs treated with miR-132 mimic electroexosome was injected subcutaneously into SCID male mice ($n = 6$) in the inguinal regions,

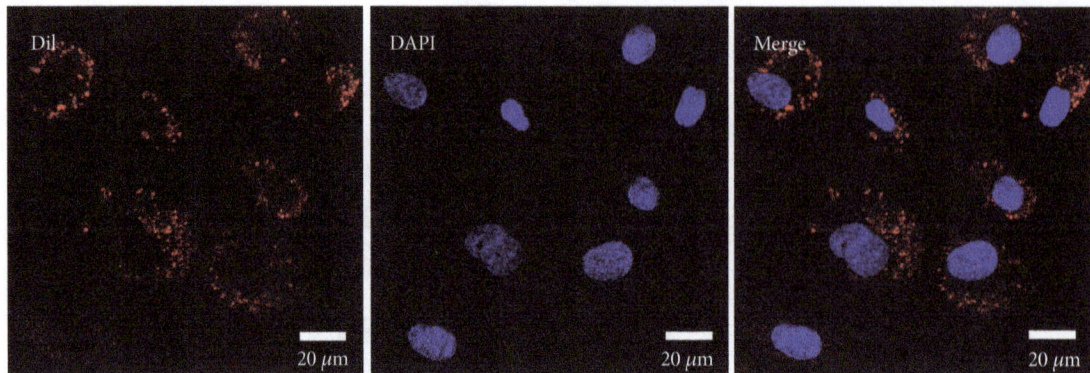

(a)

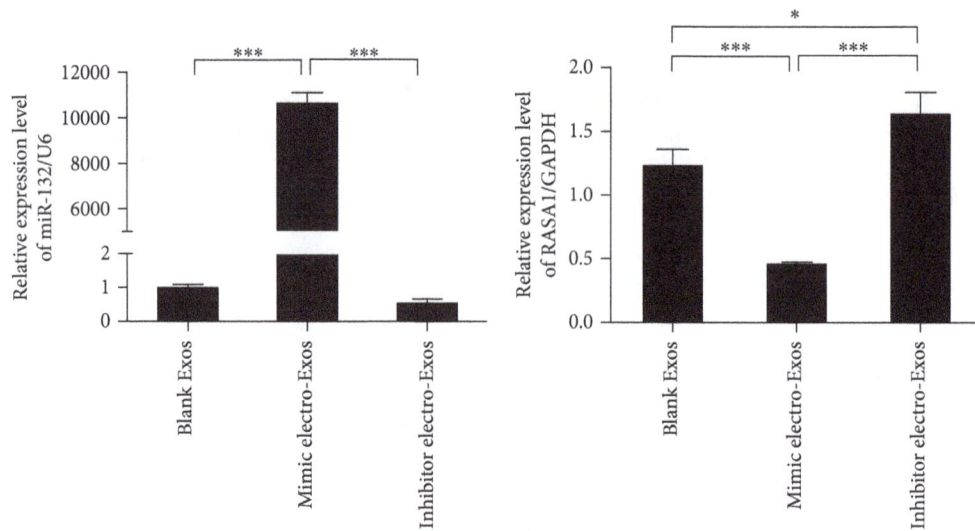

(b)   (c)

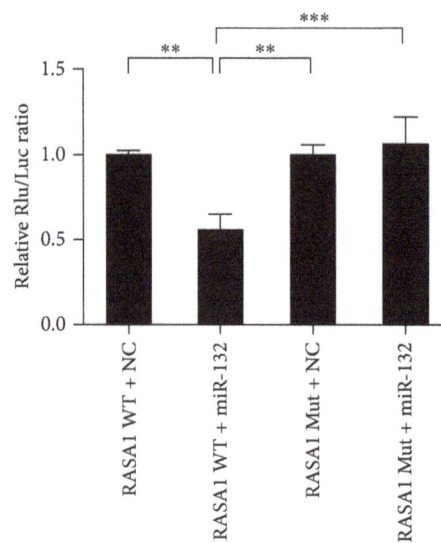

(d)

FIGURE 2: Internalization of miR-132-electroporated exosomes and detection of target gene RASA1. (a) Confocal images of DiI-labelled exosomes taken up by HUVECs. Scale bar: 20 μm. (b, c) HUVECs were incubated with miR-132 mimics or inhibitor-electroporated exosomes for 2 h. The relative expression level of miR-132 and its target gene RASA1 was detected by RT-PCR ($n = 3$). (d) 293T was cotransfected with miR-132 mimics or NC and firefly luciferase reporter plasmid containing wild-type or mutant-type 3′UTR of RASA1. After incubation for 48 h, the firefly luciferase activity of each sample was detected and normalized to the Renilla luciferase activity ($n = 3$). The data represent the mean ± SEM of triplicates. $^*P < 0.05$, $^{**}P < 0.01$, $^{***}P < 0.001$.

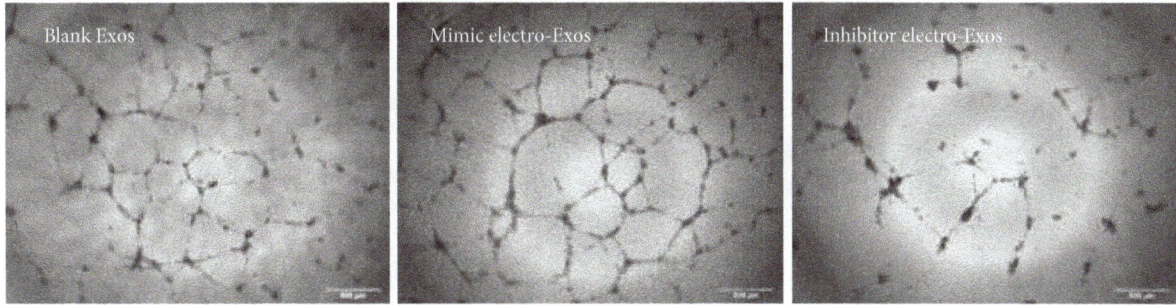

(a)

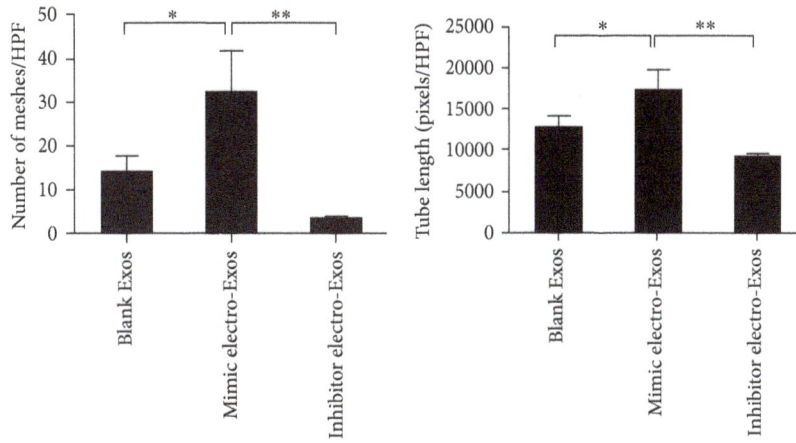

(b) (c)

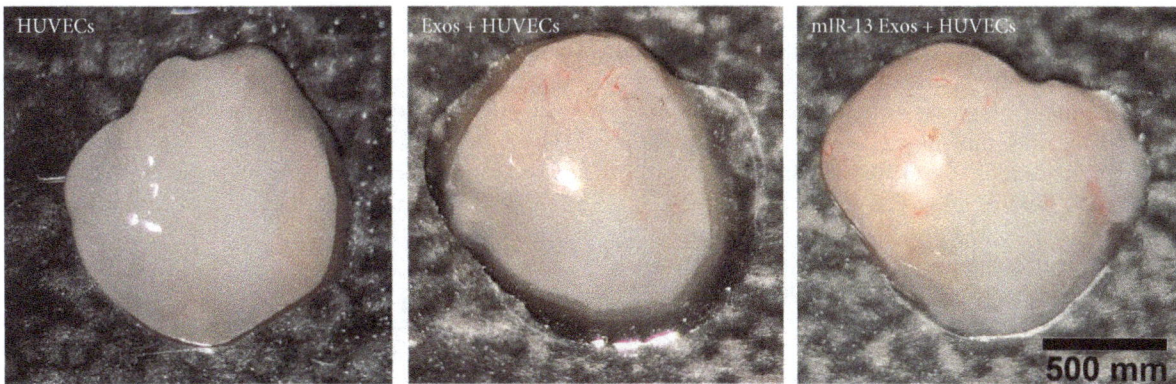

(d)

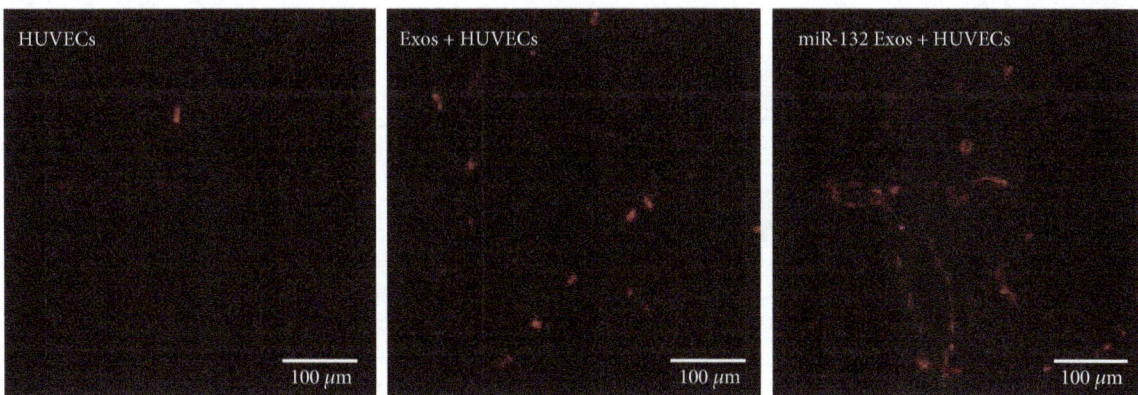

(e)

Figure 3: Continued.

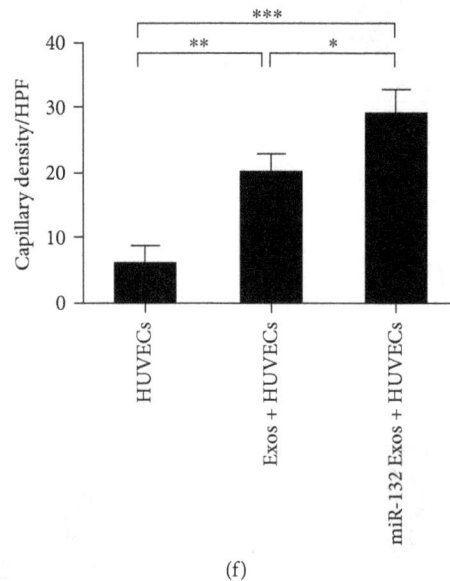

(f)

FIGURE 3: miR-132-electroporated exosomes promoted angiogenesis *in vitro* and *in vivo*. (a) Tube formation assay on Matrigel was assessed 6 h after seeding HUVECs pretreated with blank, miR-132 mimic-electroporated or miR-132 inhibitor-electroporated exosomes. Scale bar: 500 μm. (b, c) Quantitative assessment of the total number of meshes and tube length ($n = 3$). $^{*}P < 0.05$, $^{**}P < 0.01$. (d) Gross look of Matrigel plugs. (e, f) Immunofluorescence staining of vessels in the sections of Matrigel plugs and quantitative assessment of capillaries per high-power field in each group ($n = 3$). $^{*}P < 0.05$, $^{***}P < 0.001$.

respectively. After 14 days, Matrigel was excised and photographed to assess the presence of blood vessels. The Matrigel plugs containing miR-132 exosome exhibited bright red color indicating blood-perfused vessels, whereas blank exosome-containing plugs presented light yellowish color that is correlated with the limited formation of new vessels (Figure 3(d)). In addition, the immunofluorescence staining showed that the number of vessels in the plugs containing miR-132 exosomes (29.33 ± 2.86/HPF) was also significantly higher than that in the negative control (6.33 ± 2.05/HPF) and those containing blank exosomes (20.33 ± 2.05/HPF) (Figures 3(e) and 3(f)).

3.5. miR-132-Electroporated Exosomes Preserve Cardiac Function and Promote Angiogenesis in a Mouse MI Model. We assessed the *in vivo* therapeutic effects of miR-132 exosomes on a mouse MI model. Preinterventional left ventricular ejection fraction (LVEF) and fractional shortening (FS) values were similar in all groups (data not shown). Significant decreases in LVEF and FS in saline-treated mice were observed on day 7 and day 28 after MI. Compared with saline-treated mice, the miR-132 and normal exosome group partially rescued MI-induced decrease of LVEF and FS, while the miR-132-exosome group significantly increased LVEF (day 7: 30.18 ± 0.94 versus 48.04 ± 1.27, $P < 0.001$, and day 28: 31.56 ± 0.83 versus 51.97 ± 1.32, $P < 0.001$, resp.) and FS (day 7: 12.21 ± 1.16 versus 19.87 ± 1.17, $P < 0.01$, and day 28: 11.80 ± 0.25 versus 21.33 ± 0.64, $P < 0.0001$, resp.) compared with saline-treated mice on day 7 and day 28 after MI (Figures 4(a) and 4(b)). Hearts were excised on day 28 after MI. Capillary density of cardiac tissue was further examined by immunohistochemical stain. Compared with

the saline-treated group (19 ± 2.45/HPF), both the miR-132 (33.33 ± 3.40/HPF) and normal exosome groups (32.67 ± 3.09/HPF) had a higher density of vessels. More importantly, the capillary density of the infarct area was significantly increased in the miR-132 exosome group (50 ± 1.63/HPF), (Figures 4(c) and 4(d)). These data demonstrate that miR-132-electroporated exosomes could effectively preserve cardiac function and promote angiogenesis in a mouse MI model.

4. Discussion

In this paper, we demonstrated that exosomes loaded with miR-132, as a vehicle for miRNA carriage and transfer, significantly increased tube formation *in vitro* and neoangiogenesis in Matrigel plug and myocardial infarction. Mechanistically, miR-132 promotes angiogenesis by downregulating the expression level of its target gene RASA1 in HUVECs. These findings greatly extend our current understanding of exosomes on angiogenesis and indicate that exosomes give an inspiring hope as vehicles of therapeutic molecules for the treatment of ischemic diseases.

Ischemic heart disease (IHD) is the leading cause of morbidity and mortality worldwide owing to aging, obesity, diabetes, and other comorbid diseases [23]. One potent therapeutic approach for IHD is to induce revascularization, therefore, increase oxygen supply, inhibit cardiomyocyte apoptosis, and reduce myocardial fibrosis. MicroRNAs are small noncoding RNAs that act as negative regulators of protein-coding genes. It has been well established that microRNAs promote both physiological and pathological angiogenesis [4, 24]. A large number of therapeutic strategies

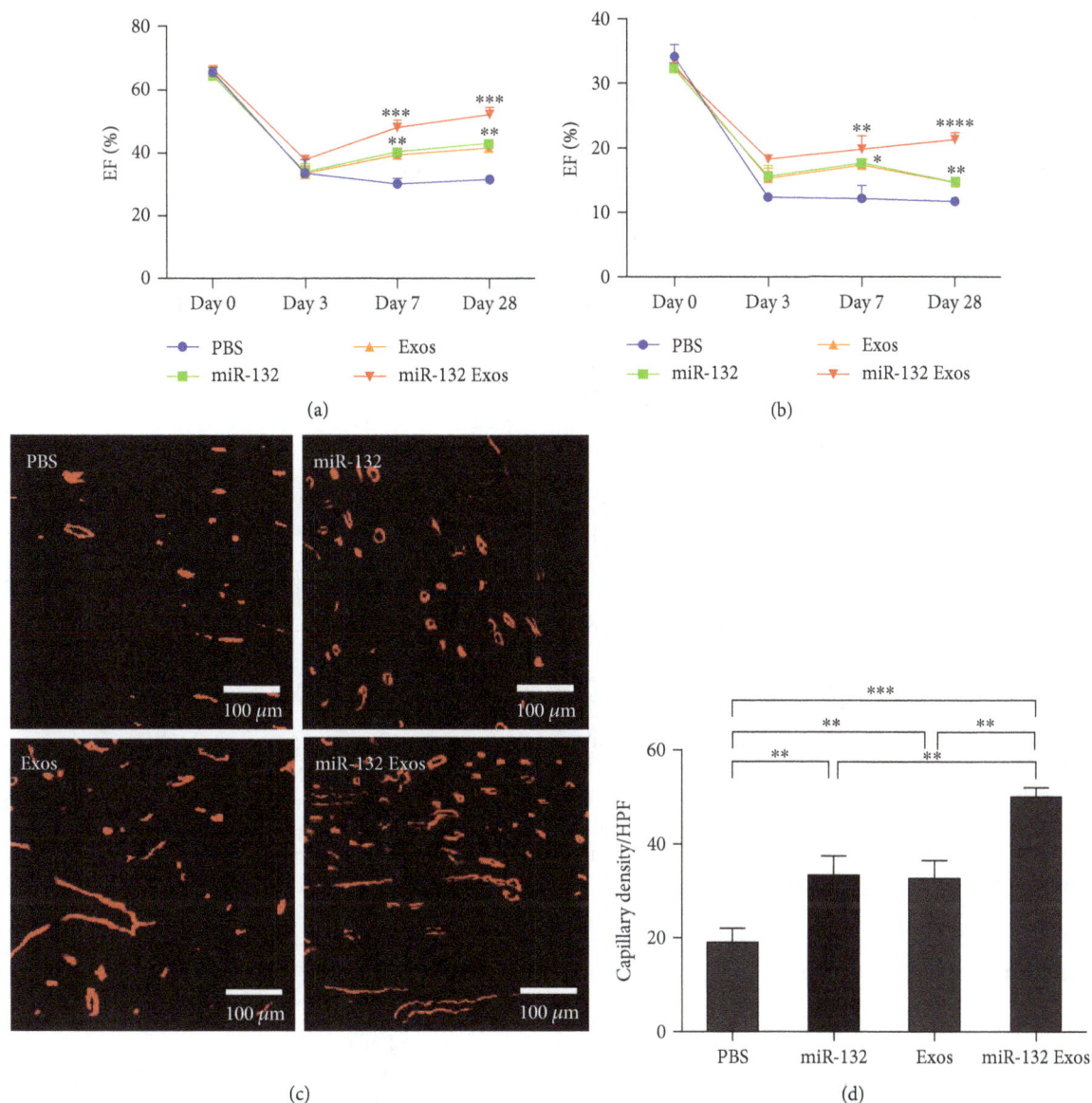

FIGURE 4: miR-132-electroporated exosomes preserve cardiac function and promoted angiogenesis in MI model. (a, b) Quantitative assessment of LVEF and FS value in each group after MI ($n = 3$). $^{*}P < 0.05$, $^{**}P < 0.01$, $^{***}P < 0.001$, $^{****}P < 0.0001$. (c, d) Immunofluorescence staining of vessels in the sections of heart tissue and quantitative assessment of capillaries per high-power field in each group. Scale bar: 500 μm ($n = 3$). $^{**}P < 0.01$, $^{***}P < 0.001$.

based on microRNAs have been carried out on the treatment of myocardial infarction and other ischemic diseases [2, 20, 22].

The intercellular communication occurs directly (between adjacent cells, via gap junctions) or indirectly (at long distances, via soluble factors and extracellular vesicles, including exosomes). These vesicles that act as the vehicles of proteins, RNA, and other molecular constituents modulate the intercellular communication. Previous studies reported that changing the miRNA expression in exosomes derived from MSCs could protect ischemia-reperfusion injury and promote angiogenesis in acute MI [10, 25]. All of these findings indicated that exosomes, as natural therapeutic delivery vehicles, play an important role in angiogenesis [10, 26]. In

addition, exosomes can be easily stored at −20°C for at least 6 months without loss of biological activity [27]. Exosomes may be easier to manufacture and standardize in terms of dosage and biological activity.

According to previous researches, we selected miR-132 for gain and loss of function in HUVECs pretreated with electroporated exosomes, to investigate the role of exosome-transferred proangiomiRs in angiogenesis. Exogenous miR-132 mimics and inhibitors were successfully electroporated into MSC-derived exosomes, and it was shown that loaded exosomes can be taken up by HUVECs. The loaded exosomes effectively delivered miR-132 mimics into HUVECs, causing increase of miR-132, and functionally promoted tube formation and neoangiogenesis in Matrigel plug and myocardial infarction. On the contrary, inhibiting the expression of miR-132 in exosomes derived from MSCs resulted in reduced angiogenesis. These findings indicate that the extracellular miR-132 was loaded into exosomes, transferred into endothelial cells, and played a critical role in angiogenesis.

Furthermore, to investigate the molecular mechanisms by which miR-132 might promote angiogenesis, we focus on its target gene RASA1. RASA1 has been reported to be an evolutionary conserved target of miR-132 [5]. Previous studies have demonstrated that RASA1 acts as a crucial negative regulator of vascular sprouting and vessel branching. Furthermore, other researches have revealed that RASA1 regulates endothelial cell behavior during angiogenesis in HUVECs by inactivating the Ras-mitogen-activated protein kinase (MAPK) signaling pathway [5]. Our results showed that increasing the expression of miR-132 led to a statistically significant decrease of RASA1 level in HUVECs. This observation is in agreement with previous data [4]. In order to confirm the interaction between miR-132 and RASA1, we performed dual-luciferase reporter assay which demonstrated that RASA1 is a real target of miR-132 in HUVECs.

In conclusion, we identified that miR-132-electroporated exosomes promoted angiogenesis *in vitro* and *in vivo*. MSC-derived exosomes could be considered as a potential candidate for therapeutic angiogenesis especially for ischemic diseases. Exosomes derived from MSCs have theoretical advantages as a medicinal product, and, in the future, exosomes may gain preference over whole cell-based therapy in the discipline of regenerative medicine.

Abbreviations

MSC:	Mesenchymal stem cells
MI:	Myocardial infarction
$3'$-UTR:	$3'$-untranslated region
VEGF-A:	Vascular endothelial growth factor A
RASA1:	p120RasGap
MeCP2:	Methyl-CpG-binding protein 2
MAPK:	Ras-mitogen-activated protein kinases
DMEM:	Dulbecco's modified eagle medium
HUVECs:	Human umbilical venous endothelial cells
TEM:	Transmission electron microscope
PFA:	Paraformaldehyde
LAD:	Left anterior descending artery
DAPI:	4,6-Diamidino-2-phenylindole
BSA:	Bovine serum albumin
WT:	Wild-type
PVDF:	Polyvinylidene difluoride
LVEF:	Left ventricular ejection fraction
FS:	Fractional shortening
IHD:	Ischemic heart disease.

Authors' Contributions

Teng Ma, Yueqiu Chen, Yihuan Chen, and Qingyou Meng contributed equally to this work. All authors have contributed to, read, and approved the final manuscript for submission.

Acknowledgments

This work was supported by the National Natural Science Foundation of China (nos. 81770260, 81400199), National Clinical Key Specialty of Cardiovascular Surgery, and Jiangsu Clinical Research Center for Cardiovascular Surgery (BL201451), and Natural Science Foundation of Jiangsu Province (BK20160346 and BK20151212).

References

[1] R. Katare, F. Riu, K. Mitchell et al., "Transplantation of human pericyte progenitor cells improves the repair of infarcted heart through activation of an angiogenic program involving micro-RNA-132," *Circulation Research*, vol. 109, no. 8, pp. 894–906, 2011.

[2] Z. Wen, W. Huang, Y. Feng et al., "MicroRNA-377 regulates mesenchymal stem cell-induced angiogenesis in ischemic hearts by targeting VEGF," *PLoS One*, vol. 9, no. 9, article e104666, 2014.

[3] J. Krol, I. Loedige, and W. Filipowicz, "The widespread regulation of microRNA biogenesis, function and decay," *Nature Reviews Genetics*, vol. 11, no. 9, pp. 597–610, 2010.

[4] S. Anand, B. K. Majeti, L. M. Acevedo et al., "MicroRNA-132–mediated loss of p120RasGAP activates the endothelium to facilitate pathological angiogenesis," *Nature Medicine*, vol. 16, no. 8, pp. 909–914, 2010.

[5] Z. Lei, A. van Mil, M. M. Brandt et al., "MicroRNA-132/212 family enhances arteriogenesis after hindlimb ischaemia through modulation of the Ras-MAPK pathway," *Journal of Cellular and Molecular Medicine*, vol. 19, no. 8, pp. 1994–2005, 2015.

[6] H. Valadi, K. Ekstrom, A. Bossios, M. Sjostrand, J. J. Lee, and J. O. Lotvall, "Exosome-mediated transfer of mRNAs and microRNAs is a novel mechanism of genetic exchange between cells," *Nature Cell Biology*, vol. 9, no. 6, pp. 654–659, 2007.

[7] R. J. Simpson, S. S. Jensen, and J. W. E. Lim, "Proteomic profiling of exosomes: current perspectives," *Proteomics*, vol. 8, no. 19, pp. 4083–4099, 2008.

[8] L. Alvarez-Erviti, Y. Seow, H. F. Yin, C. Betts, S. Lakhal, and M. J. A. Wood, "Delivery of siRNA to the mouse brain by systemic injection of targeted exosomes," *Nature Biotechnology*, vol. 29, no. 4, pp. 341–345, 2011.

[9] J. L. Hood, R. S. San, and S. A. Wickline, "Exosomes released by melanoma cells prepare sentinel lymph nodes for tumor metastasis," *Cancer Research*, vol. 71, no. 11, pp. 3792–3801, 2011.

[10] Z. Zhang, J. Yang, W. Yan, Y. Li, Z. Shen, and T. Asahara, "Pretreatment of cardiac stem cells with exosomes derived from mesenchymal stem cells enhances myocardial repair," *Journal of the American Heart Association*, vol. 5, no. 1, article e002856, 2016.

[11] M. Morigi, B. Imberti, C. Zoja et al., "Mesenchymal stem cells are renotropic, helping to repair the kidney and improve func-

tion in acute renal failure," *Journal of the American Society of Nephrology*, vol. 15, no. 7, pp. 1794–1804, 2004.

[12] A. Mokarizadeh, N. Delirezh, A. Morshedi, G. Mosayebi, A. A. Farshid, and K. Mardani, "Microvesicles derived from mesenchymal stem cells: potent organelles for induction of tolerogenic signaling," *Immunology Letters*, vol. 147, no. 1-2, pp. 47–54, 2012.

[13] H. Xin, Y. Li, B. Buller et al., "Exosome-mediated transfer of miR-133b from multipotent mesenchymal stromal cells to neural cells contributes to neurite outgrowth," *Stem Cells*, vol. 30, no. 7, pp. 1556–1564, 2012.

[14] H. Tadokoro, T. Umezu, K. Ohyashiki, T. Hirano, and J. H. Ohyashiki, "Exosomes derived from hypoxic leukemia cells enhance tube formation in endothelial cells," *Journal of Biological Chemistry*, vol. 288, no. 48, pp. 34343–34351, 2013.

[15] B. Yu, H. W. Kim, M. Gong et al., "Exosomes secreted from GATA-4 overexpressing mesenchymal stem cells serve as a reservoir of anti-apoptotic microRNAs for cardioprotection," *International Journal of Cardiology*, vol. 182, pp. 349–360, 2015.

[16] G. W. Hu, Q. Li, X. Niu et al., "Exosomes secreted by human-induced pluripotent stem cell-derived mesenchymal stem cells attenuate limb ischemia by promoting angiogenesis in mice," *Stem Cell Research & Therapy*, vol. 6, no. 1, p. 10, 2015.

[17] M. Gnecchi and L. G. Melo, "Bone marrow-derived mesenchymal stem cells: isolation, expansion, characterization, viral transduction, and production of conditioned medium," *Methods in Molecular Biology*, vol. 482, pp. 281–294, 2009.

[18] F. Momen-Heravi, S. Bala, T. Bukong, and G. Szabo, "Exosome-mediated delivery of functionally active miRNA-155 inhibitor to macrophages," *Nanomedicine: Nanotechnology, Biology and Medicine*, vol. 10, no. 7, pp. 1517–1527, 2014.

[19] P. Mocharla, S. Briand, G. Giannotti et al., "AngiomiR-126 expression and secretion from circulating CD34$^+$ and CD14$^+$ PBMCs: role for proangiogenic effects and alterations in type 2 diabetics," *Blood*, vol. 121, no. 1, pp. 226–236, 2013.

[20] W. Huang, S. S. Tian, P. Z. Hang, C. Sun, J. Guo, and Z. M. Du, "Combination of microRNA-21 and microRNA-146a attenuates cardiac dysfunction and apoptosis during acute myocardial infarction in mice," *Molecular Therapy - Nucleic Acids*, vol. 5, article e296, 2016.

[21] A. K. Horst, W. D. Ito, J. Dabelstein et al., "Carcinoembryonic antigen–related cell adhesion molecule 1 modulates vascular remodeling in vitro and in vivo," *The Journal of Clinical Investigation*, vol. 116, no. 6, pp. 1596–1605, 2006.

[22] Y. Chen, Y. Zhao, W. Chen et al., "MicroRNA-133 overexpression promotes the therapeutic efficacy of mesenchymal stem cells on acute myocardial infarction," *Stem Cell Research & Therapy*, vol. 8, no. 1, p. 268, 2017.

[23] A. Saparov, V. Ogay, T. Nurgozhin et al., "Role of the immune system in cardiac tissue damage and repair following myocardial infarction," *Inflammation Research*, vol. 66, no. 9, pp. 739–751, 2017.

[24] M. Dews, A. Homayouni, D. Yu et al., "Augmentation of tumor angiogenesis by a Myc-activated microRNA cluster," *Nature Genetics*, vol. 38, no. 9, pp. 1060–1065, 2006.

[25] W. D. Gray, K. M. French, S. Ghosh-Choudhary et al., "Identification of therapeutic covariant microRNA clusters in hypoxia-treated cardiac progenitor cell exosomes using systems biology," *Circulation Research*, vol. 116, no. 2, pp. 255–263, 2015.

Permissions

All chapters in this book were first published in SCI, by Hindawi Publishing Corporation; hereby published with permission under the Creative Commons Attribution License or equivalent. Every chapter published in this book has been scrutinized by our experts. Their significance has been extensively debated. The topics covered herein carry significant findings which will fuel the growth of the discipline. They may even be implemented as practical applications or may be referred to as a beginning point for another development.

The contributors of this book come from diverse backgrounds, making this book a truly international effort. This book will bring forth new frontiers with its revolutionizing research information and detailed analysis of the nascent developments around the world.

We would like to thank all the contributing authors for lending their expertise to make the book truly unique. They have played a crucial role in the development of this book. Without their invaluable contributions this book wouldn't have been possible. They have made vital efforts to compile up to date information on the varied aspects of this subject to make this book a valuable addition to the collection of many professionals and students.

This book was conceptualized with the vision of imparting up-to-date information and advanced data in this field. To ensure the same, a matchless editorial board was set up. Every individual on the board went through rigorous rounds of assessment to prove their worth. After which they invested a large part of their time researching and compiling the most relevant data for our readers.

The editorial board has been involved in producing this book since its inception. They have spent rigorous hours researching and exploring the diverse topics which have resulted in the successful publishing of this book. They have passed on their knowledge of decades through this book. To expedite this challenging task, the publisher supported the team at every step. A small team of assistant editors was also appointed to further simplify the editing procedure and attain best results for the readers.

Apart from the editorial board, the designing team has also invested a significant amount of their time in understanding the subject and creating the most relevant covers. They scrutinized every image to scout for the most suitable representation of the subject and create an appropriate cover for the book.

The publishing team has been an ardent support to the editorial, designing and production team. Their endless efforts to recruit the best for this project, has resulted in the accomplishment of this book. They are a veteran in the field of academics and their pool of knowledge is as vast as their experience in printing. Their expertise and guidance has proved useful at every step. Their uncompromising quality standards have made this book an exceptional effort. Their encouragement from time to time has been an inspiration for everyone.

The publisher and the editorial board hope that this book will prove to be a valuable piece of knowledge for researchers, students, practitioners and scholars across the globe.

List of Contributors

Hang Liang, Sheng Chen, Donghua Huang, Xiangyu Deng, Kaige Ma and Zengwu Shao
Department of Orthopaedics, Union Hospital, Tongji Medical College, Huazhong University of Science and Technology, 1277 Jiefang Avenue, Wuhan 430022, China

Jun Jia, Liang-yu Ma, Jia-bin Yu and Chen Wang
School of Medicine, Southeast University, 87 Ding Jia Qiao Road, Nanjing, Jiangsu 210009, China

Yu-dong Guo
Department of Orthopaedics, Zhongda Hospital, School of Medicine, Southeast University, 87 Ding Jia Qiao Road, Nanjing,Jiangsu 210009, China

Shan-zheng Wang
Department of Orthopaedics, Zhongda Hospital, School of Medicine, Southeast University, 87 Ding Jia Qiao Road, Nanjing,Jiangsu 210009, China
The First Clinical Medical School, Nanjing Medical University, 300 Guangzhou Road, Nanjing, Jiangsu 210029, China

Natalie Lee and Aishwarya Sundaresh
Wolfson Childhood Cancer Research Centre, Northern Institute for Cancer Research, Newcastle University, UK

Deepali Pal
Wolfson Childhood Cancer Research Centre, Northern Institute for Cancer Research, Newcastle University, UK
North East Stem Cell Institute, Newcastle University, UK

Jane Carr-Wilkinson
Wolfson Childhood Cancer Research Centre, Northern Institute for Cancer Research, Newcastle University, UK
North East Stem Cell Institute, Newcastle University, UK
Faculty of Health Sciences and Wellbeing, University of Sunderland, UK

Deborah A. Tweddle
Wolfson Childhood Cancer Research Centre, Northern Institute for Cancer Research, Newcastle University, UK
North East Stem Cell Institute, Newcastle University, UK
Great North Children's Hospital, Newcastle upon Tyne Hospitals NHS Trust, UK

Nilendran Prathalingam and Majlinda Lako
North East Stem Cell Institute, Newcastle University, UK
Institute of Genetic Medicine, Newcastle University, UK

Mary Herbert
North East Stem Cell Institute, Newcastle University, UK
Institute of Genetic Medicine, Newcastle University, UK
Newcastle Fertility Centre, Newcastle University, UK

Helen Forgham
Faculty of Health Sciences and Wellbeing, University of Sunderland, UK

Mohammad Moad
Northern Institute for Cancer Research, Paul O-Gorman Building, Newcastle University, UK

Peter James
Institute of Health & Society, Newcastle University, UK

Letizia De Chiara
Centro di Eccellenza DeNothe, Department of Biomedical, Experimental and Clinical Sciences, University of Florence, Viale Pieraccini 6, 50139 Firenze, Italy
Molecular Biotechnology Center, Department of Molecular Biotechnology and Health Sciences, University of Turin, Via Nizza 52,10126 Turin, Italy

Elvira Smeralda Famulari, Stefano Buttiglieri, Emanuela Tolosano, Lorenzo Silengo and Fiorella Altruda
Molecular Biotechnology Center, Department of Molecular Biotechnology and Health Sciences, University of Turin, Via Nizza 52,10126 Turin, Italy

Sharmila Fagoonee
Molecular Biotechnology Center, Department of Molecular Biotechnology and Health Sciences, University of Turin, Via Nizza 52,10126 Turin, Italy
The Institute of Biostructure and Bioimaging (CNR) c/o Molecular Biotechnology Center, Turin, Italy

Saskia K. M. van Daalen and Ans M. M. van Pelt
Center for Reproductive Medicine, Women's and Children's Hospital, Academic Medical Center, University of Amsterdam, Meibergdreef 9, 1105 AZ Amsterdam, Netherlands

Alberto Revelli
Obstetrics and Gynecology 1U, Physiopathology of Reproduction and IVF Unit, Department of Surgical Sciences, Sant'Anna Hospital, University of Turin, Corso Spezia 60, 10126 Turin, Italy

Da-Hai Hu
Department of Burns and Cutaneous Surgery, Xijing Hospital, Fourth Military Medical University, Xi'an, Shanxi 710032, China

Liang Luo
Department of Burns and Cutaneous Surgery, Xijing Hospital, Fourth Military Medical University, Xi'an, Shanxi 710032, China
Stem Cell Research Center, Neurosurgery Institute of PLA Army, Beijing 100700, China
Bayi Brain Hospital, General Hospital of PLA Army, Beijing 100700, China

James Q. Yin and Ru-Xiang Xu
Stem Cell Research Center, Neurosurgery Institute of PLA Army, Beijing 100700, China
Bayi Brain Hospital, General Hospital of PLA Army, Beijing 100700, China

Feng Jiao, He Huang, Zhaofei Zhang, Donghua Liu and Hongyi Zhang
Guangzhou Hospital of Integrated Traditional and Western Medicine, China

Wang Tang
Guangzhou University of Chinese Medicine, China

Hui Ren
The First Affiliated Hospital of Guangzhou University of Traditional Chinese Medicine, China

Lijia Guo and Yuxing Bai
Department of Orthodontics School of Stomatology, Capital Medical University, Beijing, China

Yanan Hou
Department of Orthodontics, Peking University School of Stomatology, The Third Dental Center, Beijing, China

Liang Song
Department of Stomatology, The Fifth People's Hospital of Shanghai, Fudan University, Shanghai, China

Siying Zhu and Feiran Lin
Laboratory of Tissue Regeneration and Immunology and Department of Periodontics, Beijing Key Laboratory of Tooth Regeneration and Function Reconstruction, School of Stomatology, Capital Medical University, Beijing, China

Yunpeng Shi, Chengrui Nan, Zhongjie Yan, Liqiang Liu and Zongmao Zhao
Department of Neurosurgery, The Second Hospital of Hebei Medical University, Shijiazhuang, Hebei 050000, China
Neuroscience Research Center, Hebei Medical University, Shijiazhuang, Hebei 050000, China

Jingjing Zhou and Depei Li
Department of Anesthesiology and Critical Care, The University of Texas MD Anderson Cancer Center, Houston, TX 77030, USA

Jolene Phelps
Pharmaceutical Production Research Facility, Department of Chemical and Petroleum Engineering, Schulich School of Engineering, University of Calgary, 2500 University Drive N. W., Calgary, AB, Canada T2N 1N4
Biomedical Engineering Graduate Program, University of Calgary, 2500 University Drive N. W., Calgary, AB, Canada T2N 1N4

Arindom Sen
Pharmaceutical Production Research Facility, Department of Chemical and Petroleum Engineering, Schulich School of Engineering, University of Calgary, 2500 University Drive N. W., Calgary, AB, Canada T2N 1N4
Biomedical Engineering Graduate Program, University of Calgary, 2500 University Drive N. W., Calgary, AB, Canada T2N 1N4
Center for Bioengineering Research and Education, Schulich School of Engineering, University of Calgary, 2500 University Drive N. W., Calgary, AB, Canada T2N 1N4

Amir Sanati-Nezhad
Biomedical Engineering Graduate Program, University of Calgary, 2500 University Drive N. W., Calgary, AB, Canada T2N 1N4
BioMEMS and Bioinspired Microfluidic Laboratory, Department of Mechanical and Manufacturing Engineering, Schulich School of Engineering, University of Calgary, 2500 University Drive N. W., Calgary, AB, Canada T2N 1N4
Center for Bioengineering Research and Education, Schulich School of Engineering, University of Calgary, 2500 University Drive N. W., Calgary, AB, Canada T2N 1N4

Mark Ungrin
Biomedical Engineering Graduate Program, University of Calgary, 2500 University Drive N. W., Calgary, AB, Canada T2N 1N4

Center for Bioengineering Research and Education, Schulich School of Engineering, University of Calgary, 2500 University Drive N.W., Calgary, AB, Canada T2N 1N4
Faculty of Veterinary Medicine, Heritage Medical Research Building, University of Calgary, 3330 Hospital Drive N. W., Calgary, AB, Canada T2N 4N1

Neil A. Duncan
Biomedical Engineering Graduate Program, University of Calgary, 2500 University Drive N. W., Calgary, AB, Canada T2N 1N4
Center for Bioengineering Research and Education, Schulich School of Engineering, University of Calgary, 2500 University Drive N. W., Calgary, AB, Canada T2N 1N4
Musculoskeletal Mechanobiology and Multiscale Mechanics Bioengineering Lab, Department of Civil Engineering, Schulich School of Engineering, University of Calgary, 2500 University Drive N. W., Calgary, AB, Canada T2N 1N4

Sonia Bergante, Pasquale Creo, Marco Piccoli, Andrea Ghiroldi, Alessandra Menon, Federica Cirillo and Paola Rota
Laboratory of Stem Cells for Tissue Engineering, Scientific Institute for Research, Hospitalization, and Health Care (IRCCS) Policlinico San Donato, San Donato 20097, Italy

Luigi Anastasia
Laboratory of Stem Cells for Tissue Engineering, Scientific Institute for Research, Hospitalization, and Health Care (IRCCS) Policlinico San Donato, San Donato 20097, Italy
Department of Biomedical Sciences for Health (L.I.T.A.), Università degli Studi di Milano, Segrate 20090, Italy

Michelle M. Monasky, Giuseppe Ciconte and Carlo Pappone
Arrhythmology Department, Scientific I nstitute for Research, Hospitalization, and Health Care (IRCCS) Policlinico San Donato, San Donato Milanese, Italy

Pietro Randelli
Azienda Socio Sanitaria Territoriale Centro Specialistico Ortopedico Traumatologico Gaetano Pini-CTO, Milano 20122, Italy
Department of Biomedical Sciences for Health (L.I.T.A.), Università degli Studi di Milano, Segrate 20090, Italy

Laura Hyväri, Miina Ojansivu, Miia Juntunen, Susanna Miettinen and Sari Vanhatupa
Adult Stem Cell Research Group, BioMediTech Institute and Faculty of Medicine and Life Sciences, University of Tampere, Tampere, Finland

Science Center, Tampere University Hospital, Tampere, Finland

Kimmo Kartasalo
Computational Biology Group, BioMediTech Institute and Faculty of Medicine and Life Sciences, University of Tampere, Tampere, Finland
BioMediTech Institute and Faculty of Biomedical Sciences and Engineering, Tampere University of Technology, Tampere, Finland

Yong-Heng Luo, Juan Chen, En-Hua Xiao and Qiu-Yun Li
Department of Radiology, Second Xiangya Hospital of Central South University, Changsha, Hunan 410011, China

Yong-Mei Luo
Department of safety & environmental protection, Shenzhen Zhongjin Lingnan Nonfemet Company Ltd, Shenzhen,Guangdong 518040, China

Hailong Huang, Xiaohua Han, Xin Li, Xiaolin Huang and Hong Chen
Department of Rehabilitation Medicine, Tongji Hospital, Tongji Medical College, Huazhong University of Science and Technology,Wuhan 430030, China

Kun Qian
Department of Reproductive Medicine, Tongji Hospital, Tongji Medical College, Huazhong University of Science and Technology, Wuhan 430030, China

Yifeng Zheng
Department of Neurosurgery, Tongji Hospital, Tongji Medical College, Huazhong University of Science and Technology, Wuhan 430030, China

Zhishui Chen
Institute of Organ Transplantation, Key Laboratory of the Ministry of Health and the Ministry of Education, Tongji Hospital,Tongji Medical College, Huazhong University of Science and Technology, Wuhan 430030, China
Key Laboratory of Organ Transplantation, Ministry of Education, Wuhan 430030, China
Key Laboratory of Organ Transplantation, Ministry of Health, Wuhan 430030, China

Wenjie Zhang and Xinquan Jiang
Department of Prosthodontics, Ninth People's Hospital affiliated to Shanghai Jiao Tong University, School of Medicine,639 Zhizaoju Road, Shanghai 200011, China
Shanghai Key Laboratory of Stomatology & Shanghai Research Institute of Stomatology, National Clinical Research Centerof Stomatology, 639 Zhizaoju Road, Shanghai 200011, China

Maolin Zhang
Department of Prosthodontics, Ninth People's Hospital affiliated to Shanghai Jiao Tong University, School of Medicine,639 Zhizaoju Road, Shanghai 200011, China
Shanghai Key Laboratory of Stomatology & Shanghai Research Institute of Stomatology, National Clinical Research Centerof Stomatology, 639 Zhizaoju Road, Shanghai 200011, China
Division of Molecular and Regenerative Prosthodontics, Tohoku University Graduate School of Dentistry, 4-1 Seiryo-machi, Aobaku, Sendai, Miyagi 980-8575, Japan

Kunimichi Niibe and Hiroshi Egusa
Division of Molecular and Regenerative Prosthodontics, Tohoku University Graduate School of Dentistry, 4-1 Seiryo-machi, Aobaku, Sendai, Miyagi 980-8575, Japan

Wenwen Yu
Department of Oral and Craniomaxillofacial Science & Sleep-disordered Breathing Center, Ninth People's Hospital affiliated to Shanghai Jiao Tong University, School of Medicine, 639 Zhizaoju Road, Shanghai, China

Tingting Tang
Shanghai Key Laboratory of Orthopaedic Implants, Department of Orthopaedic Surgery, Shanghai Ninth People's Hospital,Shanghai Jiaotong University, School of Medicine, Shanghai 200011, China

Zhonglong Liu, Shuiting Fu and Yue He
Department of Oral Maxillofacial & Head and Neck Oncology, Shanghai Ninth People's Hospital Affiliated to Shanghai Jiao Tong University School of Medicine, Shanghai 200011, China

Tao Li and Xiaojun Zhou
Department of Orthopedics, Shanghai Ninth People's Hospital Affiliated to Shanghai Jiao Tong University School of Medicine, Shanghai 200011, China

Si'nan Deng
Department of Stomatology, Central Hospital of Min-Hang District, Shanghai 201109, China

Teng Ma, Yueqiu Chen, Yihuan Chen, Qingyou Meng, Jiacheng Sun, Lianbo Shao, Yunsheng Yu, Haoyue Huang, Yanqiu Hu, Ziying Yang, Junjie Yang and Zhenya Shen
Department of Cardiovascular Surgery of the First Affiliated Hospital & Institute for Cardiovascular Science, Soochow University, Suzhou, China

Index

A

Adipogenic Lineages, 118

Alizarin Red, 2, 13-15, 36-37, 39, 58-60, 67, 70, 112-114, 120, 122, 124, 151, 156, 166-167

Alkaline Phosphatase, 37-39, 42, 59-60, 102, 111, 118, 120, 124, 129, 156, 167

Anoxia, 96

B

Biomolecules, 87-88, 93, 97, 102, 106

Bioprocessing, 87, 105

Blood Cell, 13

Bone Marrow, 1, 8-9, 35, 39, 41-42, 44, 53-54, 57-59, 64-65, 75-76, 82, 85-87, 90-92, 94-95, 103-109, 111, 116, 118, 128, 131, 139, 149-151, 160, 163-166, 175, 180, 182, 185, 191

Brain Ischemia Injury, 77

C

Cardiovascular Disease, 70, 104, 182

Cell Metabolism, 66, 101

Cell Sphingolipids, 111, 113

Craniofacial Skeleton, 23

Cytokines, 11-12, 16, 18-19, 46, 63, 66, 68, 88, 91-92, 94-96, 100-101, 104, 132, 136, 175

D

Dna Methylation, 47, 54, 136, 138-139

Dopamine, 23-25, 27, 31-34, 86

E

Edaravone, 77-78, 80-84, 86

Embryonic Stem Cell, 33, 35, 42, 55-56, 108, 148

Endothelial Cell, 48, 77, 103, 150, 152, 181, 190

Enzyme, 11, 31, 143, 145, 147

Epidermis, 77, 179

Extracellular Matrix, 2, 9, 11, 17-20, 56, 88, 95, 102, 112-113, 119

Extracellular Vesicles, 36, 42, 87-88, 90-93, 104-109, 182, 189

F

Flow Cytometry, 3, 17, 32, 36, 39, 51, 67-68, 70, 72, 77-78, 81, 119, 121, 132-133, 151, 153, 155, 167, 170, 182, 185

Focal Adhesion Kinase, 118-119, 128-129

G

Ganglioside, 110-114, 116-117

H

Hepatocytes, 131-139

Histone, 46-47, 54

Homeostasis, 8, 17, 47, 111, 161, 165

Human Adipose, 10, 41, 43, 52-56, 91, 100, 107-109, 118, 129-130, 164

Human Mesenchymal Stem Cells, 35, 44, 52, 64, 76, 105-106, 116, 129, 163, 180

Human Umbilical Cord, 77, 82, 85-86, 103, 107-109

Hypoxia/anoxia, 96

I

Icariin, 57, 65

Immunofluorescence, 11, 14, 17, 23, 25-27, 29-30, 36, 59, 62-64, 122-123, 131, 133, 135, 137, 167, 172-174, 183, 188-189

Inflammatory Cytokines, 16, 66, 91, 101, 175

Interleukin, 22, 70, 73, 92, 103, 129

Intervertebral Disc, 1, 8-11, 21-22, 105

Intervertebral Disc Degeneration, 9, 11

Intraparenchymal Neural Stem, 140

Ischemic Stroke, 83, 140-143, 146-149

K

Karyotype, 26-27

L

Leukemia, 53, 103-105, 191

Leukocyte, 11-13, 16-17, 19, 21-22, 102

M

Mechanical Stimuli, 94, 97

Mesenchymal Stem Cell, 13, 21, 39, 42-43, 54-55, 65, 77, 86, 103-109, 111, 117, 128, 139, 181, 190

Mononuclear Cells, 68

Morphology, 91, 95, 119

N

Neural Cells, 31, 43-44, 46-51, 53, 82, 86, 191

Neural Crest, 23-24, 26, 28-34, 55-56, 70

Neural Crest Cells, 23-24, 31-32, 34, 70

Neuroblastoma Cell, 23-24, 26, 28-29, 31-32

Neuroblastoma Pathogenesis, 23

Neurological Diseases, 43-44, 82, 182

Neuronal Differentiation, 27-29, 43, 49, 53-54, 56, 86, 111

Nucleus Pulposus, 1, 6, 8-14, 16-17, 21

O

Osteoarthritis, 10, 18, 21, 57, 65, 108

Osteoblasts, 44, 59, 110, 112-116, 118, 122, 165, 177

P

Periodontal Ligament, 66-67, 70, 75-76

Periodontitis, 66, 70, 75-76

Peripheral Nervous System, 23, 31

Phenotype, 10, 21, 26-27, 33, 38-39, 49-50, 52, 54, 56, 78, 80-81, 95, 101, 104-105, 110, 128, 132, 162, 182

Platelet-rich Plasma, 11, 21-22, 52, 110

Progenitor Cell Transplantation, 140, 149

Proinflammatory Cytokines, 11, 19, 91, 101

R

Rhodamine, 58, 60, 63, 120

Root Ganglion, 26, 28

S

Secretome, 85, 87-88, 93-97, 100-107, 191

Spermatogonial Stem Cells, 35, 42

Stem Cell Differentiation, 29, 33, 55, 64, 78, 93, 110, 118, 128-129, 131, 164

Stem Cell Homeostasis, 111

Sympathetic Neurons, 23-24, 26, 31-34

Synaptic Plasticity, 49, 77, 84-86

T

Tendon Stem Cells, 110-111, 113

Tyrosine Hydroxylase, 23-25, 27, 32-33

W

Wound Healing Assay, 2, 6-7

Z

Zebularine, 131-139

www.ingramcontent.com/pod-product-compliance
Lightning Source LLC
Chambersburg PA
CBHW050448200326
41458CB00014B/5104